Headache and Migraine Management

Headache and Migraine Management

Edited by Arabella Cross

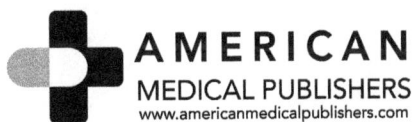

AMERICAN
MEDICAL PUBLISHERS
www.americanmedicalpublishers.com

American Medical Publishers,
41 Flatbush Avenue,
1st Floor, New York,
NY 11217, USA

Visit us on the World Wide Web at:
www.americanmedicalpublishers.com

ISBN: 978-1-63927-298-3

Cataloging-in-Publication Data

Headache and migraine management / edited by Arabella Cross.
    p. cm.
Includes bibliographical references and index.
ISBN 978-1-63927-298-3
1. Headache. 2. Migraine. 3. Headache--Treatment. 4. Migraine--Treatment.
5. Head--Diseases. I. Cross, Arabella.
RC392 .H433 2022
616.849 1--dc23

Table of Contents

Preface

Pain which is felt in the head and neck region is known as a headache. The most common causes of headache are sleep deprivation, fatigue, dehydration, stress, effects of medications and recreational drugs, common cold, head injury, loud noises and viral infections. The main types of headache include migraine, cluster headache and tension-type headache. Migraine is a headache disorder that causes moderate to severe recurrent headaches. It usually affects one half of the head. The symptoms of migraine include vomiting, nausea, and sensitivity to light, smell or sound. Headaches are commonly treated with pain medications. The management of migraine consists of three main aspects of treatment including acute symptomatic control, trigger avoidance and medication for prevention. This book contains some path-breaking studies in the fields of migraine and headache management. It presents researches and studies performed by experts across the globe. It will serve as a valuable source of reference for graduate and post graduate students.

After months of intensive research and writing, this book is the end result of all who devoted their time and efforts in the initiation and progress of this book. It will surely be a source of reference in enhancing the required knowledge of the new developments in the area. During the course of developing this book, certain measures such as accuracy, authenticity and research focused analytical studies were given preference in order to produce a comprehensive book in the area of study.

This book would not have been possible without the efforts of the authors and the publisher. I extend my sincere thanks to them. Secondly, I express my gratitude to my family and well-wishers. And most importantly, I thank my students for constantly expressing their willingness and curiosity in enhancing their knowledge in the field, which encourages me to take up further research projects for the advancement of the area.

Editor

Treatment of withdrawal headache in patients with medication overuse headache

Sabina Cevoli[1*], Giulia Giannini[1,2], Valentina Favoni[1,2], Rossana Terlizzi[1,2], Elisa Sancisi[3], Marianna Nicodemo[4], Stefano Zanigni[5,2], Maria Letizia Bacchi Reggiani[6], Giulia Pierangeli[1,2] and Pietro Cortelli[1,2]

Abstract

Background: Drug withdrawal still remains the key element in the treatment of Medication Overuse Headache (MOH), but there is no consensus about the withdrawal procedure. Still debated is the role of the steroid therapy. The aim of this study was to evaluate the effectiveness of methylprednisolone or paracetamol in the treatment of withdrawal headache in MOH.

Methods: We performed a pilot, randomized, single-blinded, placebo controlled trial. MOH patients, unresponsive to a 3 months prophylaxis, underwent withdrawal therapy on an inpatient basis. Overused medications were abruptly stopped and methylprednisolone 500 mg i.v (A) or paracetamol 4 g i.v. (B) or placebo i.v. (C) were given daily for 5 days. Patients were monitored at 1 and 3 months.

Results: Eighty three consecutive MOH patients were enrolled. Fifty seven patients completed the study protocol. Nineteen patients were randomized to each group. Withdrawal headache on the 5th day was absent in 21.0% of group A, in 31.6% of group B and in 12.5% of group C without significant differences. Withdrawal headache intensity decreased significantly after withdrawal without differences among the groups. Rregardless of withdrawal treatment, 52% MOH patients reverted to an episodic migraine and 62% had no more medication overuse after 3 months.

Conclusions: This study suggests that in a population of severe MOH patients, withdrawal headache decreased significantly in the first 5 days of withdrawal regardless of the treatment used. Methylprednisolone and paracetamol are not superior to placebo at the end of the detoxification program.

Keywords: Medication overuse headache, Detoxification, Migraine

Background

Medication Overuse Headache (MOH) is a worsening of a pre-existing primary headache associated with overuse of acute headache medication [1]. MOH has a strong social impact and represents a public-health concern given the large amount of associated disability and financial costs [2]. MOH affects between 1 and 2% of the general population [3] and 30–50% of patients seen in headache centres. In tertiary headache centres we are used to visit refractory patients with MOH and abrupt drug withdrawal is actually considered the best treatment [4]. Although stopping the acute medication may result in withdrawal symptoms such as increase of headache, nausea, vomiting, arterial hypotension, tachycardia, insomnia and anxiety [5], subsequent headache improvement usually, but not always, occurs. According to EFNS guidelines, treatment of MOH patients should include: patient's education on the nature of the disease, on risk factors and on treatment options; withdrawal including rescue medication; preventive treatment and a multimodal approach including psychological support, if necessary [6].

However, the role of detoxification programs and the possibility to use only the prophylactic therapy is still highly debated [7, 8]. Previous studies have shown that simple information about MOH may be sufficient for

* Correspondence: sabina.cevoli@unibo.it
[1]IRCCS Institute of Neurological Sciences of Bologna, UOC Clinica Neurologica, Bellaria Hospital, Via Altura 3, 40139 Bologna, Italy

some treatment-naïve patients to stop medication over-use on their own [9–11].

MOH subjects who fail withdrawal after simple advice or are complicated by a long duration of disease, multiple overuse, comorbidity or history of unsuccessful treatments have been scarcely studied [4]. However, a study showed that 49% of patients who failed to withdraw from medication overuse after simple advice, had a successful outcome after a structured detoxification program and close follow-up [12].

Another unsolved issue regards whether to begin prophylactic treatment immediately or after the effect of the detoxification, although, as recently revised, the combination of education and prophylactic treatment is superior to prophylactic treatment alone [4].

A multinational study on a large population applied a consensus protocol for the management of MOH showing that two-thirds of subjects were no longer overusers after 6 months and in 46.5% headache reverted to an episodic pattern. Dropout rate was higher in the outpatient program when compared with the inpatient approach, but both regimens were effective [13]. Moreover disability, depression and anxiety were considerably reduced in patients with MOH after a protocol based on rescue, symptomatic and prophylactic medications [14].

Treatment recommendations for the acute phase of drug withdrawal vary considerably among studies. They include fluid replacement, analgesics, anxiolytics, neuroleptics, amitriptyline, valproate, intravenous dihydroergotamine, oxygen and antiemetics. Still debated is the role of steroid therapy [15]. Two independent placebo-controlled randomized studies revealed discordant results regarding the efficacy of the oral prednisone therapy in controlling withdrawal symptoms and headache intensity in the first six and 5 days of withdrawal respectively [16, 17]. More recently, a study partly supported the hypothesis that prednisone reduces the consumption of rescue medications without decreasing the severity and duration of withdrawal headache [18], but comparisons with safer and better tolerated analgesics are lacking.

We aimed to perform a pilot study in order to evaluate the efficacy of methylprednisolone or paracetamol on withdrawal headache in MOH patients.

Methods
Standard protocol approvals and patient consents
The study was conducted in agreement with principles of good clinical practice and the study protocol was approved by the Local Ethic Committee of the local health service of Bologna, Italy (n. 504/CE). All patients gave their written informed consent to study participation.

Participants
Patients from the Headache Centre of IRCCS of Neurological Sciences of Bologna, Italy were recruited consecutively.

Patients were eligible if they were ≥18 years of age, were able to give verbal and written informed consent and met criteria for MOH as defined by the International Headache Society in 2006 [19]: headache present on ≥15 days/months, regular overuse for >3 months of ergotamine, triptans, opioids or combination analgesics on ≥10 days/months, or simple analgesics or any combination of ergotamine, triptans, combination analgesics or opioids on ≥10 days/months. Exclusion criteria included pregnancy and breast-feeding, secondary headaches, history of other types of addiction (such as alcohol, sedative, cannabis and psychoactive substances), as well as any serious ongoing physical or psychiatric illness. Patients with contraindication to use steroids or paracetamol, overusing paracetamol or using steroids for comorbidities were also excluded. Secondary headaches were ruled out by clinical examination, laboratory testing and neuroimaging studies, when indicated.

Study design and procedure
The study was a pilot, randomized, single-blind, placebo controlled trial. Fig. 1 illustrates the study design. MOH patients, unresponsive to education on the nature of the disease, simple advice to reduce the intake of medication and a prophylaxis in a three-month run-in period, underwent withdrawal therapy on an inpatient basis of 5 days. Overused medications were suddenly stopped and patients were randomized (1:1:1) to methylprednisolone (group A) or paracetamol (acetaminophen) (group B) or placebo (group C) for 5 days. Patients in group A received methylprednisolone 500 mg i.v. once a day, patients in group B received paracetamol 2000 mg at 8.00 a.m., 1000 mg at 2.00 p.m., and 1000 mg at 8.00 p.m., and patients in group C received normal saline solution i.v. All patients received lansoprazole 30 mg cap per os at 8.00 a.m. Treatment groups were scheduled in order to maintain patients blind through a double dummy design (Fig. 1). Allowed rescue therapies were: metoclopramide 10 mg i.m. and lorazepam 1 mg or 2.5 mg cap.

Subjects were assigned sequentially to group A or B or C when admitted to hospital receiving a computer-generated random medication code number. The random allocation sequence was not generated by researchers who assigned participants to interventions. Subjects were kept blind about the assigned treatment until discharge.

Study visits
Visits occurred at baseline (preliminary visit T0), 3 months after baseline (T1), 5 days after inpatient withdrawal program (T2), then at 1 month (T3) and 3 months (T4) after inpatient withdrawal program (Fig. 1). At T0 patients were educated about the MOH diagnosis and received advice to stop overused drugs; a pharmacological prophylaxis was prescribed.

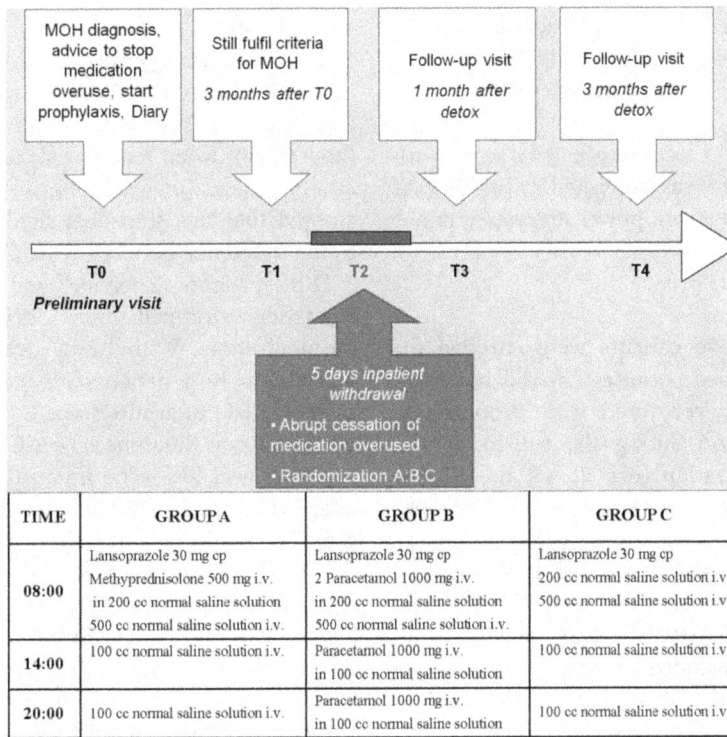

Fig. 1 Study design and treatment groups. A: Methyprednisolone group; B: Paracetamol group; C: Placebo group; *MOH* Medication Overuse Headache

Education consisted in a brief explanation about the nature of the disease and about the consequences of too frequent intake of medication to treat headache attacks. Prophylactic treatment was chosen based on the efficacy and side effects of previous treatments, comorbidity and patients' preferences. At T1, patients still fulfilling the diagnosis of MOH were planned for the inpatient 5-day withdrawal program (T2). T3 and T4 were follow-up visits.

A clinical diary in which patients recorded all headache attacks and the drugs taken for headache during all the study period was given at the preliminary visit and checked at every follow-up visit. Patients recorded the number of days of headache attacks with daytime duration of headache (number of hours), and headache intensity (classified as 1 = mild, 2 = moderate, 3 = severe). Another daily diary was used during the inpatient period to collect data about withdrawal headache and other withdrawal symptoms together with rescue medication intake. Depressive and anxious symptoms (Zung Self-Rating Anxiety Scale and Zung Self-Rating Depression Scale) [20, 21], and degree of disability (Migraine Disability Assessment Score, MIDAS) [22] were evaluated at T0. Patients were interviewed and examined by neurologists expert in headaches.

Outcome measures
The primary endpoint was to evaluate the efficacy of steroids or paracetamol i.v. in the treatment of withdrawal headache in patients with MOH (absence of headache at the fifth day of withdrawal).

Secondary endpoints were: headache intensity and associated withdrawal symptoms each day of treatment, number of rescue medications needed during hospitalization, efficacy of detoxification on headache frequency and medication overuse at follow-up (1 and 3 months after inpatient withdrawal). Associated withdrawal symptoms analysed included nausea, vomiting, arterial hypotension/hypertension, tachycardia, dizziness, photo-phonophobia and anxious symptoms.

Statistics
The normality of the distribution of the parameters was checked using a Skewness-Kurtosis test. Quantitative variables were expressed as the mean ± standard deviation (SD) or median along with interquartile ranges (IQR) when appropriate, while categorical variables were described by their absolute and/or relative frequencies. We compared categorical variables using Chi square test. Oneway Analysis of variance (ANOVA) and Kruskal-Wallis Tests were performed to compare continuous variables with a symmetrical (normal) and an asymmetrical (non-normal) distribution respectively. Post hoc test was performed when appropriate. We performed repeated measures ANOVA to compare headache intensity per day among groups (within-subjects variable time:

headache intensity on days 1–2–3–4–5; among subjects variable group: A vs. B vs. C; and interaction between days and treatment groups). Significance level was set at $p \leq 0.05$. Data analysis was performed with STATA® version 12.0.

This is a pilot study because any previous study with the same primary endpoint was published at the time of the beginning of our study, so a power analysis was not performed.

Results

At baseline, 83 consecutive patients were enrolled for the study; 26 were excluded because they did not meet the inclusion criteria: 20 recovered with prophylactic therapy and the education during the run-in period, while 6 refused hospitalization (Fig. 2). Of the 57 enrolled patients, 50 (87.7%) were females and 7 (12.3%) were males; mean age ± standard deviation (SD) was 47.3 ± 10.3 years. All participants suffered from migraine at onset, with a mean age at onset ± SD was 15.0 ± 7.1 years, and a chronification age of 36.0 ± 9.5 years (Table 1).

Overused medications included triptans (68.4%), simple analgesics (31.6%), ergots (5.3%) and combination analgesics (29.8%). No one overused opiates. Of the final sample, 24 (42.1%) patients received preventive monotherapy while 33 (57.9%) received polytherapy: 21 (36.8%) received a combination of 2 drugs and 12 (21.1%) of 3 drugs. Main prophylactic medications included amitriptyline (26.3%), beta-blockers (29.8% atenolol and 8.8% propranolol), flunarizine (7.0%), perphenazine (12.3%), topiramate (28.1%), valproic acid (8.8%). No differences in prophylactic medications were found among the three groups.

Table 1 presents the demographic and clinical characteristics of the patients randomized to the three different detoxification groups: 19 patients were randomized to A, 19 to B and 19 to C. Sociodemographic variables, headache frequency (days per month), headache

intensity, frequency of overused medications (days per month), MOH duration (years), previous detoxification and scores at Zung scales and MIDAS did not differ significantly among the three groups. Participants randomized to group C showed an increased headache duration (hours/day) when compared to those randomized to others groups (p = 0.0230): an ANOVA post hoc test showed that this statistical significance was attributable to the difference between B vs. C group (p = 0.042).

Three patients (2 females and 1 male) randomized to C group dropped out during the 3rd day of hospitalization. Withdrawal headache on the 5th day was absent in 4 patients (21.0%) of group A, in 6 patients (31.6%) of group B and 2 (12.5%) of group C without significant differences (p = 0.396) (Table 2).

Withdrawal headache intensity decreased significantly after withdrawal without differences among the three groups (headache intensity, days-effect: $p < 0.001$, F = 13.25; group effect: p = 0.103, F = 2.30; interaction days-group effects: p = 0.192, F = 1.41) (Table 2). The highest rebound headache intensity was reached during the 2nd day of withdrawal. Headache intensity was lower in A and B vs. C in the 2nd day, as showed in Table 2, without reaching a significantly difference.

According to the intention-to-treat analysis, withdrawal headache intensity decreased significantly after withdrawal with significant differences among the three groups (headache intensity, days-effect: $p < 0.001$, F = 10.00; group effect: p = 0.002, F = 6.17) without differences when considering their interaction (headache intensity, interaction days-group effects: p = 0.508, F = 0.91).

The three groups did not differ in associated withdrawal symptoms and in number of rescue medications according to the per-protocol analysis (Table 2). Any serious adverse events have not been reported.

Excluding patients chronic at T3, the median (IQR) of the withdrawal headache duration was 7 days (5–8) without differences among treatment groups (Table 2). After the hospitalization one patient randomized to group C was lost at 1 month follow-up. Of the 53 remaining patients, 33 (62.2%) returned to suffer with less than 15 migraine days in the first month after detoxification. And 39 (73.6%) stopped to overuse medications, with no detectable differences among groups. Overall headache frequency was reduced to a median (IQR) of 13.5 (8–24) while frequency of medication intake was reduced to a median (IQR) of 8 (5–13) without differences among groups (Table 3). After the 3 months of follow-up, 28 (52.8%) participants still presented an episodic migraine: 9 (50.0%) randomized to group A, 8 (42.1%) to B and 11 (68.7%) to C without significant differences. Of the final sample, 33 (62.3%) subjects were MOH-free without differences among groups: 11 (61.1%)

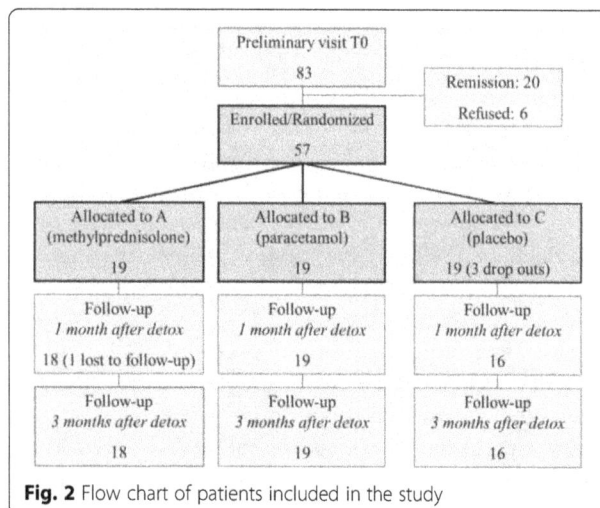

Fig. 2 Flow chart of patients included in the study

Table 1 Demographic and baseline clinical characteristics of the study sample

		Total	Withdrawal therapy groups			
			A: Methylprednisolone	B:Paracetamol	C:Placebo	p value
Sample	N (%)	57	19 (33.3)	19 (33.3)	19 (33.3)	
Age (years)	mean ± SD	47.3 ± 10.3	45.7 ± 9.5	49.8 ± 10.4	46.5 ± 11.2	0.4402
Sex						
Males	N (%)	7 (12.3)	2 (10.5)	2 (10.5)	3 (15.8)	0.850
Females	N (%)	50 (87.7)	17 (89.5)	17 (89.5)	16 (84.2)	
Marital Status						
Single	N (%)	7 (12.3)	3 (15.8)	3 (15.8)	1 (5.3)	0.842
Married	N (%)	43 (75.4)	15 (78.9)	13 (68.4)	15 (78.9)	
Separated/Divorced	N (%)	5 (8.8)	1 (5.3)	2 (10.5)	2 (10.5)	
Widower	N (%)	2 (3.5)	0 (0.0)	1 (5.3)	1 (5.3)	
Years of Education	mean ± SD	12.5 ± 4.2	12.1 ± 3.5	12.7 ± 5.4	12.8 ± 3.6	0.8575
Employment						
Unemployed	N (%)	1 (1.7)	0 (0.0)	1 (5.3)	0 (0.0)	0.859
Student	N (%)	3 (5.3)	1 (5.3)	1 (5.3)	1 (5.3)	
Employee	N (%)	34 (59.7)	13 (68.4)	9 (47.4)	12 (63.2)	
Housewife	N (%)	11 (19.3)	4 (21.0)	4 (21.0)	3 (15.8)	
Retired	N (%)	4 (7.0)	0 (0.0)	2 (10.5)	2 (10.5)	
Self-employed	N (%)	4 (7.0)	1 (5.3)	2 (10.5)	1 (5.3)	
Age at Migraine Onset (years)	mean ± SD	15.0 ± 7.1	13.8 ± 4.5	15.7 ± 8.5	15.3 ± 7.8	0.7029
Age of Migraine chronification	mean ± SD	36.0 ± 9.5	34.3 ± 8.7	39.8 ± 10.2	33.8 ± 8.9	0.0953
Duration of MOH (years)	med; IQR	10; 3–14	11; 3–15	8; 3–12	10; 3–14	0.8198
Headache frequency (days/month)	med; IQR	28.5; 21–30	29; 21–30	24.5; 20–30	30; 21–30	0.4243
Headache duration (hours/day)	mean ± SD	8.6 ± 5.8	7.0 ± 5.2	6.8 ± 4.3	12.1 ± 6.3	**0.0230**
Headache intensity (1–3 scale)	mean ± SD	1.6 ± 0.5	1.7 ± 0.5	1.7 ± 0.5	1.5 ± 0.4	0.3555
Frequency of medication intake (days/month)	mean ± SD	23.4 ± 6.7	23.4 ± 7.2	23.4 ± 5.8	23.2 ± 7.2	0.9941
Overused Drugs						
Triptans	N (%)	39 (68.4)	13 (68.4)	13 (68.4)	13 (68.4)	1
Simple analgesics and/or NSAIDs	N (%)	18 (31.6)	4 (21.0)	8 (42.1)	6 (31.6)	0.377
Ergots	N (%)	3 (5.3)	2 (10.5)	1 (5.3)	0 (0.0)	0.348
Combination analgesics	N (%)	17 (29.8)	7 (36.8)	6 (31.6)	4 (21.0)	0.556
Previous detoxification						
No	N (%)	32 (56.1)	10 (52.6)	12 (63.2)	10 (52.6)	0.180
Yes, outpatient program	N (%)	3 (5.3)	1 (5.3)	1 (5.3)	1 (5.3)	
Yes, inpatient program	N (%)	19 (33.3)	8 (42.1)	3 (15.8)	8 (42.1)	
Yes, inpatient and outpatient programs	N (%)	3 (5.3)	0 (0.0)	3 (15.8)	0 (0.0)	
Migraine disability assessment score	med; IQR	80; 35–130	59.5; 21.5–156.5	83.5; 36.5–170	69; 41–91	0.7270
Epworth Sleepiness Scale	mean ± SD	6.3 ± 3.5	7.2 ± 3.6	5.6 ± 4.1	6.2 ± 2.8	0.4303
Zung Self-Rating Anxiety Scale	med; IQR	35; 33–39	35; 32.5–42.5	33.5; 32–35	37; 34–38	0.2035
Zung Self-Rating Depression Scale	mean ± SD	44.6 ± 8.9	46.7 ± 10.1	42.9 ± 7.5	43.8 ± 8.9	0.4082

Legend: *IQR* interquartile range; *med*: median; *MOH* medication overuse headache; *N* sample size; *NSAIDs* Nonsteroidal Anti-inflammatory Drugs; *SD* standard deviation
Statistically significant *p*-values are denoted in bold

Table 2 Clinical features of patients randomized to the three different detoxification groups during the withdrawal program

		Withdrawal therapy groups			
		A:Methylprednisolone	B:Paracetamol	C:Placebo	p value
Headache Intensity (1–3 scale)					
1st day	mean ± SD	1.8 ± 0.7	1.5 ± 0.9	2.0 ± 0.7	
2nd day	mean ± SD	1.8 ± 0.5	1.9 ± 0.8	2.3 ± 0.5	**< 0.001**[a]
3rd day	mean ± SD	1.3 ± 0.7	1.5 ± 0.8	1.9 ± 0.9	0.103[b]
4th day	mean ± SD	1.4 ± 0.6	1.4 ± 0.8	1.2 ± 0.7	0.192[c]
5th day	mean ± SD	1.2 ± 0.8	1.1 ± 0.9	1.1 ± 0.6	
Headache on 5th day (yes/no)	N (%) / N (%)	15 (79.0) /4 (21.0)	13 (68.4) / 6 (31.6)	14 (87.5) / 2 (12.5)	0.396
Associated withdrawal Symptoms					
1st day	N (%)	15 (79.0)	13 (68.4)	15 (79.0)	0.685
2nd day	N (%)	18 (94.7)	14 (73.7)	15 (79.0)	0.207
3rd day	N (%)	13 (68.4)	15 (79.0)	10 (62.5)	0.554
4th day	N (%)	15 (79.0)	14 (73.8)	8 (50.0)	0.154
5th day	N (%)	12 (63.2)	10 (52.6)	6 (37.5)	0.317
Number of Medication Intake	med; IQR	3; 2–6	2; 0–3	4; 1–6	0.139
Withdrawal headache duration (days)	med; IQR	7; 5–7	6; 5–8	7; 6.5–8	0.5797

Legend: *IQR* interquartile range; *med*: median; *N* sample size; *SD* standard deviation
[a]from testing headache intensity for all patients across days
[b]from testing headache intensity among treatments
[c]from testing the interaction between treatments and days of headache intensity
Statistically significant *p*-values are denoted in bold

randomized to A, 9 (47.4%) to B and 13 (81.2%) to C group (Table 3).

Discussion

This study suggests that in a population of severe MOH patients, withdrawal headache decreased significantly in the first 5 days of withdrawal regardless of the treatment used to relieve withdrawal symptoms. No difference was found regarding associated withdrawal symptoms and in the number of rescue medications according to the per-protocol analysis, even though the number of rescue medications was lower in the two treatment groups versus placebo according to the intention-to-treat analysis. The worst headache was registered between 24 and 72 h of withdrawal program and only in the second day methylprednisolone or paracetamol indifferently

Table 3 Clinical features of patients randomized to the three different detoxification groups at follow-up visits

		Total	Withdrawal therapy groups			
			A:Methylprednisolone	B:Paracetamol	C:Placebo	p value
Sample	N (%)	53	18	19	16	
Headache frequency						
< 15 days T4	N (%)	28 (52.8)	9 (50.0)	8 (42.1)	11 (68.7)	0.481
≥ 15 days at T3	N (%)	20 (37.8)	8 (44.4)	8 (42.1)	4 (25.0)	
≥ 15 days at T4	N (%)	5 (9.4)	1 (5.6)	3 (15.8)	1 (6.3)	
Medication overused after detoxification						
< 15 days T3	N (%)	33 (62.3)	11 (61.1)	9 (47.4)	13 (81.2)	0.216
≥ 15 days at T3	N (%)	14 (26.4)	6 (33.3)	6 (31.6)	2 (12.5)	
≥ 15 days at T4	N (%)	6 (11.3)	1 (5.6)	4 (21.0)	1 (6.3)	
Headache frequency T3 (days/month)	med; IQR	13.5; 8–24	14.5; 7–26	17; 9.5–24	10; 7.5–17	0.428
Headache frequency T4 (days/month)	med; IQR	13.5; 7–20	14; 4–26	17; 7–20	12; 7–18	0.735
Frequency of Medication Intake T3 (days/month)	med; IQR	8; 5–13	8; 4–14	8.5; 6–17	7.5; 4–9.5	0.438
Frequency of Medication Intake T4 (days/month)	med; IQR	9.5; 4.5–13	10.5; 4–15	10; 5–14	9; 7–10	0.851

Legend: *IQR* interquartile range; *med*: median; *N* sample size

appeared slightly superior to placebo. Rescue therapies were requested only in the first 3 days of withdrawal program when the headache intensity was higher. Moreover, the mean duration of rebound headache was 7 days without difference between placebo and active groups.

In the intention-to-treat analysis, withdrawal headache intensity decreased significantly after withdrawal with significant differences among the three groups (headache intensity, days-effect: $p < 0.001$, F = 10.00; group effect: $p = 0.002$, F = 6.17). This statistical significance among groups is attributable to the difference in headache intensity between treatments and placebo groups. The mean headache intensity ± SD during withdrawal was 1.51 ± 0.69 in A, 1.48 ± 0.85 in B and 1.82 ± 0.83 in C, with greater difference during the second and third days of withdrawal (second day: 2.32 ± 0.50 in A, 1.93 ± 0.75 in B and 1.84 ± 0.52 in C; third day: 2.01 ± 0.87 in A, 1.53 ± 0.79 in B and 1.28 ± 0.68 in C). According to intention-to-treat analysis we considered the headache intensity of the three patients in the placebo group that dropped out exactly in the worst day and this probably explains the differences among groups. The main responsible for the three dropouts in the placebo group is probably the lack of blindness of the neurologists. However, this significance did not remain when considering the interaction between time of withdrawal and groups (headache intensity, interaction days-group effects: $p = 0.508$, F = 0.91).

Noteworthy, regardless of withdrawal treatment, more than 60% MOH patients resistant to prophylaxis reverted to an episodic migraine and 73% had no more medication overuse after 1 month. After the 3 months of follow-up, 52% of subjects still presented an episodic migraine and 62% were no longer overusers. In addition, we found that 26% of MOH patients attending a tertiary academic headache centre recovered with simple education about the negative impact of medication overuse and prophylactic therapy prescribed during the preliminary outpatient visit. Education on MOH and drug withdrawal still remain the key elements in the treatment of MOH, but there is no consensus about the withdrawal procedure [4]. Some headache specialists prefer inpatient programs, others an outpatient setting, nevertheless previous studies revealed in both a significant decrease in headache days per month and in the score of migraine disability, ruling out the superiority of one of these two methods [23, 24]. However, inpatient withdrawal resulted significantly more effective compared to both advice alone and outpatient strategy in complicated MOH patients [9].

Very few randomized controlled studies were performed in order to verify the efficacy of pharmacological treatment on withdrawal headache. Often, patients are given a short course of steroids at different dosages and route of administration. In 2008 Pageler and co-authors in a small randomized, placebo controlled, double blind study, reported that prednisone 100 mg given orally once a day for the first 5 days of inpatient withdrawal treatment reduced significantly the total number of hours with severe or moderate headache within the first 72 and 120 h [17]. In the same year Bøe and colleagues performed a randomized, double blind, placebo controlled study in order to verify whether oral prednisolone reduced headache intensity during the first 6 days after medication withdrawal. The patients were hospitalized for the first 3 days and were randomized to prednisolone 60 mg on days 1 and 2, 40 mg on days 3 and 4 and 20 mg on days 5 and 6 or placebo. One hundred MOH patients were included, 65 of whom had migraine, 13 had tension type headache and 22 had both migraine and tension type headache. Prednisolone was not effective on rebound headache in this unselected patient group [16]. More recently, Rabe and colleagues evaluated the efficacy of 100 mg of prednisone over 5 days in the treatment of withdrawal headache. This was a multicentre double blind, placebo controlled, randomized study involving 96 MOH patients with migraine or episodic tension type headache as primary headache. Prednisone reduced rescue medication intake without decreasing the number of hours with moderate or severe headache and duration of withdrawal headache [18]. Finally, Taghdiri and co-workers compared the efficacy of 400 mg/day celecoxib for the first 5 days then decreased at a rate of 100 mg every 5 days vs prednisone 75 mg/day for the first 5 days then tapered off every 5 days in 97 MOH patients. Patients treated with celecoxib had slightly lower headache intensity at the Visual Analogue Scale during the first 3 weeks after withdrawal. However, headache frequency and the demand of rescue medications, which were the primary endpoints, did not differ among groups [25].

Our study confirms that withdrawal of medication overuse is healing regardless of the treatments of rebound headache and symptoms, but it is necessary only when education and prophylaxis fail.

In this study, prophylaxis was started simultaneously with the simple advice to stop medication overuse, so we do not know the relative weight of the two procedures. Moreover, whether to begin prophylactic treatment before, immediately or after the effect of the detoxification is an important unsolved issue.

Our suggested treatment strategy is to counsel patients with MOH and start prophylaxis that may be effective in patients with chronic migraine and medication overuse as evidenced in randomised controlled trials [26]. Moreover, recent articles reported that OnabotulinumtoxinA is effective in MOH prophylaxis, also for patients who had failed previous detoxification, and shows good tolerability and few side effects, so this treatment should be taken into consideration [27, 28]. Many patients will be able to reduce their intake of medications with reduction of headache days without other more expensive and heavy treatments. However, a structured detoxification program should be offered in a short time when the first strategy fails without wasting other time.

Several limitations of our study should be discussed. First of all, this was a single blind study because a double blind design was not feasible in our neurological ward. The lack of blindness of the neurologists was probably the main responsible for the three dropouts in the placebo group exactly in the worst day, without waiting for a possible natural improvement. Moreover, the fact to be in a tertiary centre, probably contributed to pick out more severe MOH patients with previous therapeutic failures, as evidenced in the description of baseline features. In our sample, none patient was treated with OnabotulinumtoxinA before detoxification because the enrolment in this study was close to the end when our local health service approved its use. At this time, the enrolment in the study was close to the end. Placebo in this study was a rehydration treatment that appeared to be not less effective than high doses of active i.v. drugs. Zung and MIDAS scales were lost at follow-up, so they were useful only to describe baseline features of the sample. For the same reason a stratification of patients in order to analyse possible predictors of the outcome was not performed. Finally, the sample size is relatively small but for feasibility reasons we did not recruited further patients. Therefore, we cannot exclude that the absence of statistical significance between groups may be related to the small number of patients in each group. The advantage of the study was in fact, the high homogeneity of the included patients: all were complicated and all had migraine as primary headache. MOH was diagnosed according the International Headache Society 2006 criteria [19], but a chart revision confirmed that all patients included responded to chronic migraine with MOH according ICHD-3 beta criteria [1].

In conclusion, methylprednisolone 500 mg i.v. and paracetamol (acetaminophen) 4 g/die i.v. are not superior to placebo at the end of the detoxification program. Methylprednisolone and paracetamol, a well-tolerated simple analgesic, have the same efficacy in controlling withdrawal headache but might be superior to placebo (fluid replacement) in reducing the intensity of rebound headache only during the second day of withdrawal.

About 50% of patients, resistant to prophylaxis, are no longer overusers after detoxification.

In spite of being a pilot study, present data remain however important for the implementation of further studies on this topic. However, further comparative, multicentre studies among prophylaxis and detoxification programs in MOH patients are necessary to evaluate outcomes and costs [29] in order to optimize the healthcare management of people with chronic disabling headache.

Conclusions
Education on medication overuse and drug withdrawal still remain the key elements in the treatment of medication overuse headache. Our study suggest that Methylprednisolone and Paracetamol may be useful in reducing the intensity of rebound headache during the second day of withdrawal, but they are not superior to placebo at the end of the detoxification program.

Abbreviations
MIDAS: Migraine Disability Assessment Score; MOH: Medication Overuse Headache

Funding
This study was supported by RFO13COR12 – Università di Bologna.

Authors' contributions
SC conceived and design of the study, acquisition of data, analysis and interpretation of data, drafted the manuscript; GG performed analysis and interpretation of data, helped to draft the manuscript; VF acquisition of data, analysis and interpretation of data; RT acquisition of data, analysis and interpretation of data; ES participated in the conception and design of the study and acquisition of data; MN participated in the conception and design of the study and acquisition of data; SZ participated in the conception and design of the study and acquisition of data; MLBR participated in the design of the study and performed the statistical analysis; GP participated in the conception of the study, acquisition of data and interpretation of data; PC conceived of the study, and participated in its design and coordination and helped to draft the manuscript, have given final approval of the version to be published. All authors read and approved the final manuscript.

Competing interests
Dr. Cevoli, Dr. Giannini, Dr. Favoni, Dr. Terlizzi, Dr. Sancisi, Dr. Nicodemo, Dr. Zanigni, Dr. Pierangeli, Dr. Bacchi Reggiani declare that there is no competing interest. Prof. Cortelli received honoraria for speaking engagements or consulting activities from Allergan Italia, Lundbeck Italy, UCB Pharma S.p.A, Chiesi Farmaceutici, AbbVie srl.

Author details
[1]IRCCS Institute of Neurological Sciences of Bologna, UOC Clinica Neurologica, Bellaria Hospital, Via Altura 3, 40139 Bologna, Italy. [2]Department of Biomedical and NeuroMotor Sciences (DiBiNeM), Alma Mater Studiorum - University of Bologna Italy, Bologna, Italy. [3]Neurology, AUSL (Local Health Service) of Ferrara, Ferrara, Italy. [4]Division of Neurology, Maggiore Hospital, IRCCS Institute of Neurological Sciences of Bologna, Bologna, Italy. [5]Functional MR Unit, Policlinico S.Orsola-Malpighi, Bologna, Italy. [6]Department of Experimental, Diagnostic and Specialty Medicine (DIMES), Alma Mater Studiorum, University of Bologna, Bologna, Italy.

References
1. Headache Classification Committee of the International Headache Society (IHS) (2013) The international classification of headache disorders, 3rd edition (beta version). Cephalalgia 33:629–808
2. Linde M, Gustavsson A, Stovner LJ et al (2012) The cost of headache disorders in Europe: the Eurolight project. Eur J Neurol 19:703–711
3. Stovner LJ, Andree C (2010) Prevalence of headache in Europe: a review for the Eurolight project. J Headache Pain 11:289–299

4. Munksgaard SB, Jensen RH (2014) Medication overuse headache. Headache 54:1251–1257
5. Katsarava Z, Fritsche G, Muessing M et al (2001) Clinical features of withdrawal headache following overuse of triptans and other headache drugs. Neurology 57:1694–1698
6. Evers S, Jensen R, European Federation of Neurological Societies (2011) Treatment of medication overuse headache–guideline of the EFNS headache panel. Eur J Neurol 18:1115–1121
7. Diener HC (2012) Detoxification for medication overuse headache is not necessary. Cephalalgia 32:423–427
8. Olesen J (2012) Detoxification for medication overuse headache is the primary task. Cephalalgia 32:420–422
9. Rossi P, Faroni JV, Tassorelli C et al (2013) Advice alone versus structured detoxification programmes for complicated medication overuse headache (MOH): a prospective, randomized, open-label trial. J Headache Pain 14:10
10. Grande RB, Aaseth K, Benth JS et al (2001) Reduction in medication-overuse headache after short information. The Akersus study of chronic headache. Eur J Neurol 18:129–137
11. Rossi P, Di Lorenzo C, Faroni J et al (2006) Advice alone vs. structured detoxification programmes for medication overuse headache: a prospective, randomized, open-label trial in transformed migraine patients with low medical needs. Cephalalgia 26:1097–1105
12. Munksgaard SB, Bendtsen L, Jensen RH (2012) Detoxification of medication-overuse headache by a multidisciplinary treatment program is highly effective: a comparison of two consecutive treatment methods in an open-label design. Cephalalgia 32:834–844
13. Tassorelli C, Jensen R, Allena M, the COMOESTAS Consortium et al (2014) A consensus protocol for the management of medication-overuse headache: evaluation in a multicentric, multinational study. Cephalalgia 34:645–655
14. Bendtsen L, Munksgaard SB, Tassorelli C et al (2014) Disability, anxiety and depression associated with medication-overuse headache can be considerably reduced by detoxification and prophylactic treatment. Results from a multicentre, multinational study (COMOESTAS project). Cephalalgia 34:426–433
15. Halker RB, Dilli E (2013) A role for steroids in treating medication overuse headache? Cephalalgia 33:149–151
16. Bøe MG, Mygland A, Salvesen R (2007) Prednisolone does not reduce withdrawal headache: a randomized, double-blind study. Neurology 69:26–31
17. Pageler L, Katsarava Z, Diener HC et al (2008) Prednisone vs. placebo in withdrawal therapy following medication overuse headache. Cephalalgia 28:152–156
18. Rabe K, Pageler L, Gaul C et al (2013) Prednisone for the treatment of withdrawal headache in patients with medication overuse headache: a randomized, double-blind, placebo-controlled study. Cephalalgia 33:202–207
19. Committee HC, Olesen J, Bousser MG et al (2006) New appendix criteria open for a broader concept of chronic migraine. Cephalalgia 26:742–746
20. Zung WW, Richards CB, Short MJ (1965) Self-rating depression scale in an outpatient clinic: further validation of the SDS. Arch Gen Psychiatry 13:508–515
21. Zung WW (1971) A rating instrument for anxiety disorders. Psychosomatics 12:371–379
22. D'Amico D, Mosconi P, Genco S et al (2001) The migraine disability Assessment (MIDAS) questionnaire: translation and reliability of the Italian version. Cephalalgia 21:947–952
23. Grazzi L, Usai S, Prunesti A et al (2009) Behavioral plus pharmacological treatment versus pharmacological treatment only for chronic migraine with medication overuse after day-hospital withdrawal. Neurol Sci 30(Suppl 1):S117–S119
24. Rossi P, Jensen R, Nappi G, COMOESTAS Consortium et al (2009) A narrative review on the management of medication overuse headache: the steep road from experience to evidence. J Headache Pain 10:407–417
25. Taghdiri F, Togha M, Razeghi Jahromi S et al (2015) Celecoxib vs prednisone for the treatment of withdrawal headache in patients with medication overuse headache: a randomized, double blind clinical trial. Headache 55:128–135
26. Diener HC, Dodick DW, Goadsby PJ et al (2009) Utility of topiramate for the treatment of patients with chronic migraine in the presence or absence of acute medication overuse. Cephalalgia 29:1021–1027
27. Guerzoni S, Pellesi L, Baraldi C, Pini LA (2015) Increased efficacy of regularly repeated cycles with OnabotulinumtoxinA in MOH patients beyond the first year of treatment. J Headache Pain 17:48
28. Negro A, Curto M, Lionetto L, Martelletti P (2015) A two years open-label prospective study of OnabotulinumtoxinA 195 U in medication overuse headache: a real-world experience. J Headache Pain 17:1
29. Shah AM, Bendtsen L, Zeeberg P et al (2013) Reduction of medication costs after detoxification for medication-overuse headache. Headache 53:665–672

2

Modulation of inflammatory mediators in the trigeminal ganglion by botulinum neurotoxin type A: an organ culture study

Jacob Edvinsson[1], Karin Warfvinge[1,2*] and Lars Edvinsson[1]

Abstract

Background: Onabotulinumtoxin type A (BoNT-A) has been found to reduce pain in chronic migraine. The aim of the present study was to ask if BoNT-A can interact directly on sensory mechanisms in the trigeminal ganglion (TG) using an organ culture method.

Methods: To induce inflammation, rat TGs were incubated for 24 hrs with either the mitogen MEK1/2 inhibitor U0126, BoNT-A or NaCl. After this the TGs were prepared for immunohistochemistry. Sections of the TG were then incubated with primary antibodies against CGRP (neuronal transmitter), iNOS (inflammatory marker), IL-1β (Interleukin 1β), SNAP-25 (synaptic vesicle docking protein) or SV2-A (Botulinum toxin receptor element).

Results: We report that CGRP, iNOS, IL-1β, SNAP-25 and SV2-A were observed in fresh TG with a differential distribution. Interestingly, NaCl organ culture of the TG resulted in enhanced expression of CGRP and SNAP-25 in neurons and iNOS in SGCs. Co-incubation with U0126 or BoNT-A retained the increased expression of SNAP-25, while it decreased the IL-1β immunoreactivity in neurons. The iNOS expression in SGCs returned to levels observed in fresh specimens. Moreover, we observed no alteration SV2-A expression in SGCs. Thus, the overall picture is that both U0126 and BoNT-A have the ability to modify the expression of certain molecules in the TG.

Conclusion: We hypothesize that chronic migraine might be associated with some degree of inflammation in the TG that could involve both neurons and SGCs. It is clinically well recognized that treatment with corticosteroids will reduce the symptoms of chronic migraine; however this remedy is associated with long-term side effects. Understanding the mechanisms involved in the expressional alterations may suggest novel ways to modify the changes and indicate novel therapeutics. The results of the present work illustrate one way by which BoNT-A may modify these expressional alterations.

Keywords: CGRP; iNOS; IL-1β; SNAP-25; SV2-A; Monoclonal antibodies; Botulinum neurotoxin type A

Background

Migraine is a common neurological disorder that afflicts up to 16 % of the adult population in the Western countries [1]. It is characterized by episodic, often disabling headache, associated with sensory, autonomic, central nervous system (CNS) related and cognitive symptoms. The current view is that migraine is a disorder in which CNS dysfunction plays a pivotal role while various parts of the trigeminal system are necessary for the expression of peripheral symptoms and aspects of pain [2].

In a subgroup of migraine patients (1–2 %) the frequency of migraine may expand over time to multiple monthly attacks. Furthermore, these may progress to be chronic (attacks > 15 days per month) and are often associated with medication overuse [3]. These patients are very difficult to treat. Onabotulinumtoxin type A (BoNT-A) has shown efficacy in the treatment of chronic migraine [4–6], however its mechanism of action remains in this relation elusive.

The effect of BoNT-A at the neuromuscular junction is well demonstrated [7]. The C-terminal of the toxin binds to the motor neuron and mediates endocytosis of the toxin [8]. Within the vesicle of the motor endplate it

---
* Correspondence: karin.warfvinge@med.lu.se
[1]Department of Medicine, Lund University, Lund, Sweden
[2]Department of Clinical Experimental Research, Glostrup Research Institute, Glostrup Hospital, Glostrup, Denmark

cleaves the vesicular docking protein SNAP-25, which leads to inhibition of acetylcholine storing vesicles docking on the presynaptic membrane and thus reduces acetylcholine release [8]. The potential of BoNT-A in treatment of migraine was suggested 15 years ago and observed in conjunction with cosmetic treatments [9]. Since then several suggestions to explain the antimigraine effect has appeared. The most obvious would be reduction in proprioceptive signaling to the brainstem but also decreased mechanical sensitivity of nociceptors and inhibition of craniofacial muscle tone [10–12]. These mechanisms were further developed and BoNT-A was suggested to interfere with expression of mechanosensitive ion channels on meningeal nociceptors [13].

The aim of the present study was designed to ask if BoNT-A can interact directly on sensory mechanisms in the trigeminal ganglion (TG) using an organ culture method [14–16]. With this method we can study whole TG, and the interrelation between neurons and satellite glial cells (SGC). The neuronal-glial signalling in the TG might be of much relevance in migraine and in particular in the chronification pathology that develops in many patients [17]. During organ culture there is an inflammation response elicited with increased expression of cytokines and mitogen-activated protein kinases (MAPK) [14–16]. We hypothesized that BoNT-A might interfere with the expressional changes of the induced inflammation, and, in addition, the expression of SNAP-25 and the Botulinum toxin receptor element (SV2), molecules observed in the TG.

Methods

Ten Sprague Dawley rats (male, 200–250 g) were anesthetized with CO_2 and decapitated. Right and left TG were removed and either used directly for experiments (fresh), or incubated in Dulbecco's modified Eagle's medium (DMEM; Gibco, Invitrogen, Carlsbad, CA, USA) supplemented with penicillin (100 U ml^{-1}), streptomycin (100 µg mL^{-1}) and amphotericin B (0.25 µg mL^{-1}) for 24 hours at 37 °C in humidified 5 % CO_2 in air (for details on the method see Tajti et al.) [15]. Prior to start of the incubation the MEK1/2 inhibitor U0126 (LC laboratories, Boston, MA, USA) 10 µM, BoNT-A (3 units/mL, ALLERGAN) or an equal volume of NaCl (vehicle) was added. Incubation with the different substances was repeated 5–7 times. The experimental procedures were approved by the University Animal Ethics Commtttee (M43-07).

TG (either fresh or after 24 hours of incubation) were fixated in 4 % paraformaldehyde (Sigma, St Louis, USA) in phosphate buffered saline (PBS) for 2–4 hours. After fixation TG were cryoprotected using 10 % and 25 % sucrose (Sigma) in Sorensen's phosphate buffer. Subsequently, the specimens were embedded in gelatin medium (30 % egg albumin, 3 % gelatin, Sigma), cryosectioned at 12 µm and stored at −20 °C until use.

Sections were thawed in room temperature, then rehydrated in PBS containing 0.25 % Triton X-100 (PBS-T; Sigma) for 15 minutes. Sections were incubated with primary antibodies in PBS-T, containing 1 % bovine serum albumin (BSA; Sigma), overnight in +4 °C. After incubation with the primary antibody, sections were equilibrated to room temperature, rinsed in PBS-T for 2×15 min, followed by incubation with the secondary antibody for 1 hour in a dark room at room temperature (for details on antibodies, see Table 1). Sections were washed with PBST 2×15 min and mounted with anti-fading mounting medium (Vectashield, Vector Laboratories, Burlingame, CA, USA). Omission of the primary antibody served as negative control. The immune-stainings were repeated 3–5 times. For general morphology evaluation, sections were stained in hematoxylin-eosin (Htx, Sigma).

Sections were examined and images were obtained using light- and epifluorescence microscope (Nikon 80i, Tokyo, Japan) equipped with a scanning stage for upright microscope (Märzhäuser, Germany) with travel range X/Y 75 × 50 mm automatic adjustment of the Z-axis, and coupled to a Nikon DS-2 MV camera. This enabled us to take large images of TG, with high resolution. Images were taken using NIS basic research software (Nikon, Japan). We estimated the number of immunoreactive cells and the intensity in these images; however, the detailed distribution was analyzed in regular images in 20× and 40× magnification. In addition, as a complement to the analysis, fluorescence intensity was measured in three sections of CGRP, IL-1β and SNAP-25 stainings, since these showed neuronal immunoreactivity which could be measured. Mean intensity and SD were calculated. In iNOS and SV2-A stainings, the immunoreactivity was confined to the SGCs and could thereby not be used in fluorescence intensity measurements. Statistically, one-way ANOVA analysis and Bonferroni's multiple comparison test were used. $P < 0.05$ was considered as statistically significant.

Results

Morphology

The morphology of the TG was evaluated following Htx staining (Fig. 1). Neurons of different size were

Table 1 Details on primary antibodies used for immunohistochemistry

Name	Host	Dilution	Supplier
iNOS	Rabbit	1:200	Abcam; Cambridge, UK
IL1β	Rabbit	1:400	Abcam; Cambridge, UK
SNAP-25	Rabbit	1:100	Sigma-Aldrich, St. Louis, MO, USA
SV2-A	Rabbit	1:1000	Abcam; Cambridge, UK

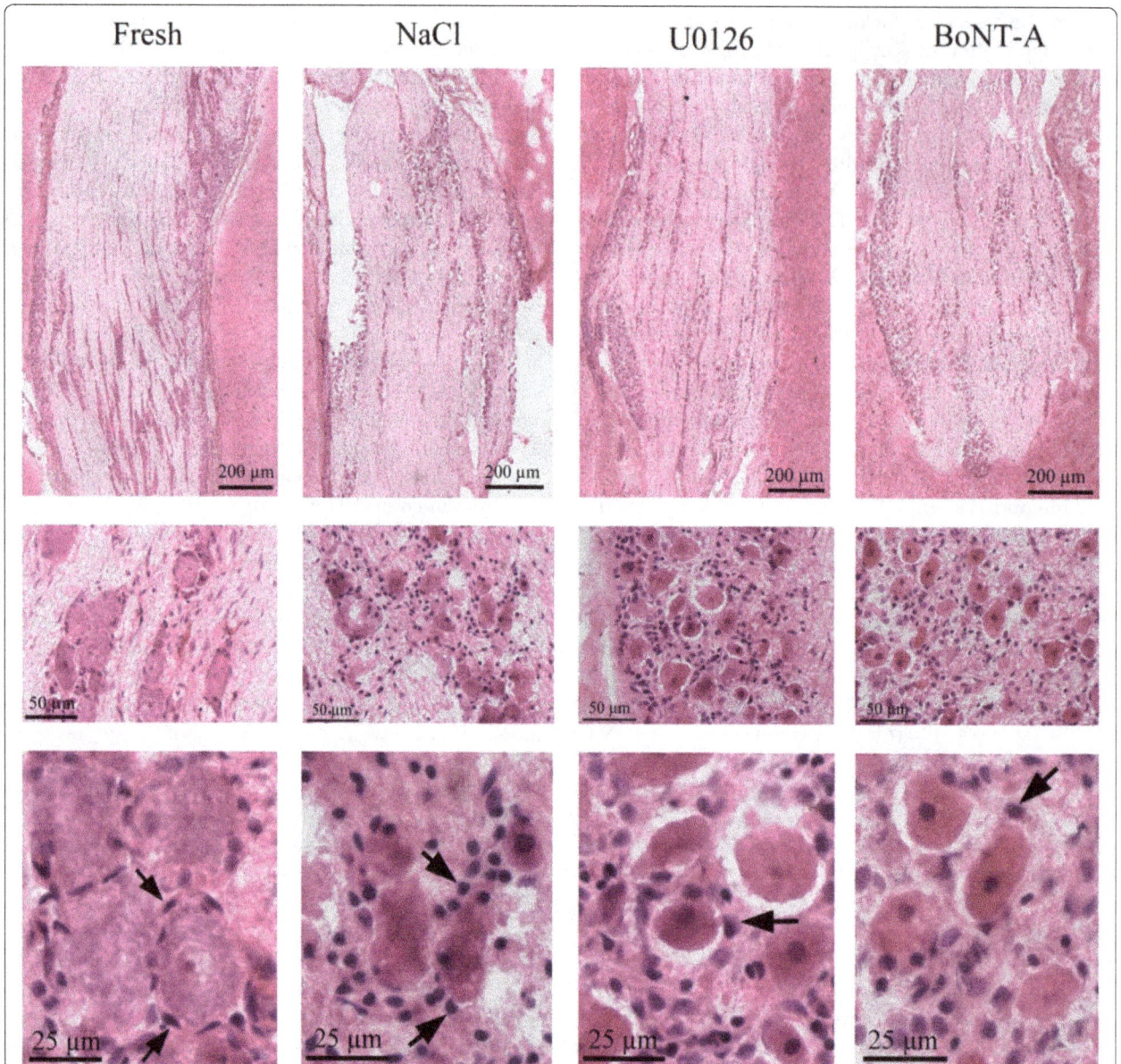

Fig. 1 Hematoxylin-Eosin staining. The column to the left shows the trigeminal ganglion in a fresh rat. The neurons were firmly enveloped by the SGC (arrows), demonstrating the close interaction between the neurons and glial cells. In comparison to a neuron, which contained a large pale nucleus and a visible nucleolus, the SGCs displayed a slender, slightly condensed nucleus. In the specimens that underwent incubation during 24 hrs, a similar morphology between the three groups was found: neurons with both condensed cytoplasm and nuclei, and enlarged rounded SGCs with highly condensed nuclei (arrows). In groups incubated with U0126 or BoNT-A, the neurons were often found in a vacuole indicating SGC detachment

firmly enveloped by SGCs, demonstrating the close interaction between the neurons and the glial cells. The neurons contained a large pale nucleus and a visible nucleolus, and the SGCs displayed a slender, slightly condensed nucleus.

In the specimens that underwent incubation during 24 hours, a similar morphology between the three groups was observed: neurons with both condensed cytoplasm and nuclei, and enlarged rounded SGCs with highly condensed nuclei. Moreover, in groups treated with U0126 or BoNT-A, the neurons were often found in a vacuole indicating cell shrinkage and SGC detachment.

Fresh TG

In the fresh TG, we observed both CGRP positive and negative neurons (Fig. 2a). The CGRP immunoreactivity was confined to the cytoplasm in a granular pattern, resembling staining of the endoplasmatic reticulum. In

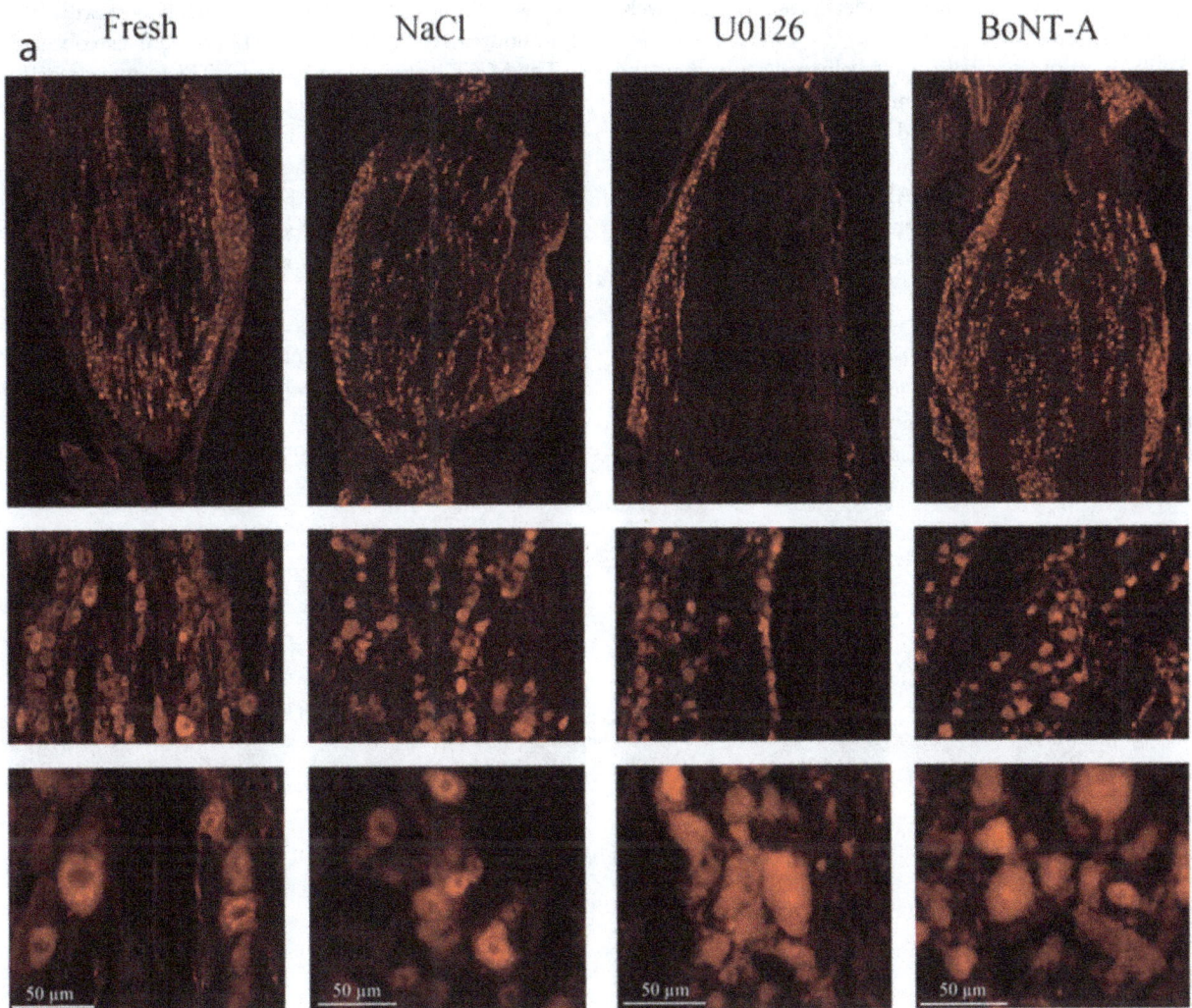

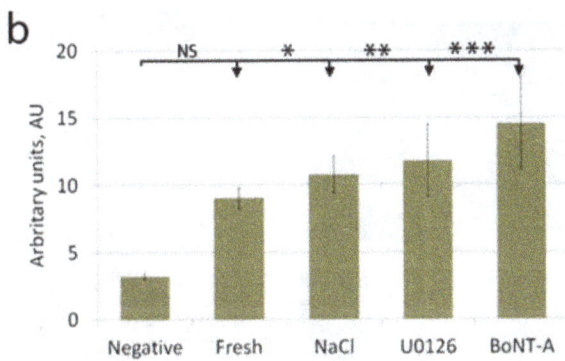

Fig. 2 CGRP immunohistochemistry. **a** Fresh TG contained both CGRP positive and negative neurons. The immunoreactivity was confined to the cytoplasm in a granular pattern, resembling staining of the endoplasmatic reticulum, and in some of the fibers. In TG incubated in medium containing saline, the number of neurons immunoreactive to CGRP seemed to be increased. The immunoreactivity was often spread in a granular matter in the entire cytoplasm as observed in the fresh TG. In the specimens incubated with U0126 or BoNT-A, the number of positive neurons increased and the immunoreactivity was found in the entire cytoplasm in almost all neurons. **b** To illustrate the microscopical findings, fluorescence intensity measurements were performed. The results confirm these findings; a tendency of intensity increase after 24 hrs of incubation with NaCl, U0126 or BoNT-A. Negative column is the same as in SNAP-25 diagram since the same secondary antibody is used in both experiments. Bars indicate SD

addition, some of the nerve fibers seen in TG were CGRP positive.

iNOS immunoreactivity was exclusively found in the SGCs (Fig. 3), and IL-1β immunoreactivity in almost all neurons, which appeared as granules in the cytoplasm (Fig. 4a).

Scattered cytoplasmatic SNAP-25 immunoreactive granules were found in most neurons (Fig. 5a) and SV2-A immunoreactivity in the cytoplasm of SGCs (Fig. 6).

Vehicle incubation for 24 hrs

In the NaCl incubated group (vehicle group), we observed no clear difference in CGRP immunoreactivity compared to fresh TG; both CGRP immunoreactive and negative neurons were observed (Fig. 2a). In addition, the granular intracytoplasmatic CGRP immunoreactivity found in fresh

TG was found after 24 hours of incubation with NaCl. Immunoreactive CGRP positive fibers were also observed.

The SCGs displayed increased iNOS immunoreactivity compared to fresh TG (Fig. 3). As for the fresh specimens, almost all neurons in the incubated groups displayed IL-1β immunoreactivity, which appeared as granules in the cytoplasm (Fig. 4a).

Compared to the fresh specimens, there was increased SNAP-25 immunoreactivity in the neurons in the NaCl incubated group, to such an extent that it was difficult to discern the distribution of immunoreactivity within the neurons (Fig. 5a). We found no difference in SV2-A immunoreactivity between the fresh specimens and the incubation group (Fig. 6), except for the rounded shape of the SGCs appearing after 24 hours of incubation, as also was seen in the Htx staining (Fig. 1).

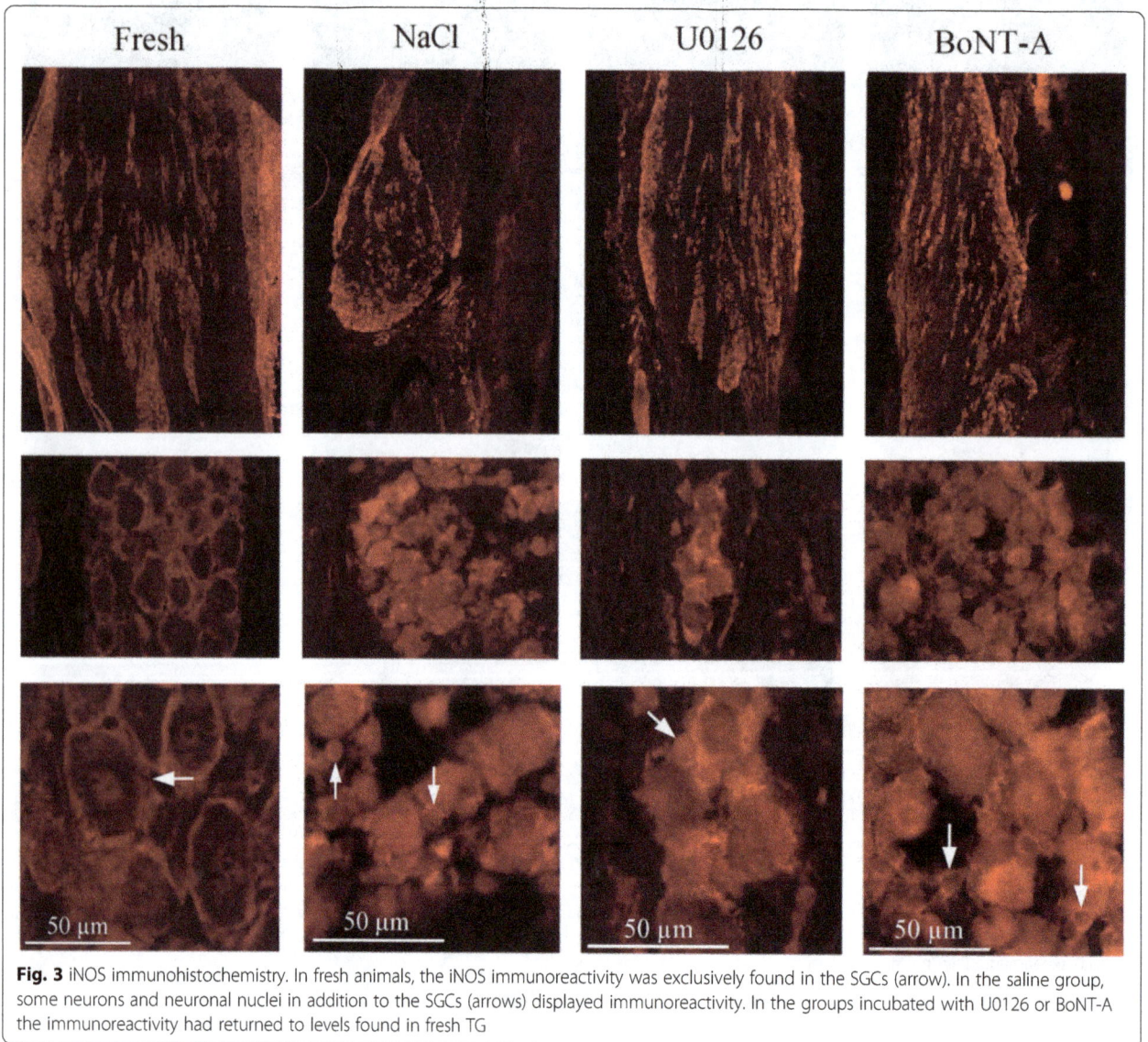

Fig. 3 iNOS immunohistochemistry. In fresh animals, the iNOS immunoreactivity was exclusively found in the SGCs (arrow). In the saline group, some neurons and neuronal nuclei in addition to the SGCs (arrows) displayed immunoreactivity. In the groups incubated with U0126 or BoNT-A the immunoreactivity had returned to levels found in fresh TG

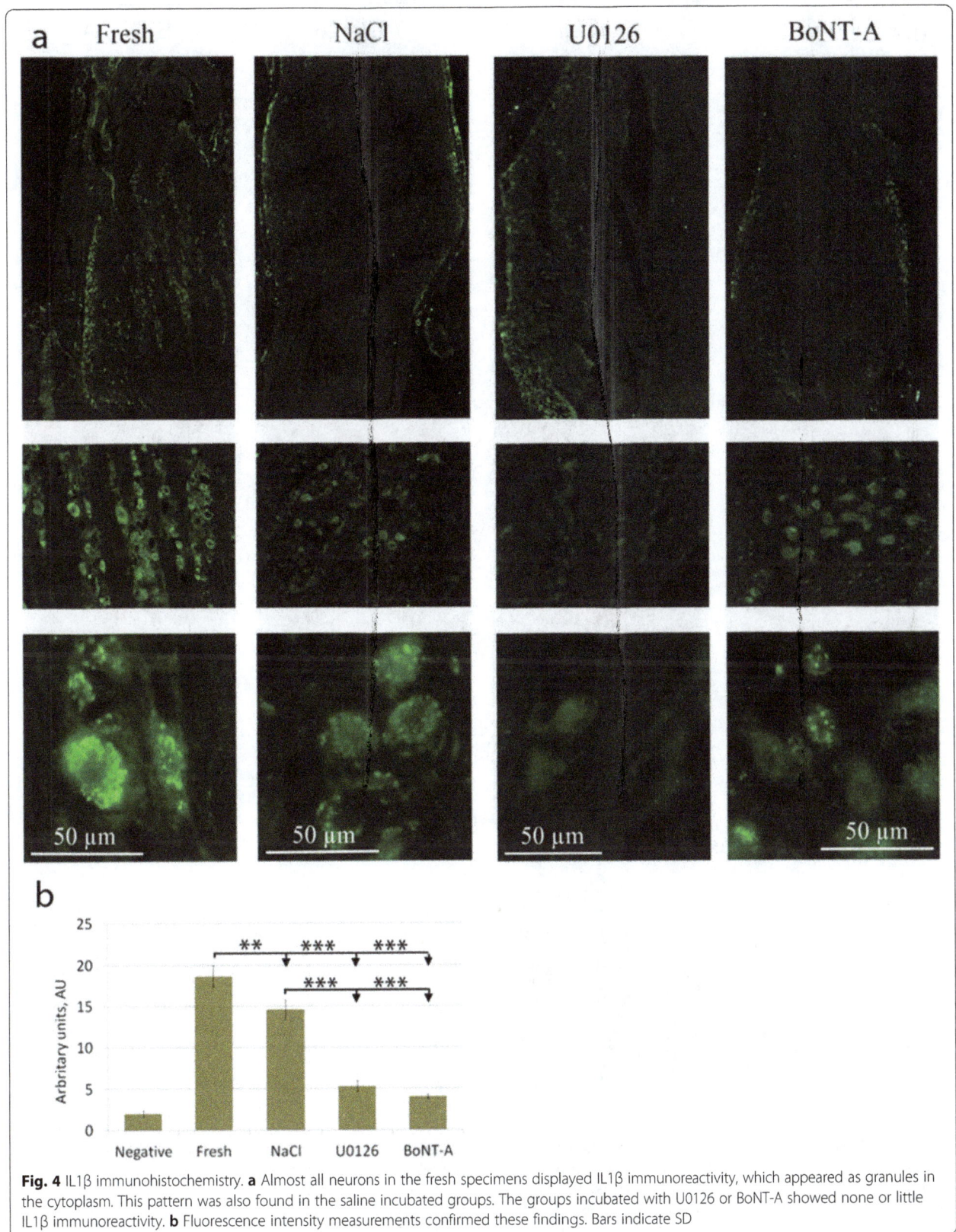

Fig. 4 IL1β immunohistochemistry. **a** Almost all neurons in the fresh specimens displayed IL1β immunoreactivity, which appeared as granules in the cytoplasm. This pattern was also found in the saline incubated groups. The groups incubated with U0126 or BoNT-A showed none or little IL1β immunoreactivity. **b** Fluorescence intensity measurements confirmed these findings. Bars indicate SD

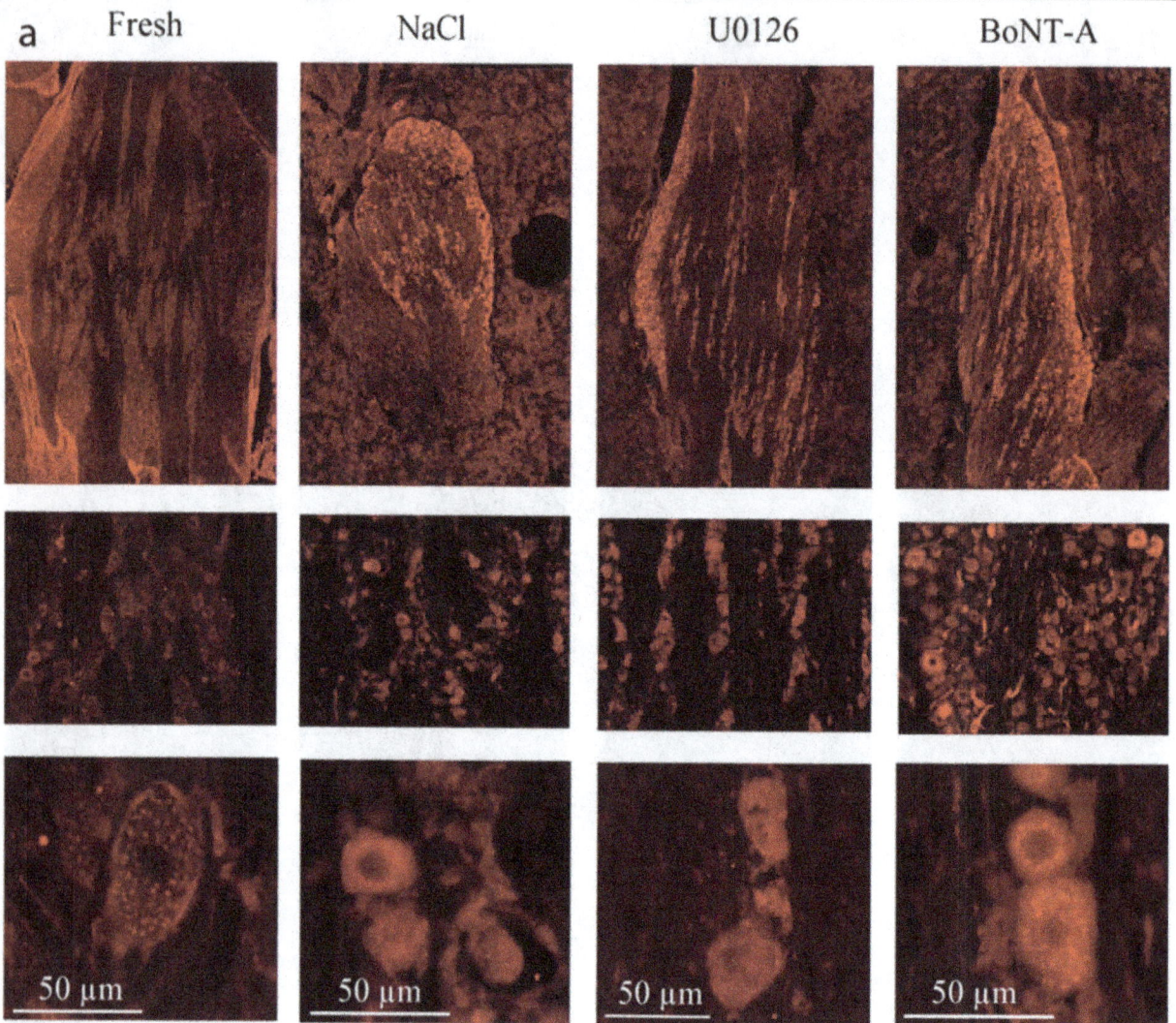

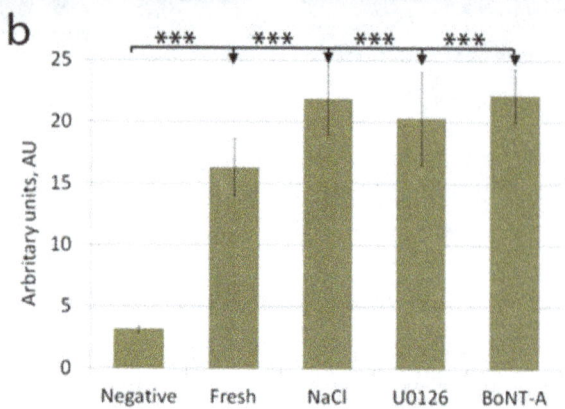

Fig. 5 SNAP-25 immunohistochemistry. **a** Scattered cytoplasmatic SNAP-25 immunoreactive granules were found in most neurons in the fresh specimens. The intensity of the staining in the incubated groups increased intensively, making it difficult to discern the distribution of immunoreactivity within the neurons. **b** Fluorescence intensity measurements confirmed these findindings. Negative column is the same as in SNAP-25 diagram since the same secondary antibody is used in both experiments. Bars indicate SD

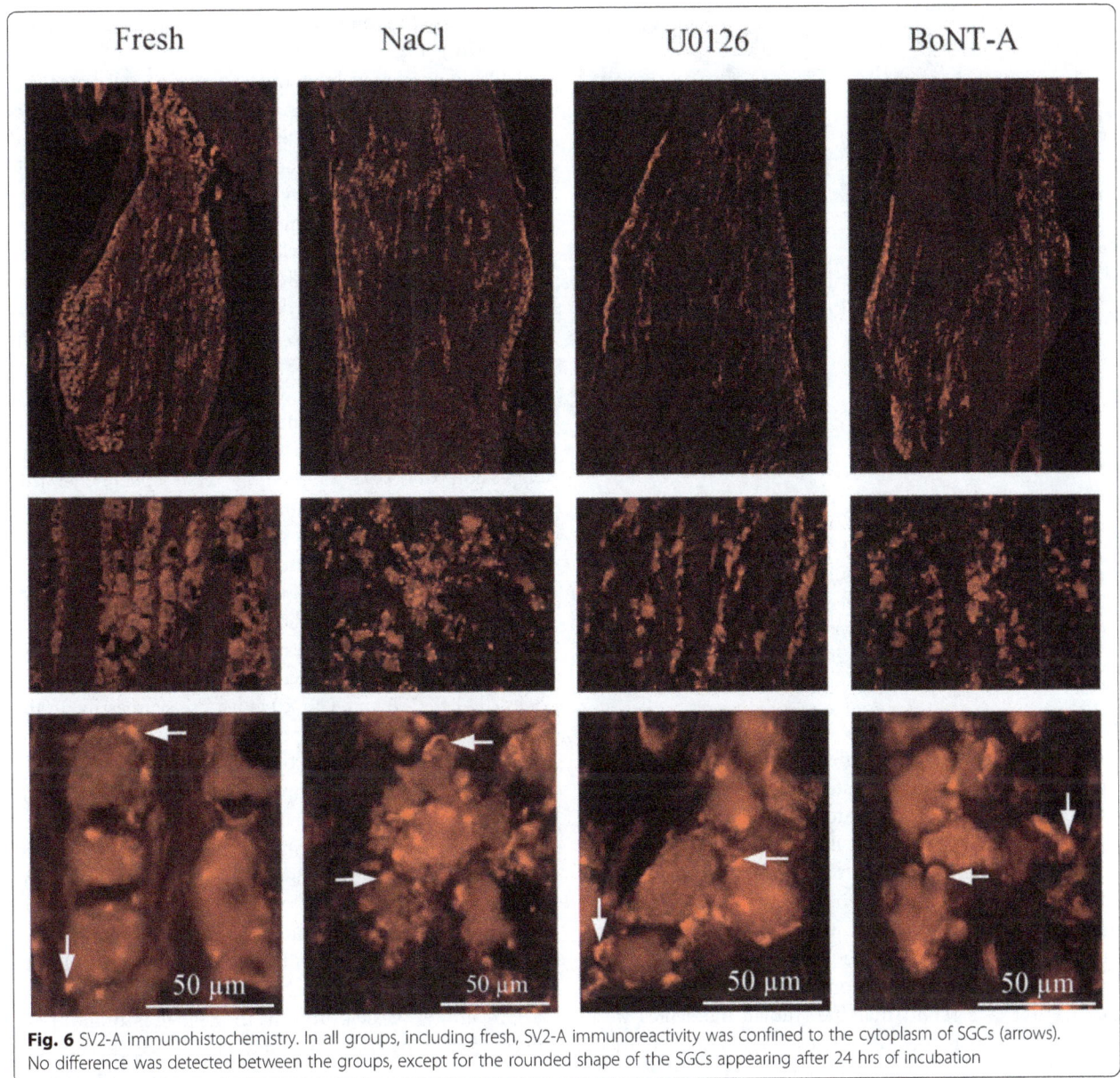

Fig. 6 SV2-A immunohistochemistry. In all groups, including fresh, SV2-A immunoreactivity was confined to the cytoplasm of SGCs (arrows). No difference was detected between the groups, except for the rounded shape of the SGCs appearing after 24 hrs of incubation

U0126 and BoNT-A incubation for 24 hrs

Compared to the fresh specimens, the number of CGRP positive cells was clearly increased in the U0126 group. This was more marked in the BoNT-A treated TG (Fig. 2a). In addition the distribution of the immunoreactivity differed compared to fresh and saline groups; the immunoreactivity was found in the entire cytoplasm in almost all neurons compared to the granular pattern observed in the other groups.

Compared to NaCl incubated group, iNOS immunoreactivity has returned to levels found in fresh TG (Fig. 3) and IL-1β immunoreactivity has decreased compared to fresh, or saline group (Fig. 4a).

The cytoplasmatic SNAP-25 immunoreactive granules found in neurons in the fresh specimens were visible again (after being hidden in the NaCl group by the high intensity of the staining), even though the intensity was considerably increased in the U0126 and BoNT-A groups compared to fresh (Fig. 5a). No difference could be seen in the SV2-A immunoreactivity between all the groups examined (Fig. 6).

Fluorescence intensity measurements of CGRP, IL-1β or SNAP-25 were performed on incubated specimens (Figs. 2b, 4b, 5b). The intensity in the neurons was measured and the mean intensity was calculated. Statistically, one-way ANOVA analysis and Bonferroni's multiple comparison test were used. The measurements confirmed the microscopical results and are presented in the illustrations.

Major findings are illustrated schematically in Fig. 7.

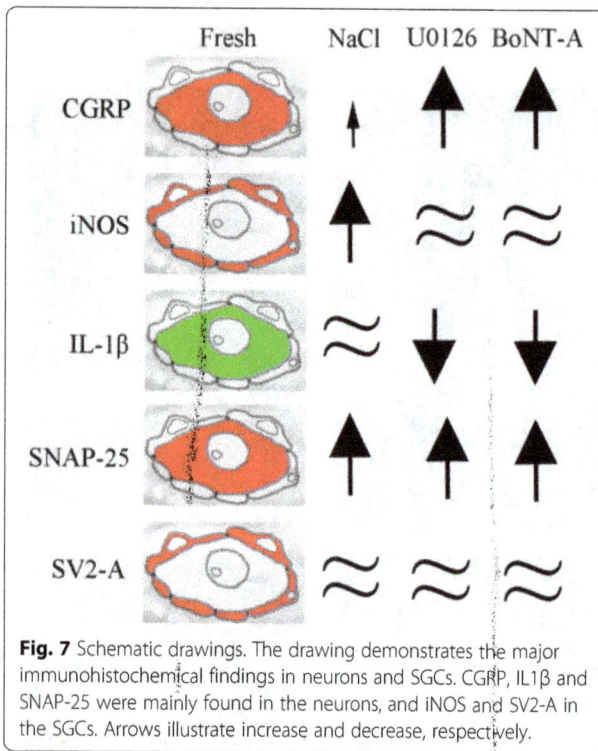

Fig. 7 Schematic drawings. The drawing demonstrates the major immunohistochemical findings in neurons and SGCs. CGRP, IL1β and SNAP-25 were mainly found in the neurons, and iNOS and SV2-A in the SGCs. Arrows illustrate increase and decrease, respectively.

Discussion

The present study was designed to examine isolated TG neurons and SGCs during different organ culture conditions as a method to illustrate possible expressional alterations of CGRP, iNOS, IL-1 β, SNAP-25 and SV2-A. The underlying hypothesis is that chronic migraine is associated with inflammation in various parts of the trigeminal system and organ culture is a way to induce an inflammatory response in the TG. The advantage of this method is the study of neurons and SGCs in their normal habitat. We report that the studied molecules were observed in fresh TG with a differential distribution. Interestingly, organ culture co-incubated with the vehicle NaCl of the TG for 24 hours resulted in enhanced expression of CGRP and SNAP-25 in neurons, and iNOS in SGCs. Co-incubation with U0126 and BoNT-A retained the increased expression of SNAP-25, while it decreased the IL-1 β immunoreactivity in neurons. The iNOS expression in SGCs returned to levels observed in fresh specimens. Moreover, we observed no alteration of SV2-A expression in SGCs. However, the overall picture is that both U0126 and BoNT-A have the ability to modify/reduce the expression of certain molecules in the TG.

CGRP was used to provide further in depth information how and if this system are involved using our method. Organ culture results in increased expression of CGRP immunoreactivity in the TG neurons at 48 hours [14, 15], but only slightly at 24 hours (present data). Although we did not perform any detailed cell counting in the present

study, the localization resembles that described by Eftekhari et al. (2010) [18].

iNOS is expressed by a wide variety of cell types, including neurons and SGCs [19]. We show that iNOS is expressed exclusively in SGCs of the TG. Increased iNOS expression in glial cells is implicated in the etiology of CNS diseases by causing inflammation and cytotoxicity [20, 21]. Inflammatory stimuli, in our case incubation for 24 hours with saline, revealed increased expression of iNOS in SGCs as compared to non-incubated TG. It has been demonstrated that there is increased expression of iNOS in isolated cultured SGCs in response to CGRP and this is mediated by activation of the MAPKs ERK1/2, JNK and p38 [22]. In the present study, we extended the findings to provide evidence that co-incubation with U0126 or BoNT-A show the same expression of iNOS as seen in fresh specimens; this means that these treatments reduced the organ culture induced increase in iNOS expression.

There is IL-1β immunoreactivity expressed in many neurons in fresh TG. Co-incubation with saline did not change this pattern of expression, however, the MEK1/2 inhibitor U0126 and BoNT-A decreased the expression of IL-1β. There is increasing evidence that proinflammatory cytokines (IL-1 β, IL-6 and TNF-α) either are synthesized in the central (CNS) or in the peripheral nervous system (PNS) by resident cells, or imported by immune blood cells. These are involved in several pathophysiological functions, including an unexpected impact on synaptic transmission and neuronal excitability. Targeting these cytokines, and related signalling molecules, is considered a novel option for the development of therapies in various CNS or PNS disorders associated with an inflammatory component [23].

BoNTs is known to inhibit the release of excitatory neurotransmitters from both motor and sensory neurons by preventing vesicle fusion to cell membrane [24]. Under pathophysiological conditions, BoNTs prevent neurotransmission from almost every type of neuron suggesting common targets present in the majority of neurons. BoNTs specifically and exclusively attack pre-synaptic nerve terminals. The fusion of a secretory vesicle with the cell membrane is a highly regulated process with the formation of t-SNARE complex playing a pivotal role. The light chain of BoNTs acts to cleave SNAP-25, which inhibits synaptic exocytosis, and therefore, disables neural transmission [25]. We report that the level of expression of SNAP-25 increased after incubation with BoNT-A, but also after NaCl and U0126 incubation. This indicates accumulation of SNAP-25 in the cytosol of the neurons, as a suggestion regarding BoNT-A incubated TG, from cleavage of SNAP-25 inhibiting exocytosis. However, other mechanisms may be involved when it comes to TG incubated with NaCl or U0126.

Synaptic vesicles (SVs), present in all types of neurons [26, 27], are secretory organelles of presynaptic nerve terminals that accumulate high quantities of neurotransmitters and secrete them by fusion with the presynaptic plasma membrane. BoNT-A may enter neurons by binding to synaptic vesicle protein SV2 (isoforms A, B or/and C) [18]. The details of the BoNT-A binding to SV2 has been clarified in hippocampus from knockout mice, demonstrating that those that lacked the isoforms displayed reduced sensitivity to BoNT-A. It was concluded that SV2 acts as the protein receptor for BoNT-A [19]. We showed that the SV2-A isoform is expressed in the SGCs of rat TG, but not in the neurons. This would point towards these cells as a possible site for a putative action of BoNT-A.

The SGCs surround the TG neurons like a pearl necklace, outnumber the neurons in a 10:1 manner, and are joined by gap junctions [20, 28]. The space between the SGCs and the neurons is 20 nm, which allows for an effective control of the extracellular environment by both neurons and SGCs [20]. The role of the SGCs in the function of the trigeminovascular system is poorly known and has by and large received little attention over the years [20]. In previous work, we observed that the SGCs stored CGRP receptor components (RAMP1, CLR) [18]. In the present study we demonstrate the presence of the inflammation marker iNOS. Vast evidence exists for interaction between the SGCs and the TG neurons. Hence these may be activated via peripheral nociceptors such as those within the dura mater (20, 21) and from the temporomandibular joint (TMJ) [23, 29], as well as from central connections in the trigeminal nucleus caudalis (TNC) [13, 30].

The organ culture method has been used in various reports from our laboratory [14–16]. It has been shown that the method could be used to investigate inflammatory events and neuropeptide expression in the TG. In the present study we show that 24 hours of incubation results in condensed nuclear chromatin and compacted cytoplasm in neurons, and enlarged rounded SGCs with highly condensed nuclear chromatin. Moreover, in groups treated with U0126 or BoNT-A, the neurons were often found in a vacuole indicating cell shrinkage and SGC detachment. The impact of these findings in correlation with the expressional alterations of CGRP, iNOS, IL-1 β, SNAP-25 and SV2-4 can only be speculated upon. Pannese (2010) highlighted the striking morphological changes that SGCs undergo after nerve injury, which includes hypertrophy and formation of bridges with other SGCs, which contain numerous newly formed gap junctions [31]. Obviously, SGCs can sense injury-related changes in the neurons, which might have influenced some of the expressional alterations demonstrated here.

Recently, we asked if a chronic inflammation elicited with injection into the TMJ of CFA [32] or CGRP [33], of CFA on the dura mater (Lukács M, Haanes KA, Majláth Z, Tajti J, Vécsei L, Warfvinge K, Edvinsson L. Exposure of the rat dura mater to inflammatory soup or Complete Freund's Adjuvant induces an inflammatory response in the rat trigeminal ganglion.) might result in altered expression of various markers in the TG. We feel it is of particular importance to maintain the cellular organization because activation of trigeminal neurons leads to changes in adjacent glia that may involve communication through gap junctions and paracrine signaling [17]. The animals were followed for a week and during this time there was a successive increase in inflammation mediators in SGCs and neurons. Interestingly, this enhanced expression could be modified by mitogen-activated protein kinase (MAPK) inhibition in vivo or modified by interacting with the glutamatergic system. In the present method of organ culture we found activation of some of these molecules. The MAPK inhibitor U0126 could modify the expression of CGRP and IL-β. On the other hand the inhibition of a single molecule such as CGRP receptor telcagepant did not change the expression (data not shown). Interestingly, BoNT-A had the same effect as for U0126.

Conclusion

We hypothesize that chronic migraine might be associated with some degree of inflammation in the TG that could involve both neurons and SGCs. It is a clinically well recognized that treatment with corticosteroids will reduce the symptoms of chronic migraine; however this remedy is associated with long-term side effects. Understanding the mechanisms involved in the expressional alterations in the trigeminal system may suggest novel ways to modify the changes and indicate novel therapeutics. The results of the present work illustrate one way by which BoNT-A could modify these expressional alterations in the sensory TG.

Abbreviations
TG: Trigeminal ganglion; SGC: Satellite glial cells, PBS, Phosphate buffered saline; BSA: Bovine serum albumin; MAPK: Mitogen-activated protein kinases; CGRP: Calcitonin gene-related peptide; U0126: Mitogen activated kinase kinase (EK1/2) inhibitor; BoNT-A: Onabotulinumtoxin type A; iNOS: Inducible nitric oxide synthase; IL-1β: Interleukin 1β; SNAP-25: Synaptosome-associated protein of 25 kDa; SV2-A: Synaptic vesicle protein 2.

Competing interests
Dr. Edvinsson reports grants and Botox donation from Allergan during the conduct of the study. In addition, Dr. Edvinsson is consulting on CGRP for Lilly and Teva Pharmaceuticals. JE and KW report no competing interests.

Authors' contribution
JE, KW and LE participated in the design of the study. JE and KW carried out the immunohistochemistry and all three authors participated in the analysis of the results. KW and LE wrote the manuscript. All three authors read and approved the final manuscript.

Acknowledgments
Supported by grants from the Swedish Research Council (no 5958) and the Swedish Heart and Lung Foundation.

Disclosures
The author collaborates have received an unrestricted grant from Allergan and samples of Botox for this preclinical project.

References
1. Lipton RB, Bigal ME, Diamond M, Freitag F, Reed ML, Stewart WF, AMPP Advisory Group (2007) Migraine prevalence, disease burden, and the need for preventive therapy. Neurology 68(5):343–9
2. Akerman S, Holland PR, Goadsby PJ (2011) Diencephalic and brainstem mechanisms in migraine. Nat Rev Neurosci 12(10):570–84
3. Diener HC, Dodick DW, Goadsby PJ, Lipton RB, Olesen J, Silberstein SD (2011) Chronic migraine–classification, characteristics and treatment. Nat Rev Neurol 8(3):162–71
4. Aurora SK, Dodick DW, Turkel CC, DeGryse RE, Silberstein SD, Lipton RB et al. (2010) OnabotulinumtoxinA for treatment of chronic migraine: results from the double-blind, randomized, placebo-controlled phase of the PREEMPT 1 trial. Cephalalgia 30(7):793–803
5. Diener HC, Dodick DW, Aurora SK, Turkel CC, DeGryse RE, Lipton RB et al (2010) OnabotulinumtoxinA for treatment of chronic migraine: results from the double-blind, randomized, placebo-controlled phase of the PREEMPT 2 trial. Cephalalgia 30(7):804–14
6. Dodick DW, Turkel CC, DeGryse RE, Aurora SK, Silberstein SD, Lipton RB et al. (2010) OnabotulinumtoxinA for treatment of chronic migraine: pooled results from the double-blind, randomized, placebo-controlled phases of the PREEMPT clinical program. Headache 50(6):921–36
7. Dolly JO, Lawrence GW, Meng J, Wang J, Ovsepian SV (2009) Neuro-exocytosis: botulinum toxins as inhibitory probes and versatile therapeutics. Curr Opin Pharmacol 9(3):326–35
8. Meunier FA, Schiavo G, Molgo J (2002) Botulinum neurotoxins: from paralysis to recovery of functional neuromuscular transmission. J Physiol Paris 96(1–2):105–13
9. Binder WJ, Brin MF, Blitzer A, Schoenrock LD, Pogoda JM (2000) Botulinum toxin type A (BOTOX) for treatment of migraine headaches: an open-label study. Otolaryngol Head Neck Surg 123(6):669–76
10. Dougherty CO, Silberstein SD (2012) OnabotulinumtoxinA in the treatment of migraine headache. Reg Anesth Pain Manag 16:41–6
11. Gazerani P, Pedersen NS, Staahl C, Drewes AM, Arendt-Nielsen L (2009) Subcutaneous Botulinum toxin type A reduces capsaicin-induced trigeminal pain and vasomotor reactions in human skin. Pain 141(1–2):60–9
12. Gazerani P, Au S, Dong X, Kumar U, Arendt-Nielsen L, Cairns BE (2010) Botulinum neurotoxin type A (BoNTA) decreases the mechanical sensitivity of nociceptors and inhibits neurogenic vasodilation in a craniofacial muscle targeted for migraine prophylaxis. Pain 151(3):606–16
13. Burstein R, Zhang X, Levy D, Aoki KR, Brin MF (2014) Selective inhibition of meningeal nociceptors by botulinum neurotoxin type A: therapeutic implications for migraine and other pains. Cephalalgia 34(11):853–69
14. Kuris A, Xu CB, Zhou MF, Tajti J, Uddman R, Edvinsson L (2007) Enhanced expression of CGRP in rat trigeminal ganglion neurons during cell and organ culture. Brain Res 1173:6–13
15. Tajti J, Kuris A, Vécsei L, Xu CB, Edvinsson L (2011) Organ culture of the trigeminal ganglion induces enhanced expression of calcitonin gene-related peptide via activation of extracellular signal-regulated protein kinase 1/2. Cephalalgia 31(1):95–105
16. Kristiansen KA, Edvinsson L (2010) Neurogenic inflammation: a study of rat trigeminal ganglion. J Headache Pain 11(6):485–95
17. Thalakoti S, Patil VV, Damodaram S, Vause CV, Langford LE, Freeman SE et al. (2007) Neuron-glia signaling in trigeminal ganglion: implications for migraine pathology. Headache 47(7):1008–23, discussion 24–5
18. Eftekhari S, Salvatore CA, Calamari A, Kane SA, Tajti J, Edvinsson L (2010) Differential distribution of calcitonin gene-related peptide and its receptor components in the human trigeminal ganglion. Neuroscience 169(2):683–96
19. Fiebich BL, Lieb K, Engels S, Heinrich M (2002) Inhibition of LPS-induced p42/44 MAP kinase activation and iNOS/NO synthesis by parthenolide in rat primary microglial cells. J Neuroimmunol 132(1–2):18–24
20. Murphy S (2000) Production of nitric oxide by glial cells: regulation and potential roles in the CNS. Glia 29(1):1–13
21. Paakkari I, Lindsberg P (1995) Nitric oxide in the central nervous system. Ann Med 27(3):369–77
22. Vause CV, Durham PL (2009) CGRP stimulation of iNOS and NO release from trigeminal ganglion glial cells involves mitogen-activated protein kinase pathways. J Neurochem 110(3):811–21
23. Vezzani A, Viviani B. Neuromodulatory properties of inflammatory cytokines and their impact on neuronal excitability. Neuropharmacology. 2014(96):70-82. Epub 2014 Nov 8. Review.PMID: 25445483
24. Durham PL, Cady R (2011) Insights into the mechanism of onabotulinumtoxinA in chronic migraine. Headache 51(10):1573–7
25. Sutton RB, Fasshauer D, Jahn R, Brunger AT (1998) Crystal structure of a SNARE complex involved in synaptic exocytosis at 2.4 A resolution. Nature 395(6700):347–53
26. Bajjalieh SM, Scheller RH (1994) Synaptic vesicle proteins and exocytosis. Adv Second Messenger Phosphoprotein Res 29:59–79
27. Janz R, Sudhof TC (1999) SV2C is a synaptic vesicle protein with an unusually restricted localization: anatomy of a synaptic vesicle protein family. Neuroscience 94(4):1279–90
28. Hanani M (2010) Satellite glial cells in sympathetic and parasympathetic ganglia: in search of function. Brain Res Rev 64(2):304–27
29. Durham PL, Garrett FG (2010) Development of functional units within trigeminal ganglia correlates with increased expression of proteins involved in neuron-glia interactions. Neuron Glia Biol 6(3):171–81
30. Dong M, Yeh F, Tepp WH, Dean C, Johnson EA, Janz R et al. (2006) SV2 is the protein receptor for botulinum neurotoxin A. Science 312(5773):592–6
31. Pannese E (2010) The structure of the perineuronal sheath of satellite glial cells (SGCs) in sensory ganglia. Neuron Glia Biol 6(1):3–10
32. Eftekhari S, Warfvinge K, Blixt FW, Edvinsson L (2013) Differentiation of nerve fibers storing CGRP and CGRP receptors in the peripheral trigeminovascular system. J Pain 14(11):1289–303
33. Cady RJ, Glenn JR, Smith KM, Durham PL (2011) Calcitonin gene-related peptide promotes cellular changes in trigeminal neurons and glia implicated in peripheral and central sensitization. Mol Pain 7:94

3

Methylprednisolone blocks interleukin 1 beta induced calcitonin gene related peptide release in trigeminal ganglia cells

Lars Neeb[1*], Peter Hellen[2], Jan Hoffmann[1,3], Ulrich Dirnagl[1] and Uwe Reuter[1]

Abstract

Background: Methylprednisolone (MPD) is a rapid acting highly effective cluster headache preventive and also suppresses the recurrence of migraine attacks. Previously, we could demonstrate that elevated CGRP plasma levels in a cluster headache bout are normalized after a course of high dose corticosteroids. Here we assess whether MPD suppresses interleukin-1β (IL-1β)- and prostaglandin E_2 (PGE_2)-induced CGRP release in a cell culture model of trigeminal ganglia cells, which could account for the preventive effect in migraine and cluster headache. Metoprolol(MTP), a migraine preventive with a slow onset of action, was used for comparison.

Methods: Primary cultures of rat trigeminal ganglia were stimulated for 24 h with 10 ng/ml IL-1β or for 4 h with 10 μM PGE_2 following the exposure to 10 or 100 μM MPD or 100 nM or 10 μM MTP for 45 min or 24 h. CGRP was determined by using a commercial enzyme immunoassay.

Results: MPD but not MTP blocked IL-1β-induced CGRP release from cultured trigeminal cells. PGE_2-stimulated CGRP release from trigeminal ganglia cell culture was not affected by pre-stimulation whether with MPD or MTP.

Conclusion: MPD but not MTP suppresses cytokine (IL-1β)-induced CGRP release from trigeminal ganglia cells. We propose that blockade of cytokine mediated trigeminal activation may represent a potential mechanism of action that mediates the preventive effect of MTP on cluster headache and recurrent migraine attacks.

Keywords: Cluster headache, Migraine, Trigeminal ganglia cells, Calcitonin gene related peptide, Methylprednisolone, Metoprolol, Interleukin-1β, Prostaglandin E_2

Background

The trigeminal system and the neuropeptide calcitonin gene-related peptide (CGRP) are key players in migraine and cluster headache pathophysiology. Activation of perivascular trigeminal nerves within the meninges causes the release of CGRP [1, 2]. CGRP plasma levels were elevated during migraine and cluster headache attacks and effective attack treatment led to the normalization of CGRP levels [3, 4]. The release of CGRP contributes to vasodilatation, neurogenic inflammation, transmission of pain signals and central sensitization [5]. These mechanisms seem to be of significance in migraine pathophysiology and might also be involved in cluster headache pathophysiology.

CGRP plasma levels may also serve as biomarkers for primary headaches. Patients with episodic and chronic migraine demonstrate elevated CGRP plasma levels between attacks [6]. Recently, we could demonstrate that CGRP plasma levels are elevated interictally in episodic cluster headache patients in the bout and that these levels are reduced after short term prophylaxis with corticosteroids [7]. We hypothesized that elevated CGRP plasma levels in a cluster bout might represent a hyperactive state of the trigeminal nervous system. Suppression of trigeminal hyperactivity could be a consequence of corticosteroid therapy, which in turn leads to the suppression of cluster headache attacks. However, our study could not exclude that altered CGRP levels were rather a consequence than the cause of the reduced attack frequency.

Previously, we observed in cultured trigeminal ganglia cells that interleukin 1β (IL-1β) and prostaglandin E_2

---

* Correspondence: lars.neeb@charite.de
[1]Department of Neurology and Experimental Neurology, Charité Universitätsmedizin Berlin, Charitéplatz 1, 10117 Berlin, Germany

(PGE$_2$) induce CGRP release in a cyclooxygenase-2 dependent pathway [8]. Cytokines and especially IL-1β have been linked to migraine [9, 10] and cluster headache [11] and an involvement of pro-inflammatory cytokines in the pathophysiology of primary headaches is probable.

To determine whether corticosteroids may influence trigeminal activation directly, we studied the effects of corticosteroids on CGRP release in this trigeminal ganglia cell model using IL-1β and PGE$_2$ for stimulation. In addition to short-term cluster headache prophylaxis methylprednisolone (MPD) is also used to abort a migrainous state or to prevent the recurrence of migraine attacks [12]. Therefore, we compared the effects of MPD, a drug with rapid onset of action, with the slowly acting migraine preventive metoprolol (MTP) on CGRP release in this model.

Methods
Animals
We used 3-day-old male and female Sprague Dawley rats (Charles River, Sulzheim, Germany). All animals were kept under standard laboratory housing conditions with a 12 h light–dark cycle and with an adult female Sprague Dawley rat (Charles River, Sulzheim, Germany) with free access to food and water. For cell culture procedures newborn animals were anaesthetized with an isoflurane vaporizer (4 %) and decapitated. All animal work was carried out in accordance with the European Communities Council Directive of 24 November 1986 (86/609/EEC) regarding the care and use of animals for experimental procedures. The sacrifice of the rats and extraction of their brains was approved by and reported to the Landesamt für Gesundheit und Soziales Berlin (LaGeSo; T0322/96).

Cell culture
Trigeminal ganglia cell culture was established as previously described by our group [8]. In brief, trigeminal ganglia were dissected from 3 day old male and female Sprague Dawley rats (Charles River, Sulzheim, Germany). The cells were incubated for 90 min at 37 °C in 10 ml dissociation medium (modified eagles medium; Biochrom, Berlin, Germany; with 10 % bovine serum, 10 mM HEPES, 44 mM glucose, 100 U penicillin + streptomycin, 2 mM glutamine, 100 IE insulin/l) containing collagenase/dispase (final concentration 100 μg/ml) (Boehringer Mannheim, Germany), rinsed twice with phosphate buffered saline (PBS) 0.1 M and again incubated with trypsin/EDTA (0.05 %/0.02 % w/v in PBS) for 30 min for dissociation. Subsequently, cells were rinsed twice with PBS and once with dissociation medium, dissociated by Pasteur pipette and pelleted by centrifugation at 2100 x g for 2 min at 21 °C. After suspension in starter medium (Invitrogen, Karlsruhe, Germany) plus 1 % penicillin/streptomycin, 0,25 % L-glutamine, 2 % B27-supplement, 0,1 % 25 mM glutamate, 2.5 mM calcium chloride and 100 ng/ml nerve growth factor-β, cells were plated in 24 well plates and filled to 500 μl with starter medium at a density of 0.5 x 10^{-6} cells/cm^2 (equates approximately 2 ganglia/well). Wells were pretreated by incubation with poly-l-lysin (5 % w/v in PBS) for 90 min at 4 °C, then rinsed with PBS, followed by incubation with coating medium (dissociation medium with 1 % w/v collagen G) for 90 min at 37 °C in the incubator. After that, the wells were rinsed twice with PBS and filled with starter medium in which cells were seeded. Cytosine arabinoside (final concentration 10 μM; Sigma Aldrich, Munich, Germany) was added at day 1 and day 3 to minimize growth of non-neuronal cells. Cultures were kept at 37 °C and 5 % CO$_2$ and fed with neurobasal medium + B27 medium every second day by replacing 50 % of the medium. Condition of cultures was assessed by light microscopy. Stimulation experiments were performed on day 6.

CGRP determination by enzyme immunoassay
After 6 days in culture the medium was gently removed and replaced with fresh medium without nerve growth factor to exclude effects of nerve growth factor on protein release. 1 h later cells were stimulated for 24 h with IL-1β (10 ng/ml), 4 h with PGE$_2$ (10 μM) or equal volume of vehicle (PBS 0.1 M). For inhibition studies cells were pre-incubated with MPD (10 μM or 100 μM), MTP (100 nM or 10 μM) or PBS 45 min or 24 h prior to simulation with vehicle (PBS), IL-1β or PGE$_2$. Immediately before the stimuli 50 μl supernatant of each well were removed to assess baseline CGRP levels. At the end of the stimulation supernatants of two dishes were pooled and used for CGRP determination with a specific CGRP enzyme immunoassay (SPIbio, Montigny le Bretonneux, France) as recommended by the manufacturer. For each experiment, one set of wells was treated with 60 mM KCl to determine the responsiveness of the cultures to an established depolarizing stimulus [13]. Cultures that exhibited a response less than 2-fold on CGRP release after the depolarizing stimulus were not analyzed. CGRP release was determined in pg/ml as absolute increase over baseline values in the corresponding two wells (CGRP levels after stimulation – baseline CGRP levels before stimulation). All samples were measured in duplicates. Each experimental condition was repeated in at least seven independent experiments.

Statistical analysis
Due to small sample size nonparametric statistics were used. Differences of CGRP values between groups were analysed with the Kruskal-Wallis H test. If this test showed statistical significance pairwise comparison was performed using the Mann–Whitney U test. Resulting

p-values were adjusted for multiple comparisons using the Bonferroni-Holm method. Corrected $p < 0.05$ was considered statistically significant. All statistical tests were performed with the SPSS 20 statistical software (SPSS, Chicago, IL, USA). Data are shown as mean ± standard error of the mean (SEM).

Results

In a first step we investigated the effect of MPD on basal and stimulated CGRP release in cultures of rat trigeminal ganglia cells. Cultures were pretreated with vehicle (PBS) or MPD (10 or 100 µM) for 45 min followed by stimulation with PBS or IL-1β (10 ng/ml) for 24 h.

A Kruskal-Wallis H test showed that there was a statistically significant difference in CGRP levels between the different stimulations (χ^2 (3) = 10.270, $p = 0.016$). Pairwise comparison using the Mann–Whitney U test with correction for multiple comparison (Bonferroni-Holm method) revealed that stimulation of trigeminal ganglia cells with IL-1β led to a significantly increased CGRP release compared to control (PBS) (IL-1β: 638 ± 189 SEM pg/ml vs. PBS: 295 ± 48 SEM pg/ml; $n = 9$; $p = 0.031$). Administration of 10 µM or 100 µM MPD into the culture (45 min before stimulation with IL-1β) led to a statistical significant suppression of IL-1β-stimulated CGRP release (310 ± 47 SEM pg/ml; $p = 0.022$ (10 µM) and 264 ± 74 SEM pg/ml; $p = 0.012$ (100 µM); $n = 9$). In contrast, pretreatment of cultures with MPD for 45 min itself without adding IL-1β did not significantly change the amount of CGRP release in controls (PBS exposure solely) (Fig. 1).

Subsequently we tested if PGE_2-induced CGRP release is also altered by pre-stimulation with MPD. There was a statistically significant difference in the CGRP levels between different stimulations as determined by a Kruskal-Wallis H test (χ^2 (3) = 10.318, $p = 0.016$) Stimulation of cultured trigeminal ganglia cells with PGE_2 (10 µM) for 4 h led to significantly increased CGRP levels in the supernatant compared to PBS (324 ± 93 vs. 33 ± 7 pg/ml SEM; $n = 8$, $p < 0.0001$). However, the administration of MPD 10 µM ($n = 8$) or 100 µM ($n = 7$) to trigeminal ganglia cells 45 min prior to PGE_2 stimulation did not alter CGRP release compared to pre-stimulation with vehicle (PBS) ($p > 0.05$). The extension of MPD exposure to 24 h did neither affect PGE_2-induced CGRP release ($n = 8$) (Fig. 2).

In a second step we assessed whether the exposure to MTP had any effect on IL-1β- or PGE_2-induced CGRP release. In contrast to MPD, MTP did not change significantly the amount of stimulus-induced CGRP release in this model. There was a trend towards lower CGRP levels in cultures pretreated with MTP 45 min prior to PGE_2 exposure. However, the results did not reach statistical significance ($p = 0.14$; $n = 9$), (Figs. 3 and 4). In

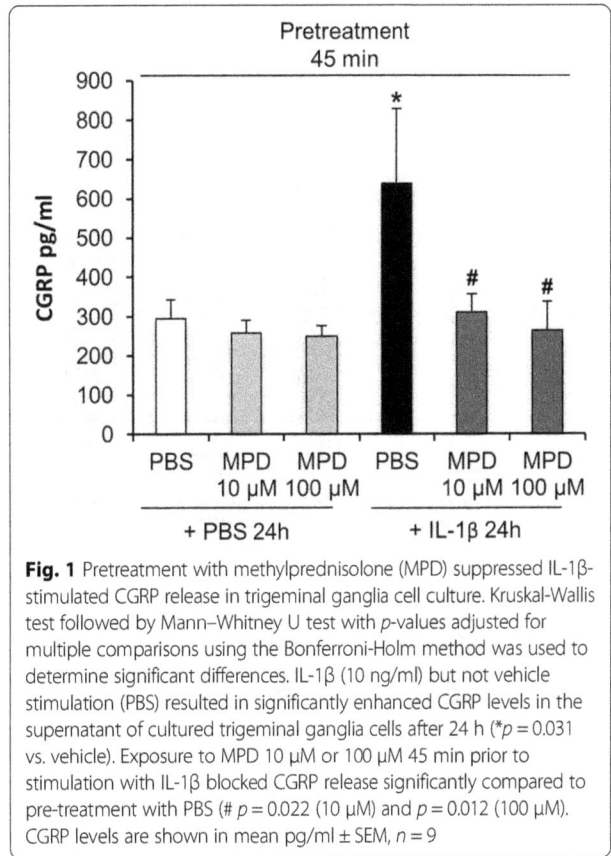

Fig. 1 Pretreatment with methylprednisolone (MPD) suppressed IL-1β-stimulated CGRP release in trigeminal ganglia cell culture. Kruskal-Wallis test followed by Mann–Whitney U test with p-values adjusted for multiple comparisons using the Bonferroni-Holm method was used to determine significant differences. IL-1β (10 ng/ml) but not vehicle stimulation (PBS) resulted in significantly enhanced CGRP levels in the supernatant of cultured trigeminal ganglia cells after 24 h (*$p = 0.031$ vs. vehicle). Exposure to MPD 10 µM or 100 µM 45 min prior to stimulation with IL-1β blocked CGRP release significantly compared to pre-treatment with PBS (# $p = 0.022$ (10 µM) and $p = 0.012$ (100 µM). CGRP levels are shown in mean pg/ml ± SEM, $n = 9$

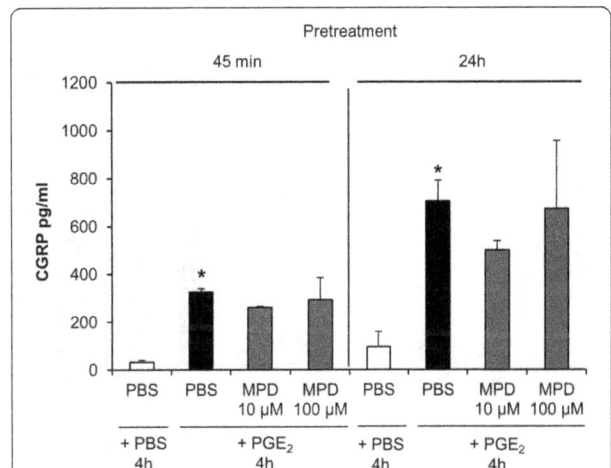

Fig. 2 Pretreatment with methylprednisolone (MPD) did not affect PGE_2-stimulated CGRP release in trigeminal ganglia cell culture. CGRP secretion was determined after pretreatment with PBS or MPD (10 µM or 100 µM) for 45 min or 24 h followed by stimulation with PGE_2 (10 µM) or vehicle for 4 h. CGRP release was significantly enhanced after PBS + PGE_2 (* $p < 0.0001$, compared to PBS + PBS). CGRP levels were not altered by pre-stimulation with MPD for 45 min or 24 h ($p > 0.05$, compared to pre-treatment with PBS). CGRP levels are shown in mean pg/ml ± SEM, $n = 7$–8

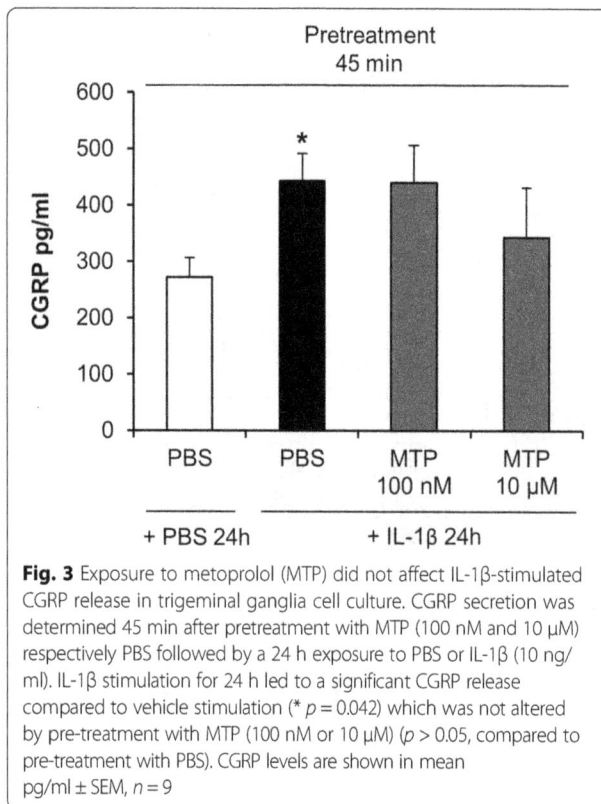

Fig. 3 Exposure to metoprolol (MTP) did not affect IL-1β-stimulated CGRP release in trigeminal ganglia cell culture. CGRP secretion was determined 45 min after pretreatment with MTP (100 nM and 10 µM) respectively PBS followed by a 24 h exposure to PBS or IL-1β (10 ng/ml). IL-1β stimulation for 24 h led to a significant CGRP release compared to vehicle stimulation (* $p = 0.042$) which was not altered by pre-treatment with MTP (100 nM or 10 µM) ($p > 0.05$, compared to pre-treatment with PBS). CGRP levels are shown in mean pg/ml ± SEM, $n = 9$

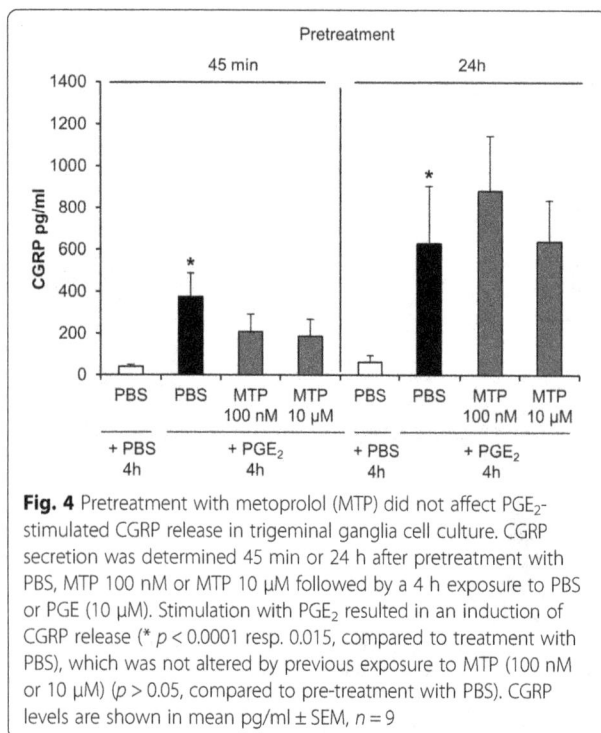

Fig. 4 Pretreatment with metoprolol (MTP) did not affect PGE₂-stimulated CGRP release in trigeminal ganglia cell culture. CGRP secretion was determined 45 min or 24 h after pretreatment with PBS, MTP 100 nM or MTP 10 µM followed by a 4 h exposure to PBS or PGE (10 µM). Stimulation with PGE₂ resulted in an induction of CGRP release (* $p < 0.0001$ resp. 0.015, compared to treatment with PBS), which was not altered by previous exposure to MTP (100 nM or 10 µM) ($p > 0.05$, compared to pre-treatment with PBS). CGRP levels are shown in mean pg/ml ± SEM, $n = 9$

preliminary experiments ($n = 4$) higher concentrations of MTP (100 µM) did neither alter CGRP release in this model.

Discussion

In this study MPD blocked IL-1β-induced CGRP secretion in a trigeminal ganglion cell culture model. MPD had no effect on PGE₂-stimulated CGRP release. Vehicle treated CGRP release in cultured trigeminal ganglia cells was not affected by MPD. The migraine preventive MTP had no effect on IL-1β- or PGE₂-stimulated CGRP release. In contrast, previous studies in a similar cell culture model showed that the migraine preventives topiramate and botulinum toxin type A blocked CGRP release in cultured trigeminal ganglia cells when stimulated with KCl, capsaicin, protons or nitric oxide [14, 15].

Concentrations and time points for stimulation with IL-1β or PGE₂ were determined by previous results in this model with maximum CGRP release at these values [8]. Doses for MPD (10 or 100 µM) and MTP (100 nM and 10 µM) used in this experimental study were derived from human data on serum concentrations after applying therapeutically beneficial doses of the drugs. Intake of 80 mg oral methylprednisolone leads to a serum concentration of 7 µM [16]. Intravenous administration of 1000 mg methylprednisolone results in serum concentrations between 16 and 77 µM [17]. Mean serum concentrations of metoprolol after oral application of 100 mg were stated with 136 nM [18]. To assess a maximal effect we chose the higher metoprolol dose equal to the effective dose of methylprednisolone (10 µM).

For pre-stimulation with MTP and MPD we chose 45 min and 24 h before the exposure to PGE₂ (4 h) to assess the acute effect of stimuli as well as effects that may be mediated through longer acting mechanisms (e.g. gene expression). Due to the long exposure to IL-1β (24 h) prestimulation was restricted to 45 min in these experiments.

Primary trigeminal afferents are a major source of CGRP release into the extracerebral circulation [19]. Activation of trigeminal ganglia afferents and subsequent release of CGRP is thought to play a prominent role in the pathophysiology of migraine [20] and cluster headache [21, 22] pathophysiology. The pro-inflammatory cytokine IL-1β and other cytokines are elevated in migraine [9, 10] and cluster headache patients [11, 23, 24]. The cytokines IL-1β and tumor necrosis factor alpha induce CGRP release in cultured trigeminal ganglia cells [8, 25]. The involvement of immunological mechanisms in primary headaches is possible but the role of cytokines in headache pathophysiology remains incompletely understood.

Cytokines are proteins that are released by glial cells in proximity to peripheral and central neurons. They are involved in pro-inflammatory signaling pathways and represent key elements in the induction and mainten- ance of pain [26–30]. Increased cytokine expression and pro-inflammatory protein synthesis are both patho- physiological components for the development and maintenance of peripheral and central sensitization. Both mechanisms are important in the pathophysi- ology of migraine [26, 31, 32]. CGRP itself differen- tially regulates cytokine secretion from cultured trigeminal ganglion glia cells. In CGRP treated cultures secreted levels of some cytokines (e.g. IL-β) increased while others such as tumor necrosis factor alpha decreased. These results point to a paracrine trigeminal activation due to CGRP release from tri- geminal ganglia neurons and glial cytokine secretion that may lead to an inflammatory loop, which could account for sustained sensitization of second-order trigeminal neu- rons [33]. Chronically sensitized central nociceptive neu- rons are supposed to contribute to the development of chronic migraine and its resistance to treatment [34].

In contrast to IL-1β-induced CGRP release, PGE$_2$-in- duced CGRP release was not affected by prior exposure to MPD. Previously, we demonstrated that IL-1β in- duced CGRP release in trigeminal ganglia cells is dependent on COX-2 induction [8]. Methylprednisolone prevents PGE$_2$ formation by suppression of COX-2 activity [35]. If inhibition of CGRP release by methyl- prednisolone is mediated through the prevention of PGE$_2$ formation, it is feasible that direct induction of CGRP release by PGE$_2$ cannot be blocked by methyl- prednisolone. In a recent clinical study, we demonstrated the effect of MPD on CGRP release in episodic cluster headache patients in an active bout. A three day pulse therapy with 1000 mg MPD per day led to the normalization of interictally elevated CGRP plasma levels in parallel to the suppression of headache attacks [7]. We extend this observation with our experimental findings in a cell culture of trigeminal ganglia cells. This data support the hypotheses that corticosteroids might exert their preventive action in migraine and cluster headache by the inhibition of trigeminal activation, which is necessary for the initiation of a headache attack. Blockade of trigeminal neurotransmitter secretion could account for prevention of central sensitization and trig- gering of headache attacks.

Metoprolol, a migraine preventive with slow onset of action had no effect in this experimental model. MTP seems to mediate its prophylactic effect through an alternative mode of action on possible non- inflammatory mechanisms and not on a cellular level in the trigeminal ganglion. The precise mechanism of action of metoprolol in migraine prophylaxis is not known, but modification of cortical excitability by inhibiting central β-receptors most likely contributes to its preventative effects [36–38].

Conclusions

Pretreatment with MPD blocked IL-1β-, but not PGE$_2$- induced CGRP release in cultured primary trigeminal ganglia cells. Based on our findings, we propose that MPD used for short-term cluster headache prophylaxis or prevention of migraine recurrence might act via the suppression of cytokine mediated trigeminal activation.

Abbreviations
CGRP: Calcitonin gene related peptide; IL-1β: Interleukin-1β; MDP: Methylprednisolone; MTP: Metoprolol; PGE$_2$: Prostaglandin E$_2$.

Competing interests
The authors declare that they have no competing interests.

Authors' contributions
LN and UR designed the study. LN, PH and JH performed the experiments and analyzed the data. UR and UD supervised the study. LN wrote the manuscript, and all authors read and approved the final draft of the manuscript.

Acknowledgements
This work was supported by a grant from the Bundesministerium für Bildung und Forschung (BMBF 01EM 0515). The BMBF had no role in the study design, data collection and analysis, decision to publish, or preparation of the manuscript. We are grateful to Sonja Blumenau for excellent technical assistance.

Author details
[1]Department of Neurology and Experimental Neurology, Charité Universitätsmedizin Berlin, Charitéplatz 1, 10117 Berlin, Germany. [2]Department of Neuroradiology, Universitätsmedizin Göttingen, Robert-Koch-Straße 40, 37075 Göttingen, Germany. [3]Department of Systems Neuroscience, University Medical Center Hamburg-Eppendorf, Martinistrasse 52, D-20246 Hamburg, Germany.

References
1. Uddman R, Edvinsson L, Ekman R, Kingman T, McCulloch J (1985) Innervation of the feline cerebral vasculature by nerve fibers containing calcitonin gene-related peptide: trigeminal origin and co-existence with substance P. Neurosci Lett 62(1):131–136
2. Edvinsson L, Hara H, Uddman R (1989) Retrograde tracing of nerve fibers to the rat middle cerebral artery with true blue: colocalization with different peptides. J Cereb Blood Flow Metab 9(2):212–218
3. Goadsby PJ, Edvinsson L (1994) Human in vivo evidence for trigeminovascular activation in cluster headache. Neuropeptide changes and effects of acute attacks therapies. Brain 117(Pt 3):427–434
4. Goadsby PJ, Edvinsson L, Ekman R (1990) Vasoactive peptide release in the extracerebral circulation of humans during migraine headache. Ann Neurol 28(2):183–187. doi:10.1002/ana.410280213
5. Bigal ME, Walter S, Rapoport AM (2013) Calcitonin gene-related peptide (CGRP) and migraine current understanding and state of development. Headache 53(8):1230–1244. doi:10.1111/head.12179
6. Cernuda-Morollon E, Larrosa D, Ramon C, Vega J, Martinez-Camblor P, Pascual J (2013) Interictal increase of CGRP levels in peripheral blood as a biomarker for chronic migraine. Neurology. doi:10.1212/WNL. 0b013e3182a6cb72.
7. Neeb L, Anders L, Euskirchen P, Hoffmann J, Israel H, Reuter U (2015) Corticosteroids alter CGRP and melatonin release in cluster headache episodes. Cephalalgia 35(4):317–326. doi:10.1177/0333102414539057
8. Neeb L, Hellen P, Boehnke C, Hoffmann J, Schuh-Hofer S, Dirnagl U, Reuter U (2011) IL-1beta stimulates COX-2 dependent PGE synthesis and CGRP release in rat trigeminal ganglia cells. PLoS One 6(3):e17360. doi:10.1371/journal.pone.0017360
9. Perini F, D'Andrea G, Galloni E, Pignatelli F, Billo G, Alba S, Bussone G, Toso V (2005) Plasma cytokine levels in migraineurs and controls. Headache 45(7): 926–931. doi:10.1111/j.1526-4610.2005.05135.x

10. Sarchielli P, Alberti A, Baldi A, Coppola F, Rossi C, Pierguidi L, Floridi A, Calabresi P (2006) Proinflammatory cytokines, adhesion molecules, and lymphocyte integrin expression in the internal jugular blood of migraine patients without aura assessed ictally. Headache 46(2):200–207. doi:10.1111/j.1526-4610.2006.00337.x

11. Martelletti P, Granata M, Giacovazzo M (1993) Serum interleukin-1 beta is increased in cluster headache. Cephalalgia 13(5):343–345, discussion 307–348

12. Huang Y, Cai X, Song X, Tang H, Huang Y, Xie S, Hu Y (2013) Steroids for preventing recurrence of acute severe migraine headaches: a meta-analysis. Eur J Neurol 20(8):1184–1190. doi:10.1111/ene.12155

13. Durham PL, Russo AF (1999) Regulation of calcitonin gene-related peptide secretion by a serotonergic antimigraine drug. J Neurosci 19(9):3423–3429

14. Durham PL, Niemann C, Cady R (2006) Repression of stimulated calcitonin gene-related peptide secretion by topiramate. Headache 46(8):1291–1295. doi:10.1111/j.1526-4610.2006.00538.x

15. Durham PL, Cady R (2004) Regulation of calcitonin gene-related peptide secretion from trigeminal nerve cells by botulinum toxin type A: implications for migraine therapy. Headache 44(1):35–42. doi:10.1111/j.1526-4610.2004.04007.x, discussion 42–33

16. Rohatagi S, Barth J, Mollmann H, Hochhaus G, Soldner A, Mollmann C, Derendorf H (1997) Pharmacokinetics of methylprednisolone and prednisolone after single and multiple oral administration. J Clin Pharmacol 37(10):916–925

17. Baylis EM, Williams IA, English J, Marks V, Chakraborty J (1982) High dose intravenous methylprednisolone "pulse" therapy in patients with rheumatoid disease. Plasma methylprednisolone levels and adrenal function. Eur J Clin Pharmacol 21(5):385–388

18. Oosterhuis B, Jonkman JH, Kerkhof FA (1988) Pharmacokinetic and pharmacodynamic comparison of a new controlled-release formulation of metoprolol with a traditional slow-release formulation. Eur J Clin Pharmacol 33(Suppl):S15–18

19. Hoffmann J, Wecker S, Neeb L, Dirnagl U, Reuter U (2012) Primary trigeminal afferents are the main source for stimulus-induced CGRP release into jugular vein blood and CSF. Cephalalgia 32(9):659–667. doi:10.1177/0333102412447701

20. Ho TW, Edvinsson L, Goadsby PJ (2010) CGRP and its receptors provide new insights into migraine pathophysiology. Nat Rev Neurol 6(10):573–582. doi:10.1038/nrneurol.2010.127

21. Fanciullacci M, Alessandri M, Figini M, Geppetti P, Michelacci S (1995) Increase in plasma calcitonin gene-related peptide from the extracerebral circulation during nitroglycerin-induced cluster headache attack. Pain 60(2):119–123

22. Fanciullacci M, Alessandri M, Sicuteri R, Marabini S (1997) Responsiveness of the trigeminovascular system to nitroglycerine in cluster headache patients. Brain 120(Pt 2):283–288

23. Empl M, Forderreuther S, Schwarz M, Muller N, Straube A (2003) Soluble interleukin-2 receptors increase during the active periods in cluster headache. Headache 43(1):63–68

24. Steinberg A, Sjostrand C, Sominanda A, Fogdell-Hahn A, Remahl AI (2011) Interleukin-2 gene expression in different phases of episodic cluster headache–a pilot study. Acta Neurol Scand 124(2):130–134. doi:10.1111/j.1600-0404.2010.01434.x

25. Bowen EJ, Schmidt TW, Firm CS, Russo AF, Durham PL (2006) Tumor necrosis factor-alpha stimulation of calcitonin gene-related peptide expression and secretion from rat trigeminal ganglion neurons. J Neurochem 96(1):65–77. doi:10.1111/j.1471-4159.2005.03524.x

26. Miller RJ, Jung H, Bhangoo SK, White FA (2009) Cytokine and chemokine regulation of sensory neuron function. Handb Exp Pharmacol 194:417–449. doi:10.1007/978-3-540-79090-7_12

27. White FA, Jung H, Miller RJ (2007) Chemokines and the pathophysiology of neuropathic pain. Proc Natl Acad Sci U S A 104(51):20151–20158. doi:10.1073/pnas.0709250104

28. Uceyler N, Schafers M, Sommer C (2009) Mode of action of cytokines on nociceptive neurons. Exp Brain Res 196(1):67–78. doi:10.1007/s00221-009-1755-z

29. Boettger MK, Weber K, Grossmann D, Gajda M, Bauer R, Bar KJ, Schulz S, Voss A, Geis C, Brauer R, Schaible HG (2010) Spinal tumor necrosis factor alpha neutralization reduces peripheral inflammation and hyperalgesia and suppresses autonomic responses in experimental arthritis: a role for spinal tumor necrosis factor alpha during induction and maintenance of peripheral inflammation. Arthritis Rheum 62(5):1308–1318. doi:10.1002/art.27380

30. Schafers M, Sommer C, Geis C, Hagenacker T, Vandenabeele P, Sorkin LS (2008) Selective stimulation of either tumor necrosis factor receptor differentially induces pain behavior in vivo and ectopic activity in sensory neurons in vitro. Neuroscience 157(2):414–423. doi:10.1016/j.neuroscience.2008.08.067

31. Zhang XC, Kainz V, Burstein R, Levy D (2011) Tumor necrosis factor-alpha induces sensitization of meningeal nociceptors mediated via local COX and p38 MAP kinase actions. Pain 152(1):140–149. doi:10.1016/j.pain.2010.10.002

32. Yan J, Melemedjian OK, Price TJ, Dussor G (2012) Sensitization of dural afferents underlies migraine-related behavior following meningeal application of interleukin-6 (IL-6). Mol Pain 8:6. doi:10.1186/1744-8069-8-6

33. Thalakoti S, Patil VV, Damodaram S, Vause CV, Langford LE, Freeman SE, Durham PL (2007) Neuron-glia signaling in trigeminal ganglion: implications for migraine pathology. Headache 47(7):1008–1023. doi:10.1111/j.1526-4610.2007.00854.x, discussion 1024–1005

34. Mathew NT (2011) Pathophysiology of chronic migraine and mode of action of preventive medications. Headache 51(Suppl 2):84–92. doi:10.1111/j.1526-4610.2011.01955.x

35. Santini G, Patrignani P, Sciulli MG, Seta F, Tacconelli S, Panara MR, Ricciotti E, Capone ML, Patrono C (2001) The human pharmacology of monocyte cyclooxygenase 2 inhibition by cortisol and synthetic glucocorticoids. Clin Pharmacol Ther 70(5):475–483

36. Gerwig M, Niehaus L, Stude P, Katsarava Z, Diener HC (2012) Beta-blocker migraine prophylaxis affects the excitability of the visual cortex as revealed by transcranial magnetic stimulation. J Headache Pain 13(1):83–89. doi:10.1007/s10194-011-0401-x

37. Maertens de Noordhout A, Timsit-Berthier M, Timsit M, Schoenen J (1987) Effects of beta blockade on contingent negative variation in migraine. Ann Neurol 21(1):111–112. doi:10.1002/ana.410210125

38. Diener HC, Scholz E, Dichgans J, Gerber WD, Jack A, Bille A, Niederberger U (1989) Central effects of drugs used in migraine prophylaxis evaluated by visual evoked potentials. Ann Neurol 25(2):125–130. doi:10.1002/ana.410250204

4

Valproate ameliorates nitroglycerin-induced migraine in trigeminal nucleus caudalis in rats through inhibition of NF-κB

Yuanchao Li, Qin Zhang, Dandan Qi, Li Zhang, Lian Yi, Qianqian Li and Zhongling Zhang[*]

Abstract

Background: As a complex nervous system disease, migraine causes severe healthy and social issues worldwide. Valproate (VPA) is a widely used treatment agent against seizures and bipolar disorder, and its function to alleviate damage due to migraine has also been verified in clinical investigations. However, the mechanism underlying the protective effect of VPA against migraine remains poorly revealed. In the current study, the major purpose was to uncover the mechanism which drove VPA to antagonize migraine.

Methods: Nitroglycerin (NTG) was employed to induce a migraine model in rats and the migraine animals were exposed to treatment of VPA of different doses. Thereafter, the levels of indicators related to oxidative stress were measured and used to evaluate the anti-oxidant potential of VPA. The expression of calcitonin gene-related peptide (CGRP) and c-Fos was also quantified with ELISA and immunohistochemistry, respectively. Western blotting and electrophoretic mobility shift assays (EMSA) were conducted to explore the effect of VPA treatment on NF-κB pathway.

Results: NTG induced the activation of oxidative stress and led to migraine in model animals, but pre-treatment with VPA attenuated the damage due to migraine attack in brain tissues. The level of lipid peroxidation was significantly reduced while the prodcution of anti-oxidant factors was restored. Furthermore, expressions of CGRP and c-Fos, which represented the neuronal activation, were also down-regulated by VPA. The results of western blotting and EMSA demonstrated that the above mentioned effect of VPA acted through the inhibition of NF-κB pathway.

Conclusions: Although controversies on the effect of VPA on NF-κB pathway existed, our study revealed an alternative mechanism of VPA in protecting against migraine, which would promote the development of therapeutic strategies of migraine.

Keywords: Anti-oxidant, Migraine, NF-κB, Nitroglycerin, Valparoate

Background

As a complicated nervous system disease, migraine is characterized by the disability of components in the trigeminal pain pathway. Patients with migraine are attacked by disabling headache associated with sensitivity to afferent inputs, including gastrointestinal inputs, light, sound, and head movement [1]. Based on the investigation in 2002, over 20 % of the world population are affected by migraine at some stage of their entire lives [2], casting severe healthy and social issues to the public health. Although the pathophysiological mechanism which drives the onset of migraine remains poorly understood, compelling evidence infers that nitric oxide (NO) plays a critical role in the pathogenesis of migraine [3–6]. The genes related to NO pathway, including genes encoding endothelial NO synthase (eNOS), inducible NO synthase (iNOS), and vascular endothelial growth factor (VEGF) all increased patients' susceptibility to migraine [3]. The pathways involved in the induction of migraine by NO may depend on the activation of NF-κB [7], associated with the up-regulation of some

* Correspondence: zhongl_zhang67@sina.com
Department of Neurology, The First Affiliated Hospital of Harbin Medical University, No. 23 Youzheng Road, Harbin 150001, People's Republic of China

key molecules in neuronal activation, i.e., c-Fos [7, 8]. In the normal state, NF-κB is mainly located within the cytoplasm and the subunits of NF-κB, p50 and p65, are complexed with IκBα in an inactive form. Upon stimulation, IκBα is degraded and free NF-κB subunits to enter the nucleus and subsequently cause the expression of inflammatory genes which are the main regulatory enzymes for NO [9]. Thus, some therapies targeting these relevant pathways have been widely investigated regarding their potential to attenuate the damage caused by migraine [10, 11].

Among types of anti-migraine therapies, the protective function of valproate (VPA) against migraine with mild side effects has drawn lots of attention [12]. VPA is achieved by reacting valproic acid (2-Propylpentanoic acid) with a base such as sodium hydroxide and rapidly absorbed in human bodies. VPA reaches peak plasma concentration within one to four hours and thereafter maintains the concentration for four to 14 hours [12]. In clinic, VPA has been widely used as a treatment for seizures and bipolar disorder. Additionally, in many animal models, VPA has improving effect on symptoms associated with stroke, amyotrophic lateral sclerosis, Parkinson's disease, and Alzheimer's disease [13–16]. Regarding migraine, researchers in Cochrane Collaboration have affirmed the protective effect of VPA against this disorder in their review in 2015 [12]. However, even with this solid evidence that verifies the potential of VPA in antagonizing migraine, few studies have explicitly revealed the pathways which may be involved in this treatment process. Therefore, the underlying mechanism which drives the action of VPA on migraine remains poorly explained.

In this study, a rat migraine model was established via intraperitoneal injection of nitroglycerin (NTG). As a donor of NO, NTG has been successfully used as an experimental agent to induce migraine in many studies [3, 17, 18]. Administration of NTG can induce activation of cGMP and NF-κB, and further lead to pathogenesis of migraine [6, 19]. The electroencephalogram (EEG) of the experimental animals and the synthesis of oxidative stress molecules which are involved in numerous neurological diseases [20] were detected to assess the effect of VPA on the brain function. The expression of calcitonin gene-related peptide (CGRP) which is closely related to the migraine disorder and headache generation [21], and c-Fos were measured using ELISA, immunohistochemistry, and western blotting assay, respectively. To further explain the pathways involved in the treatment of VPA, the activities of IκBα and NF-κB were determined with western blotting assay and electrophoretic mobility shift assay (EMSA). We hoped that our findings in the present study would provide a preliminary explanation on the mechanism of VPA against migraine and help to promote the application of VPA in clinic.

Methods

Chemicals and animals

VPA was purchased from Melonepharma (Catal. No. MB1627, Dalian, China) and dissolved in saline. NTG was purchased from Yimin Pharmaceutical Co., Ltd (Catal. No. H11021022, Beijing, China). Antibodies against c-Fos, p65, IκBα, phosphorylated IκBα (p-IκBα), and Histone H3 were purchased from Beijing Biosynthesis Biotechnology Co., LTD (Catal. No. bs-10172R, bs-5515R, bs-1287R, bs-17422R, Beijing, China). Antibody against NF-κB subunit p65 was purchased from Boster (Catal. No. BA0610. China). Antibody against β-actin was purchased from Santa Cruz Biotechnology, Inc. (Catal. No. sc-47778. USA). Vitamin A standard was purchased from Sigma-Aldrich Co. (Catal. No. R7632, St. Louis, MO, USA). Male Sprague-Dawley rats (weighting ca. 200 g) were provided by Experimental Animal Center of China Medical University. All the animals were housed at 20-25 °C with humidity of 55 ± 5 % and had free access to food and water before experimental use. The animal experiments were conducted in accordance with the Institutional Animal Ethics Committee and Animal Care Guidelines of The First Affiliated Hospital of Harbin Medical University.

Migraine model establishment and pre-administration of VPA

Fifty SD rats were randomly divided into five groups (ten for each group): A) control group, SD rats received an intraperitoneal injection of saline. B) VPAH group, SD rats received intraperitoneal injection of 200 mg/(kg body weight) VPA for five days; C) NTG group, SD rats received intraperitoneal injection of vehicle of VPA each day for five days followed by intraperitoneall injection of 10 mg/(kg body weight) NTG. D) NTG-VPAL group, SD rats received intraperitoneal injection of 100 mg/(kg body weight) VPA for five days followed by injection of 10 mg/(kg body weight) NTG. E) NTG-VPAH group, SD rats received intraperitoneal injection of 200 mg/(kg body weight) VPA for five days followed by injection of 10 mg/(kg body weight) NTG. Four hours after NTG injection, three rats were randomly selected from each group for electroencephalogram (EEG) recording and the left animals were sacrificed for sampling of peripheral blood in jugular vessel and brain tissues.

Determination of the effect of VPA pre-treatment on the oxidative stress response in brain tissues

The lipid peroxidation was measured with the thiobarbituric-acid reaction with brain homogenate samples, which was determined by comparing the absorption to the standard curve of malondialdehyde (MDA) according to the method proposed by Placer et al. [22] using MDA detection kit according to the manufacturers' instruction (Catal. No. A003-1, Nanjing Jiangcheng Bioengineering

Institute, Nanjing, China). Additionally, the activities of glutathione (GSH) and glutathione peroxidase (GSH-x) in brain homogenate samples were measured according to the manufacturers' introductions of the assay kits (Catal. No. A006-2, A005, Nanjing Jiancheng Bioengineering Institute, China). Moreover, the concentrations of vitamin A in brain homogenate samples were quantified according to the previously described methods [23–25]. Level of vitamin C and vitamin E in brain homogenate samples were measured using detection kits according to the manufacturers' introduction (Catal. No. A009, A008, Nanjing Jiangcheng Bioengineering Institute, Nanjing, China).

Enzyme-linked immuno sorbent assay
The level of CGRP in jugular blood [26, 27] was determined with ELISA method using CGRP detection kit (Catal. No. CEA876Ra USCN, China) according to the manufacturer's instructions. For jugular blood collection, 1 mL blood samples in each group was drawn from the jugular vessel and stored in Eppendorf tubes containing EDTA (1 mg/ml blood) and the protease inhibitor Aprotinin (0.55 TIU/ml blood).

Immunohistochemical detection
For immunohistochemical assay, sections were made from trigeminal nucleus caudalis (TNC) tissues from different groups and incubated at 60 °C overnight before dewaxed with dimethylbenzene. The slides were hydrated with alcohol followed by washed with H_2O_2 for 5 min, fixed using methanol solution with 3 % H_2O_2, and blocked with 1 % goat serum for 15 min at room temperature. They were then incubated with primary anti-c-Fos antibody (1:200) at 37 °C for 30 min before incubated at 4 °C overnight. After four cycles of 0.01 M PBS wash, 5 min for each cycle, secondary antibody (1:200) was added to the slides and placed at 37 °C for 30 min before another four cycles of PBS wash. Slides were incubated with HRP at 37 °C for 30 min before three cycles of 5-min PBS washing. Then DAB was added to the slides and reacted for 3–10 min until the reaction was stopped by ddH_2O. Slides were re-stained using haematoxylin and dehydrated. Percentage of positively stained cells and the staining intensity of the different groups were determined by observation under a microscope at 400× magnification by experimenters blind to the experiments.

Western blotting assay
The protein product of c-Fos, IκBα, and p-IκBα in TNC of different groups was extracted using the Total Protein Extraction Kit according to the manufacturer's instructions (Catalog No. WLA019, Wanleibio, China). Nuclear NF-κB subunit p65 was extracted using Nuclear and Cytoplasm Protein Extraction kit (Catal. No. WLA020, Wanleibio, China). β-actin and Histone H3 were used as

internal reference proteins for different molecules. Concentrations of protein samples were determined using the BCA method and western blotting was performed as described previously with some modification [10]: 40 μg protein in 20 μL volume was subjected to 10 % sodium dodecylsulfate polyacrylamide gel electrophoresis (SDS-PAGE). After transferring the proteins onto polyvinylidene difluoride (PVDF) membranes, the membranes were washed with TTBS for 5 min and then incubated with skim milk powder solution for 1 h. Primary antibody against c-Fos (1:500), IκBα (1:500), p-IκBα (1:500), and nuclear NF-κB subunit p65 (1:400), β-actin (1:1000) or Histone H3 (1:500) was added and the membranes were incubated at 4 °C overnight. Following washing with TTBS, the membranes were incubated with HRP-conjugated IgG secondary antibodies (1:5000) for 45 min at 37 °C. After washing, the blots were developed using Beyo ECL Plus reagent and scanned in the Gel Imaging System. The relative expression levels of the target proteins were calculated with Gel-Pro-Analyzer (Media Cybernetics, USA).

Electrophoretic Mobility Shift Assay (EMSA)
The nuclear protein in TNC samples were extracted using Nuclear and Cytoplasm Protein Extraction kit (Catal. No. WLA020, Wanleibio, China). The DNA binding ability of NF-κB was quantified by EMSA using NF-κB EMSA kit (Viagene, China) according to the manufacturer's instruction: briefly, the TNC samples were diluted using PBS into 5 μg/μL and subjected to the reaction solution before addition of biotin-labelled NF-κB probe. The blots were developed using Beyo ECL Plus reagent and the results were detected in the Gel Imaging System.

Statistical analysis
All the data were expressed in the form of mean ± SD and n number for each analysis for each group was five. Post-doc multiple comparisons were conducted by LSD (least significant difference) method using general liner model with a significant level of 0.05. All the statistical analysis and graph manipulation were conducted using R language version 3.2.1 [28].

Results
Results of EEG recording
Rats in control group had normal baseline EEGs without any evidence of paroxysmal activity (Fig. 1a). The injection of NTG induced an increase of theta and delta activity in EEG record (Fig. 1b). After administration of VPA, the increase of the slow activity was restored to relatively normal pattern. Moreover, the effect of VPA on NTG-induced migraine was dose-dependent with the EEG in VPAH group performing better than that in VPAL group (Fig. 1c and Fig. 1d). However, there was

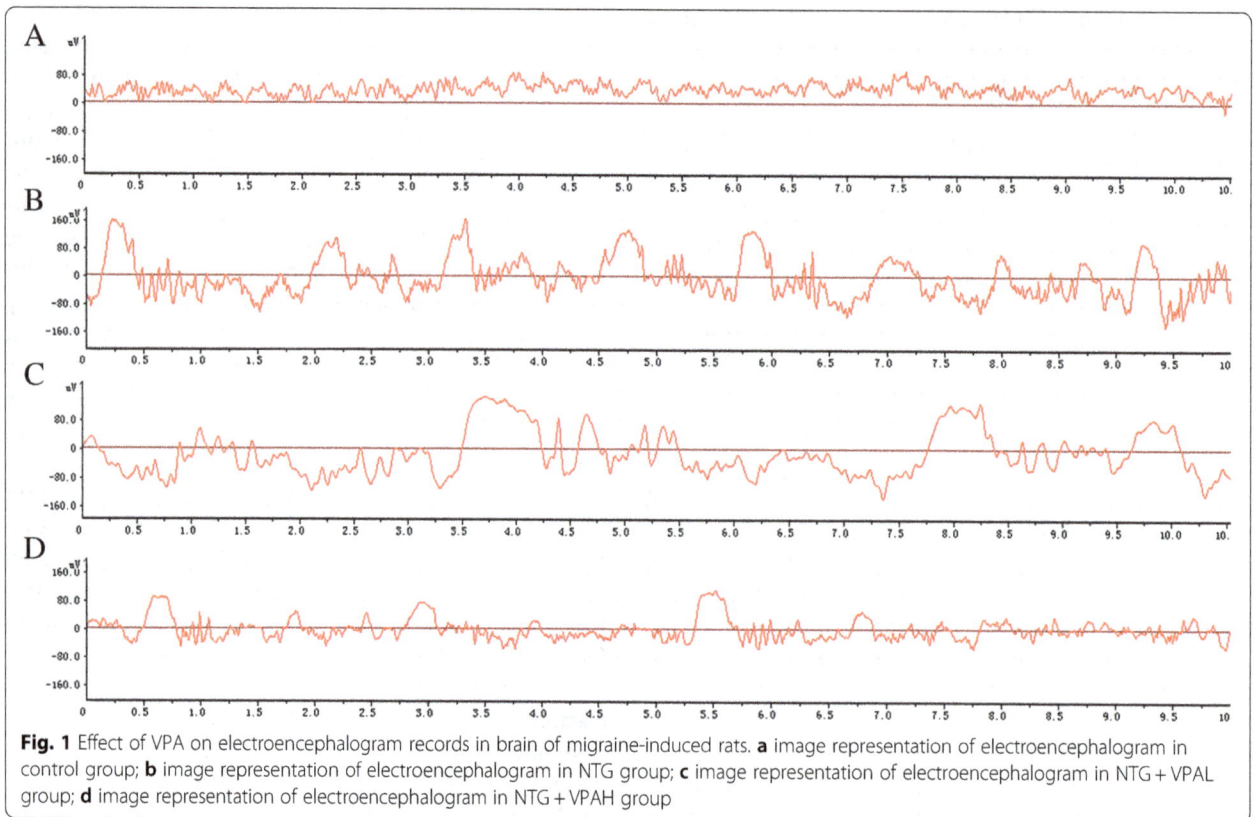

Fig. 1 Effect of VPA on electroencephalogram records in brain of migraine-induced rats. **a** image representation of electroencephalogram in control group; **b** image representation of electroencephalogram in NTG group; **c** image representation of electroencephalogram in NTG + VPAL group; **d** image representation of electroencephalogram in NTG + VPAH group

no significant change in the amplitude of the EEG waves in the four groups. Although our results didn't provide solid evidence in differentiating migraine from non-migraine cases, it might suggest some difference in the posterior background activity in the EEG in migraine rats as compared to the controls.

Pre-administration of VPA improved the oxidative stress response induced by NTG injection

Detecting results of MDA, GSH, GSH-x, vitamin A, vitamin C, and vitamin E were shown in Table 1. It was confirmed that sole treatment of VPA of 200 mk/(kg body weight) had no effect on the expression of the six indicators. MDA was representative of the lipid

peroxidation and the level was up-regulated by NTG injection, indicating an increase in the lipid peroxidation in brain tissues. Contrary to the change pattern of MDA, the content of GSH and GSH-x were both reduced by NTG injection (Table 1). GSH is the most abundant thiol andioxidant in mammalian cells and maintains the thiol redox in the cells. GSH-x is critical for the reduction of hydro- and organic peroxides with the presence of GSH. The production of three indicators was restored to relatively normal levels in the VPA pre-treated groups, representing the anti-oxidation effect of VPA on brain tissues. The effect of VPA on NTG-induced dys-expression of the three indicators was dose-dependent but there was no significant difference

Table 1 The effect of VPA on the oxidative stress response in NTG-induced migraine rats (mean ± SD)

Indicators	Group				
	Control	VPAH	NTG	NTG-VPAL	NTG-VPAH
MDA (nmol/mg protein)	10.8 ± 1.9	8.5 ± 2.8	25.3 ± 6.7*,**	21.8 ± 4.2*,**	13.5 ± 3.5***,****
GSH (nmol/mg protein)	8.9 ± 1.2	8.4 ± 1.9	5.2 ± 0.9*,**	6.2 ± 1.5*	8.2 ± 1.5***
GSH-x (U/g protein)	17.8 ± 0.6	16.3 ± 3.4	7.8 ± 2.0*,**	10.8 ± 3.0*,**	15.1 ± 2.1***,****
Vitamin A (μmol/g brain)	3.3 ± 0.7	3.2 ± 0.5	1.6 ± 0.3*,**	2.1 ± 0.3*,**	2.9 ± 0.4***,****
Vitamin C (μmol/g brain)	71.0 ± 16.6	69.2 ± 11.7	33.8 ± 8.0*,**	44.0 ± 6.6***	62.5 ± 9.6***
Vitamin E (μmol/g brain)	11.0 ± 1.5	11.8 ± 2.0	5.8 ± 1.5*,**	7.4 ± 1.1*,**	9.0 ± 1.6***

"*", significantly different from the control group, $P < 0.05$; "**", significantly different from the VPAH group, $P < 0.05$; "***", significantly different from the NTG group, $P < 0.05$; "****", significantly different from the NTG-VPAL group, $P < 0.05$

between NTG and NTG-VPAL groups, and only the difference between NTG group and NTG-VPAH group was statistically significant ($P < 0.05$). The change patterns of the content of vitamin A, vitamin C, and vitamin E in different groups were similar to those of GSH and GSH-x (Table 1), which was also indicative of the anti-oxidative potential of VPA as well.

Pre-administration of VPA inhibited the increase of CGRP level in jugular blood and reduced the number of c-Fos positive neurons in TNC

As show in Fig. 2a, the synthesis of CGRP was also induced by NTG injection, but pre-administration of VPA suppressed the increase and the effect was dose-dependent: the inhibiting effect of 200 mg/(kg body weight) VPA on CGRP was stronger than that of 100 mg/(kg body weight) dose, but only the level of CGRP in NTG + VPAH group was significantly different from that of NTG group ($P < 0.05$). The expression of c-Fos in TNC was assessed using immunohistochemistry (Fig. 2b). c-Fos positive neurons were determined as the brown granules labeled in the cell nucleus. The NTG injection increased the number of c-Fos positive neurons. In VPA pre-treated groups, the densities of brown granules obviously reduced

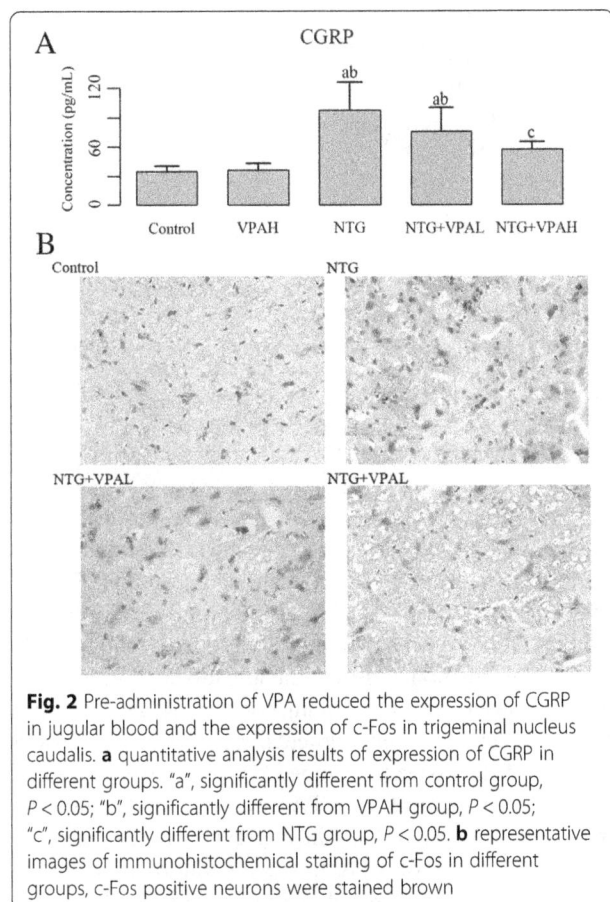

Fig. 2 Pre-administration of VPA reduced the expression of CGRP in jugular blood and the expression of c-Fos in trigeminal nucleus caudalis. **a** quantitative analysis results of expression of CGRP in different groups. "a", significantly different from control group, $P < 0.05$; "b", significantly different from VPAH group, $P < 0.05$; "c", significantly different from NTG group, $P < 0.05$. **b** representative images of immunohistochemical staining of c-Fos in different groups, c-Fos positive neurons were stained brown

under the observation with a microscope at 400× magnification. Additionally, the expression of c-Fos production illustrated by western blotting exhibited a similar pattern to that of immunohistochemistry (Fig. 3a), and the levels of c-Fos in both NTG + VPAL and NTG + VPAH groups were significantly different from that of NTG group ($P < 0.05$).

VPA protect brain tissue against the NTG-induced migraine via the inhibition of NF-κB pathway

The expressions of protein product of IκBα, p-IκBα, and NF-κB subunit p65 were quantified using western blotting assay. Production of p-IκBα and nuclear NF-κB subunit p65 was closely related to the activation of NF-κB pathway. After the injection of NTG, it was found the levels of these two molecules were up-regulated (Fig. 3b and 3c), and the differences between control groups and NTG groups were statistically significant ($P < 0.05$). The activation of NF-κB pathway was also verified by the increase of NF-κB's DNA binding ability detected by EMSA (Fig. 4). Opposite to the expression of p-IκBα and p65, the expression of IκBα was inhibited by NTG injection. IκBα in cytoplasm would bind to NF-κB and inhibit its activation. Our results confirmed that NTG-induced migraine could be initiated by the activation of the NF-κB pathway. Then pre-administration of VPA reversed the expression pattern of NF-κB pathway members due to migraine attack. Both doses of VPA significantly reduced the expressions of p-IκBα and NF-κB subunit p65 (Fig. 3b and 3c), and corresponding to the decreased level of p65, the DNA binding activity of NF-κB was also inhibited (Fig. 4). In addition, the level of cytoplasmic IκBα was restored by pre-administration of VPA. The effect of VPA on the NF-κB pathway was dose-dependent as well, and the difference between the two doses of VPA was statistically significant ($P < 0.05$).

Discussion

Trigeminovascular system is believed to play a crucial role in the attacks of migraine in classical neuroscience field [29]. The signal that will finally lead to migraine is transmitted to the ventroposterior thalamus from the so-called trigeminocervical complex (or TNC) [30]. In addition, central sensitization associated with activation of NF-κB in the TNC is reported to be involved in the pathogenesis of migraine as well [11]. NF-κB is believed to be implicated in multiple signaling pathways in variable physiological and pathological settings [31], and numerous therapies targeting the NF-κB pathways has been developed to protect patients against migraine [7, 11]. The results of the current study showed that pre-administration of VPA alleviated the impairments due to NTG-induced migraine by inhibiting the activation of NF-κB signal transduction pathway.

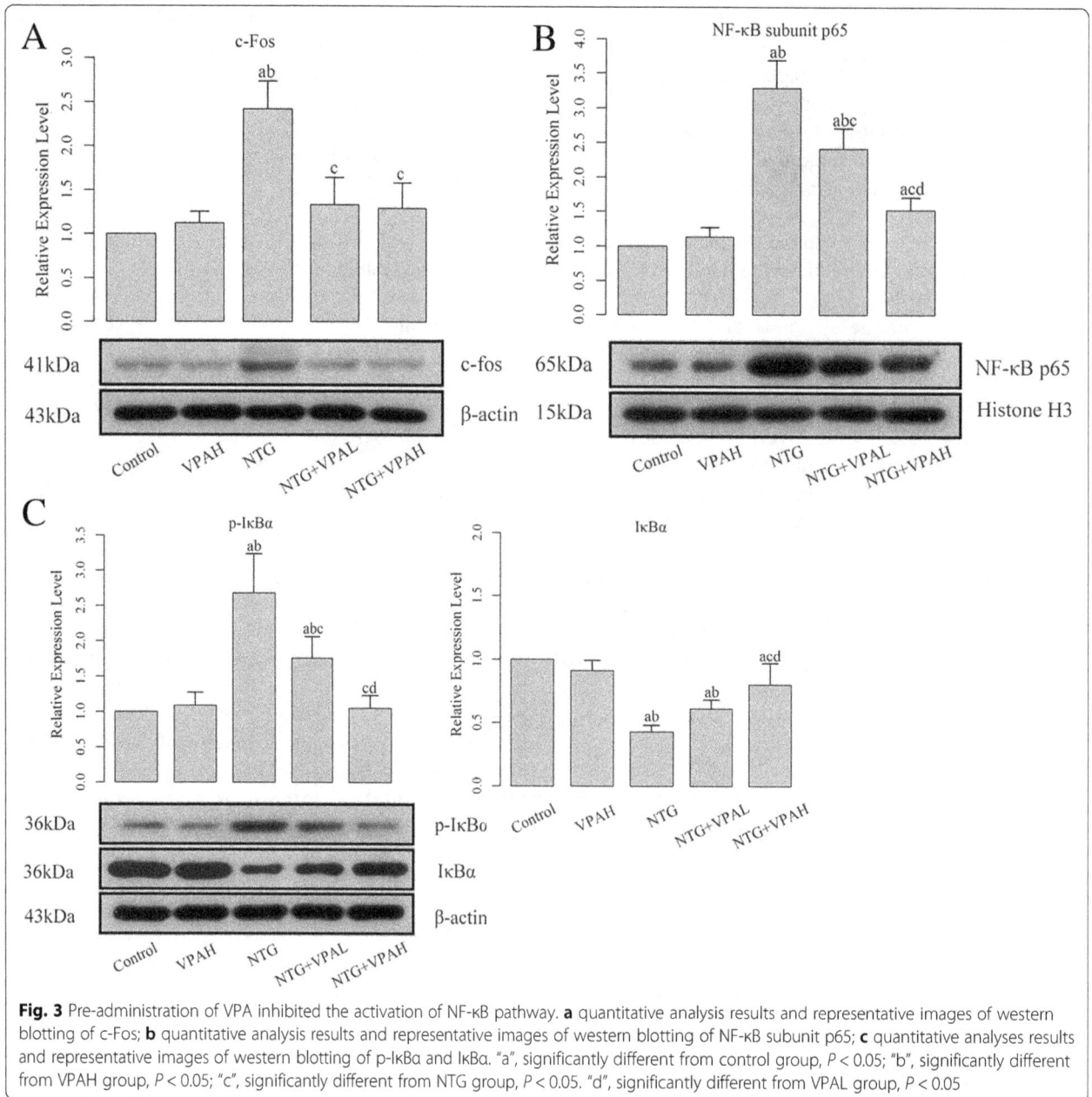

Fig. 3 Pre-administration of VPA inhibited the activation of NF-κB pathway. **a** quantitative analysis results and representative images of western blotting of c-Fos; **b** quantitative analysis results and representative images of western blotting of NF-κB subunit p65; **c** quantitative analyses results and representative images of western blotting of p-IκBα and IκBα. "a", significantly different from control group, $P < 0.05$; "b", significantly different from VPAH group, $P < 0.05$; "c", significantly different from NTG group, $P < 0.05$. "d", significantly different from VPAL group, $P < 0.05$

Experimental models of migraine induced by NTG injection reflect the inflammatory response with the contribution to the activation of iNOS and cytokines at the meningeal level [19]. Moreover, NTG is evidently proved to trigger the activation of NF-κB in the TNC [7]. In our findings, after injection of NTG, the level of MDA in NTG group was significantly up-regulated compared with control group. It is believed that oxidative stress-induced lipid peroxidation is involved in numerous neurological diseases including migraine [20]. Associated with the increase of lipid peroxidation, significant decrease in antioxidant effectors was also recorded. For GSH and GSH-x, down-regulated of these two molecules in NTG group represented an overload production of reactive oxygen species (ROS) due to NTG-induced migraine attack Also, levels of vitamin A, vitamin E, and vitamin C, which are capable of inhibiting mitochondria-induced ROS production [32], were also significantly inhibited in the brain tissues The low levels of antioxidant vitamins resulted from NTG injection would facilitate oxidative damage in the experimental rats. All the expression patterns of the above mentioned molecules were reversed by the pre-treatment of VPA, evidently indicating the anti-oxidant ability of VPA in migraine. Interestingly, the antioxidant effect of VPA has been found in other research models, including idiopathic epilepsy and primary

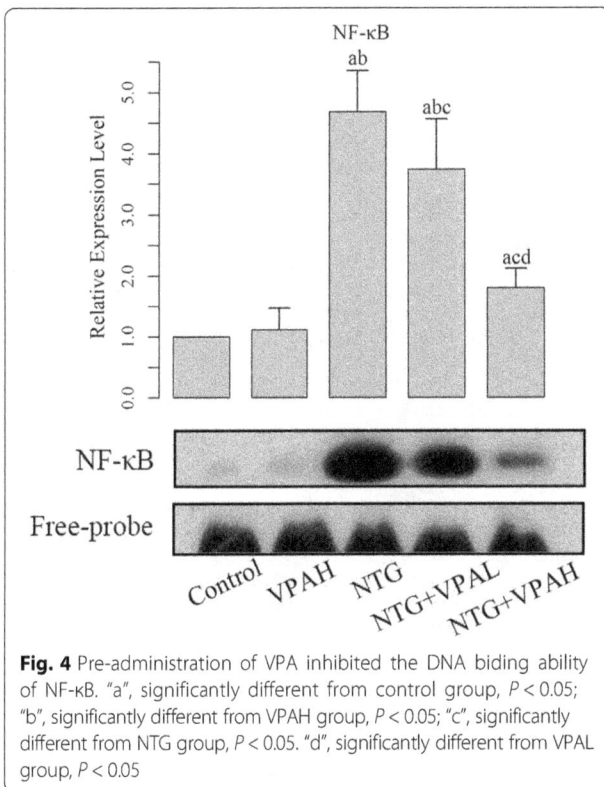

Fig. 4 Pre-administration of VPA inhibited the DNA biding ability of NF-κB. "a", significantly different from control group, $P < 0.05$; "b", significantly different from VPAH group, $P < 0.05$; "c", significantly different from NTG group, $P < 0.05$. "d", significantly different from VPAL group, $P < 0.05$

cultured rat cerebral cortical cells [33–35]. Therefore, we speculated that the protective role of VPA in NTG-induced migraine might be associated with its alleviative effects on oxidative stress damages instead of inhibition of trigeminal neuronal firing.

The migraine antagonizing capability of VPA was also verified by the decrease of jugular blood CGRP which inhibits the synaptic release of various neurotransmitters and is closely related headache generation [26, 36]. Furthermore, the decrease of c-Fos in TNC also supported antioxidant effect of VPA. c-Fos is a sensitive marker of neuronal activation following noxious stimulation, and expression of c-Fos has been widely used to identify areas of neuronal activation and to study neural correlates of nociception as well [37]. As being reported previously, VPA has an inducing effect on g-aminobutyric acid (GABA) in migraine [38]. GABA is a neutral amino acid which binds to one of at least 2 receptor subtypes [39, 40]. Metabolism of GABA is disordered during the attack of migraine [41]. Previous study indicates that administration of VPA restores brain GABA levels and suppresses migraine related events in the cortex [42]. The induction in GABA by VPA results in the inhibition of neuron activation [43], which might affect CGRP and c-fos expression via central and/or peripheral sites of action. However, more than a single GABAergic mechanism might influence the expression of CGRP and

c-fos. Thus, experiments targeting GABA based on neural progenitor cells are prepared in our lab to comprehensively explore the mechanism through which VPA exerts its function on CGRP and c-Fos.

The findings in the current study strongly suggested the inductive effect of NTG on NF-κB. NF-κB is a transcriptional factor that regulates the apoptosis and inflammation in various diseases [31]. The inactive form of NF-κB is sequestered in the cytoplasm by binding with IκBα. Once IκBα is phosphorylated into p-IκBα, NF-κB subunits will be translocated into nucleus and activate the transcriptional of the targeted genes. After being treated with NTG, the expressions of p-IκBα and nuclear NF-κB subunit p65 were all enhanced and further led to the activation of NF-κB related pathways. To the opposite, level of IκBα was reduced, which would further result in the release of active form of NF-κB in cytoplasm. Combined with the results of ELISA and immunohitochemical detection, our study was in consistence with the emerging studies that report the activity of NF-κB in regulating the plasticity of neurons and synapsis [31, 44]. In the work of Yin et al., the authors suggest that atorvastatin attenuated the NTG-induced NF-κB activation in TNC in a dose-dependent manner [11]. Furthermore, in the study of Reuter et al., the results infer that NTG promotes NF-κB activity and inflammation, and administration of parthenolide can alleviate the impairment by deactivating the activation of NF-κB and expression of iNOS [45]. Regarding the effect of VPA on NF-κB pathway, Go et al. [46] reported that VPA possesses the ability to inhibit neural progenitor cell death via the activation of NF-κB. However, the results of Go's study is exactly contrary to ours which indicated that pre-treatment with VPA significantly attenuated the activity of NF-κB pathways and led to the protective effect on nervous system. Although many studies suggest that VPA inhibits NF-κB activity possibly by increasing acetylation on NF-κB [46], at least one study reports that VPA protects neuron from oxidative stress-induced cell death by acetylation-induced activation of NF-κB. Additionally, Rao and his colleague inferred that VPA could inhibit the activation of NF-κB by decreasing the p50 protein levels and had no effect on the phosphorylation state of IκBα, level of total IκBα protein, or protein level of cytosolic p65 in cytosol [47]. But in the current study, solid evidence showed that VPA influenced the activity of both IκBα and p65. These contradictions of the effect of VPA on the NF-κB pathway has been raised by several other studies as well [48–51], which suggest the possibility that the differential regulating pattern of VPA on NF-κB activity in different experimental conditions may be due to the dose- and time window-sensitive characteristics of VPA. Thus, the application of the VPA to modulate NF-κB related pathways should be carefully assessed before being brought into practice.

Conclusions

In summary, our current work investigated the potential of VPA as a therapy against migraine. Based on a NTG-induced migraine model, it was found that pre-administration with VPA would alleviate the damage due to migraine attack. Through the inhibition of NF-κB pathway in TNC, VPA could reduce the production of ROS in brain tissues. However, the explicit mechanism of VPA acting on NF-κB pathway is still complex. Given the contrary conclusions of ours and previous studies [48–51], application of VPA in clinic should be carefully assessed based on certain conditions. What can be told is that defining the role of VPA in protecting against diseases such as migraine will provide more insights into the pathogenesis and therapeutic strategies of nervous system disorders.

Competing interests
The authors declare that they have no competing interests.

Authors' contributions
YL participated in the experiment design, carried out the model establishment and molecular studies, and drafted the manuscript. QZ carried out the ELISA. DQ carried out the immunohistochemitry. LZ participated in statistical analysis. LY carried out the EEG records. QL participated in the design of the experiment and help to draft the manuscript. ZZ revised the manuscript and approved the final submission of the work. All authors read and approved the final manuscript.

Acknowledgements
This study was supported by a grant from the Science and Technology Project of Department of Education, Heilongjiang Province (No.: 12531309).

References
1. Schurks M, Diener HC, Goadsby P (2008) Update on the prophylaxis of migraine. Curr Treat Option Ne 10(1):20–29
2. Welch KM, Goadsby PJ (2002) Chronic daily headache: nosology and pathophysiology. Curr Opin Neurol 15(3):287–295
3. Neeb L, Reuter U (2007) Nitric oxide in migraine. CNS Neurol Disord-Dr drug targets 6(4):258–264
4. Sarchielli P, Alberti A, Russo S, Codini M, Panico R, Floridi A, Gallai V (1999) Nitric oxide pathway, Ca2+, and serotonin content in platelets from patients suffering from chronic daily headache. Cephalalgia 19(9):810–816
5. Stepien A, Chalimoniuk M (1998) Level of nitric oxide-dependent cGMP in patients with migraine. Cephalalgia 18(9):631–634
6. Olesen J (2008) The role of nitric oxide (NO) in migraine, tension-type headache and cluster headache. Pharmacol Therapeut 120(2):157–171
7. Tassorelli C, Greco R, Morazzoni P, Riva A, Sandrini G, Nappi G (2005) Parthenolide is the component of tanacetum parthenium that inhibits nitroglycerin-induced Fos activation: studies in an animal model of migraine. Cephalalgia 25(8):612–621
8. Knyihar-Csillik E, Toldi J, Mihaly A, Krisztin-Peva B, Chadaide Z, Nemeth H, Fenyo R, Vecsei L (2007) Kynurenine in combination with probenecid mitigates the stimulation-induced increase of c-fos immunoreactivity of the rat caudal trigeminal nucleus in an experimental migraine model. J Neural Transm (Vienna) 114(4):417–421. doi:10.1007/s00702-006-0545-z
9. Wang S, Liu Z, Wang L, Zhang X (2009) NF-kappaB signaling pathway, inflammation and colorectal cancer. Cell Mol Immunol 6(5):327–334. doi:10.1038/cmi.2009.43
10. Di W, Zheng ZY, Xiao ZJ, Qi WW, Shi XL, Luo N, Lin JW, Ding MH, Zhang AW, Fang YN (2015) Pregabalin alleviates the nitroglycerin-induced hyperalgesia in rats. Neuroscience 284:11–17. doi:10.1016/j.neuroscience.2014.08.056
11. Yin Z, Fang Y, Ren L, Wang X, Zhang A, Lin J, Li X (2009) Atorvastatin attenuates NF-κB activation in trigeminal nucleus caudalis in a rat model of migraine. Neurosci Lett 465(1):61–65
12. Linde M, Mulleners WM, Chronicle EP, McCrory DC (2013) Valproate (valproic acid or sodium valproate or a combination of the two) for the prophylaxis of episodic migraine in adults. Cochrane DB Syst Rev 6:CD010611. doi:10.1002/14651858.CD010611
13. Chen PS, Peng GS, Li G, Yang S, Wu X, Wang CC, Wilson B, Lu RB, Gean PW, Chuang DM, Hong JS (2006) Valproate protects dopaminergic neurons in midbrain neuron/glia cultures by stimulating the release of neurotrophic factors from astrocytes. Mol Psychiatr 11(12):1116–1125. doi:10.1038/sj.mp.4001893
14. Feng HL, Leng Y, Ma CH, Zhang J, Ren M, Chuang DM (2008) Combined lithium and valproate treatment delays disease onset, reduces neurological deficits and prolongs survival in an amyotrophic lateral sclerosis mouse model. Neuroscience 155(3):567–572
15. Kim HJ, Rowe M, Ren M, Hong JS, Chen PS, Chuang DM (2007) Histone deacetylase inhibitors exhibit anti-inflammatory and neuroprotective effects in a rat permanent ischemic model of stroke: multiple mechanisms of action. J Pharmacol Exp The 321(3):892–901. doi:10.1124/jpet.107.120188
16. Qing H, He G, Ly PT, Fox CJ, Staufenbiel M, Cai F, Zhang Z, Wei S, Sun X, Chen CH, Zhou W, Wang K, Song W (2008) Valproic acid inhibits Abeta production, neuritic plaque formation, and behavioral deficits in Alzheimer's disease mouse models. J Exp Med 205(12):2781–2789. doi:10.1084/jem.20081588
17. Pardutz A, Hoyk Z, Varga H, Vecsei L, Schoenen J (2007) Oestrogen-modulated increase of calmodulin-dependent protein kinase II (CamKII) in rat spinal trigeminal nucleus after systemic nitroglycerin. Cephalalgia 27(1):46–53
18. Varga H, Pardutz A, Vamos E, Bohar Z, Bago F, Tajti J, Bari F, Vecsei L (2009) Selective inhibition of cyclooxygenase-2 attenuates nitroglycerin-induced calmodulin-dependent protein kinase II alpha in rat trigeminal nucleus caudalis. Neurosci Lett 451(2):170–173
19. Reuter U, Bolay H, Jansen-Olesen I, Chiarugi A, Sanchez del Rio M, Letourneau R, Theoharides TC, Waeber C, Moskowitz MA (2001) Delayed inflammation in rat meninges: implications for migraine pathophysiology. Brain 124(Pt 12):2490–2502
20. Erol I, Alehan F, Aldemir D, Ogus E (2010) Increased vulnerability to oxidative stress in pediatric migraine patients. Pediatr Neurol 43(1):21–24. doi:10.1016/j.pediatrneurol.2010.02.014
21. Messlinger K, Lennerz JK, Eberhardt M, Fischer MJM (2012) CGRP and NO in the trigeminal system: mechanisms and role in headache generation. Headache 52(9):1411–1427
22. Placer ZA, Cushman L, Johnson BC (1966) Estimation of products of lipid peroxidation (malonyl dialdehyde) in biological fluids. Anal Biochem 16:359–364
23. Desai ID (1984) Vitamin E analysis methods for animal tissues. Method Enzymol 105:138–147
24. Suzuki J, Katoh N (1990) A simple and cheap method for measuring vitamin A in cattle using only a spectrophotometer. The Japanese Journal of Veterinary Science 52:1282–1284
25. Jagota SK, Dani HM (1982) A new colorimetric technique for the estimation of vitamin C using Folin phenol reagent. Anal Biochem 127(1):178–182
26. Fehrenbacher JC, Taylor CP, Vasko MR (2003) Pregabalin and gabapentin reduce release of substance P and CGRP from rat spinal tissues only after inflammation or activation of protein kinase C. Pain 105(1-2):133–141
27. Offenhauser N, Zinck T, Hoffmann J, Schiemann K, Schuh-Hofer S, Rohde W, Arnold G, Dirnagl U, Jansen-Olesen I, Reuter U (2005) CGRP release and c-fos expression within trigeminal nucleus caudalis of the rat following glyceryltrinitrate infusion. Cephalalgia 25(3):225–236
28. Team RC (2014) R (2012) A language and environment for statistical computing. R Foundation for Statistical Computing, Vienna, Austria. ISBN 3-900051-07-0
29. Moskowitz MA (1992) Neurogenic versus vascular mechanisms of sumatriptan and ergot alkaloids in migraine. Trends Pharmacol Sci 13(8):307–311
30. Link AS, Kuris A, Edvinsson L (2008) Treatment of migraine attacks based on the interaction with the trigemino-cerebrovascular system. J Headache Pain 9(1):5–12. doi:10.1007/s10194-008-0011-4
31. Mattson MP (2005) NF-kappaB in the survival and plasticity of neurons. Neurochem Res 30(6-7):883–893. doi:10.1007/s11064-005-6961-x
32. Martinez-Cruz F, Osuna C, Guerrero JM (2006) Mitochondrial damage induced by fetal hyperphenylalaninemia in the rat brain and liver: its prevention by melatonin, Vitamin E, and Vitamin C. Neurosci Lett 392(1-2):1–4. doi:10.1016/j.neulet.2005.02.073

33. Varoglu AO, Yildirim A, Aygul R, Gundogdu OL, Sahin YN (2010) Effects of valproate, carbamazepine, and levetiracetam on the antioxidant and oxidant systems in epileptic patients and their clinical importance. Clin neuropharmacol 33(3):155–157

34. Wang JF, Azzam JE, Young LT (2003) Valproate inhibits oxidative damage to lipid and protein in primary cultured rat cerebrocortical cells. Neuroscience 116(2):485–489

35. Zhang YJ, Zhang M, Wang XC, Yu YH, Jin PJ, Wang Y (2011) Effects of sodium valproate on neutrophils' oxidative metabolism and oxidant status in children with idiopathic epilepsy. Zhonghua er ke za zhi Chinese Journal of pediatrics 49(10):776–781

36. Taylor CP, Angelotti T, Fauman E (2007) Pharmacology and mechanism of action of pregabalin: the calcium channel α 2–δ (alpha 2–delta) subunit as a target for antiepileptic drug discovery. Epilepsy Res 73(2):137–150

37. Harris JA (1998) Using c-fos as a neural marker of pain. Brain Res Bull 45(1):1–8

38. Cutrer FM, Limmroth V, Ayata G, Moskowitz MA (1995) Attenuation by valproate of c-fos immunoreactivity in trigeminal nucleus caudalis induced by intracisternal capsaicin. Brit J Pharmacol 116(8):3199–3204

39. Macdonald RL, Olsen RW (1994) GABAA receptor channels. Annu Rev Neurosci 17(1):569–602

40. Bonanno G, Raiteri M (1993) Multiple GABAB receptors. Trends Pharmacol Sci 14(7):259–261

41. Welch KM, Chabi E, Bartosh K, Achar VS, Meyer JS (1975) Cerebrospinal fluid gamma aminobutyric acid levels in migraine. Brit Med J 3(5982):516–517

42. Cutrer FM, Limmroth V, Moskowitz MA (1997) Possible mechanisms of valproate in migraine prophylaxis. Cephalalgia 17(2):93–100

43. Morgan JI, Cohen DR, Hempstead JL, Curran T (1987) Mapping patterns of c-fos expression in the central nervous system after seizure. Science 237(4811):192–197

44. Meberg PJ, Kinney WR, Valcourt EG, Routtenberg A (1996) Gene expression of the transcription factor NF-κ B in hippocampus: regulation by synaptic activity. Molr Brain Res 38(2):179–190

45. Reuter U, Chiarugi A, Bolay H, Moskowitz MA (2002) Nuclear factor-κB as a molecular target for migraine therapy. Ann Neurol 51(4):507–516

46. Go HS, Seo JE, Kim KC, Han SM, Kim P, Kang YS, Han SH, Shin CY, Ko KH (2011) Valproic acid inhibits neural progenitor cell death by activation of NF-B signaling pathway and up-regulation of Bcl-XL. J Biomed Sci 18(1):48

47. Rao JS, Bazinet RP, Rapoport SI, Lee HJ (2007) Chronic treatment of rats with sodium valproate downregulates frontal cortex NF-κB DNA binding activity and COX-2 mRNA1. Bipolar Disord 9(5):513–520

48. Wang Z, Leng Y, Tsai L-K, Leeds P, Chuang D-M (2011) Valproic acid attenuates blood–brain barrier disruption in a rat model of transient focal cerebral ischemia: the roles of HDAC and MMP-9 inhibition. J Cerebr Blood F Met 31(1):52–57

49. Faraco G, Pittelli M, Cavone L, Fossati S, Porcu M, Mascagni P, Fossati G, Moroni F, Chiarugi A (2009) Histone deacetylase (HDAC) inhibitors reduce the glial inflammatory response in vitro and in vivo. Neurobiol Di 36(2):269–279

50. Ichiyama T, Okada K, Lipton JM, Matsubara T, Hayashi T, Furukawa S (2000) Sodium valproate inhibits production of TNF-α and IL-6 and activation of NF-κB. Brain Res 857(1):246–251

51. Li Y, Yuan Z, Liu B, Sailhamer EA, Shults C, Velmahos GC, Alam HB (2008) Prevention of hypoxia-induced neuronal apoptosis through histone deacetylase inhibition. J Trauma Acute Care 64(4):863–871

5

The effect of 1 mg folic acid supplementation on clinical outcomes in female migraine with aura patients

Saras Menon[1], Bushra Nasir[1], Nesli Avgan[1], Sussan Ghassabian[2], Christopher Oliver[3], Rodney Lea[1], Maree Smith[2] and Lyn Griffiths[1*] (iD)

Abstract

Background: Migraine is a common neurovascular condition that may be linked to hyperhomocysteinemia. We have previously provided evidence that reduction of homocysteine with a vitamin supplementation can reduce the occurrence of migraine in women. The current study examined the occurrence of migraine in response to vitamin supplementation with a lower dose of folic acid.

Methods: This was a 6 month randomised, double blinded placebo controlled trial of daily vitamin supplementation containing 1 mg of folic acid, 25 mg of Vitamin B_6 and Vitamin B_{12}, on reduction of homocysteine and the occurrence of migraine in 300 female patients diagnosed with migraine with aura.

Results: Vitamin supplementation with 1 mg of folic acid, did not significantly decrease homocysteine levels ($P = 0.2$). The treatment group did not show a significant decrease in the percentage of participants with high migraine disability, severity or frequency at the end of the 6 month intervention ($P > 0.1$).

Conclusion: 1 mg of folic acid in combination with vitamin B_6 and B_{12} is less effective in reducing migraine associated symptoms compared to the previously tested dosage of 2 mg folic acid in combination with 25 mg of vitamin B_6 and 400 μg of vitamin B_{12}.

Keywords: Migraine, Folate, Folic acid, Vitamin B_6, Vitamin B_{12}

Background

Migraine is a very common episodic neurological disorder which is typically characterised by attacks of 4 to 72 h of severe headache and associated with autonomic and neurological symptoms [1]. The International Headache Society (IHS) has classified migraine into migraine with aura (MA) and migraine without aura (MO) [2]. The incidence of migraine is much higher in females (70 %) than in males (30 %) and is at its highest during the peak reproductive years (between the ages of 25 and 55 years) [3]. Despite the high prevalence of migraine, its pathophysiology is not completely understood. The activation of the trigeminovascular system which results in vasodilation of pain producing intracranial blood vessels is thought to be responsible for the typical pain migraineurs experience [4]. Family and twin studies have shown that both common and rare migraine subtypes have a significant genetic basis with environmental interactions also playing an important role in disease manifestation [1]. Previous studies have identified neurological, vascular and hormonal pathways to be involved in migraine susceptibility and pathophysiology [5, 6].

The human methylenetetrahydrofolate reductase (MTHFR) gene is involved in the remethylation of homocysteine to methionine. The C677T allele (rs1801133), a common variant of the MTHFR gene has a frequency of approximately 23–41 % in the Caucasian population [7]. The TT genotype of the MTHFR C677T SNP has been shown to be associated with a 50 % reduction in enzyme activity and consequently moderately increased levels of circulating homocysteine [7–10]. This variant and elevated homocysteine levels have been associated with the risk of

* Correspondence: lyn.griffiths@qut.edu.au
[1]Genomics Research Centre, Institute of Health and Biomedical Innovation, Queensland University of Technology, Kelvin Grove, QLD, Australia

several neurological conditions including migraine [11, 12]. Homocysteine related endothelial dysfunction might be involved in the initiation and maintenance of a migraine attack. Several studies have shown the TT genotype of the MTHFRC677T variant to significantly increase the risk of MA [8, 9].

Our laboratory has previously investigated the homocysteine-lowering effects of vitamin supplementation in MA patients and the modifying effect of C677T genotype on treatment response. In the Phase 1 trial, the effects of 2 mg folic acid, 25 mg vitamin B_6 and 400 μg vitamin B_{12} were examined in 52 MA sufferers [13]. The major finding of this study was that vitamin supplementation reduced plasma homocysteine levels and migraine disability significantly in this migraine group. This study also provided some evidence that the effect of vitamin supplementation on reduction of homocysteine levels and migraine disability was influenced by the MTHFRC677T genotype, whereby carriers of the C allele experienced a greater response compared to TT genotypes [13].

In the Phase 2 trial we replicated the treatment options in an independent and larger sample of MA sufferers and examined the genotypic effects of both the MTHFR and MTRR (5-Methyltetrahydrofolate-Homocysteine Methyltransferase Reductase) gene on the reduction of homocysteine and migraine disability in response to vitamin supplementation [14]. The Phase 2 trial provided further evidence that the MTHFR variant influences treatment response and that the MTRR variant may also be acting independently to influence vitamin treatment response in migraineurs. Despite improvements in some participants, the more functionally affected MTHFR T allele and MTRR G carriers seemed to resist homocysteine reduction and did not respond as well in terms of alleviation of migraine symptoms [14]. The purpose of this study was to determine if a lower folic acid dosage (1 mg) that lies within the currently recommended daily intake range was also effective in reducing homocysteine levels and migraine disability. This would enable the development of safe, personalised treatment and prophylactic regimes for migraine in the community.

Methods
Patient group
The study recruited female Caucasian adult participants. European descents living in Australia, having emigrating ancestors within the last 160 years from various locations within the British Isles and other parts of Europe were recruited from East Coast of Australia and were interviewed and completed a detailed questionnaire that was administered through the Genomics Research Centre (GRC).

As migraine is more prevalent in females and this prevalence reduces drastically in males only females between the ages of 18 and 60 were recruited. Participants were included if they had suffered migraine for over > 5 years and had a current diagnosis of MA (>90 % of their migraine attacks were associated with aura), and a 1-year history of severe, long lasting attacks (at least 4 attacks lasting more than 48 h), had a family history of migraine. Confirmation of migraine diagnosis was carried out using the IHS criteria. As this hypothesised that the outcome variable, the response to vitamin therapy is influenced by inherited factors, genetic independence of participants was given important attention. Thus it was made sure that only participants that are not related by first degree were included in the study. Participants who were currently taking vitamin supplementation, were pregnant, or had been diagnosed with a clinically recognised co-morbid disease such as vascular disease, depression or epilepsy were excluded from the trial to reduce clinical and pathological heterogeneity. Participants that had taken part in another clinical trial or had received any experimental therapy within the last one month were also excluded from the trial. The patient group was not selected on the basis of pre-existing folic acid, B_{12} or B_6 deficiency. This study was originally approved by Griffith University Human Research Ethics Committee (HREC), approval number MSC/09/05/HREC.

Randomisation and blinding
Three hundred female patients meeting the inclusion criteria were randomly assigned into either the placebo or the treatment group. A blocked random allocation sequence was generated using nQuery Advisor (Statistical Solutions, Cork, [Ireland]). Patients and everyone involved in this trial were blinded to randomisation and group allocation. One hundred random female patients were assigned to the placebo group and 200 random female patients were assigned to the vitamin tablet. The numbers in the treatment group were higher to increase the power for genotype comparisons in relation to treatment response.

Treatment
Patients received either vitamin tablets containing 1 mg of folic acid, 25 mg of vitamin B_6 and 400 μg of vitamin B_{12} or the placebo tablet. Both the vitamin and placebo tablets were produced by Blackmores (Warriewood, New South Wales, Australia) and were indistinguishable in appearance. Patients were instructed to take one tablet daily for 6 months.

Baseline and follow-up assessment
Before the treatment all participants were assessed for migraine disability using the Migraine Disability Assessment

Score (MIDAS) instrument, which provides a measure of productive days lost to migraine headache in previous 3 months (i.e. migraine disability), as well as headache frequency and pain severity [13, 15]. Patients were asked to complete a daily diary during the trial period to record the details of their migraine symptoms (duration, frequency and severity) and treatment compliance. Patients were also instructed to take their usual migraine treatment for acute attacks. A blood sample was collected for baseline measurement of plasma homocysteine (μmol/l), folate (nmol/l), vitamin B_6 and B_{12} (pmol/l) concentration. 2 ml of venous blood was collected for Genomic DNA extraction and genotyping purposes.

Patients were contacted after 3 months for headache diary and compliance checking. At the end of the 6 month trial the patients were reassessed at the GRC clinic. They were questioned about their migraine history in the last 6 months since the start of the trial. A second collection of blood samples was done for measurement of homocysteine, folate, B_6 and B_{12} concentrations.

Clinical outcome measures

Migraine disability measured by the MIDAS instrument was the primary clinical outcome in this trial. Studies have shown that the MIDAS instrument is a valid and clinically useful instrument for assessing health-related quality of life in migraineurs. Based on the 5-question MIDAS rating, participants were arbitrarily categorised into a 'low' disability group if they had a MIDAS rating of 0–10 and into a 'high' disability group if they had a MIDAS rating greater than 11 [13, 15, 16]. Secondary outcome variables, which are partly captured within the primary outcome, were migraine frequency and head pain severity. These were measured as number of days with headache (over a 3 month period) and a pain score (based on a scale of 1–10), respectively [13, 15, 16].

Predictor variables

The primary predictor variable for this study was the treatment groups (Vitamin vs placebo). The secondary predictor variables include plasma homocysteine levels and the C677T polymorphism of the MTHFR gene, grouped by TT and CT and CC genotypes. The C677T polymorphism was genotyped in the patient group in the GRC laboratory using previously published methods [9]. The Plasma homocysteine, folate, B_6 and B_{12} levels were measured in an accredited pathology laboratory (TetraQ, University of Queensland, Brisbane) [17, 18].

Statistical analysis

The analysis for the trial was conducted on a modified intention-to-treat (ITT) principle. The modified ITT cohort was composed of all randomised participants who started the trial and consumed study supplements on at least one occasion, excluding those who withdrew from the trial after the randomisation process had taken place but before the commencement of study supplement consumption. At baseline and follow-up time points, unpaired samples t-tests were used to test the group means and proportions were compared using the χ^2 test of independence. The significance threshold was set at α level of 0.05. All analyses were performed using the Statistical Package for Social Sciences (SPSS version 18.0; International Business Machines, Chicago, Illinois, USA).

Results

Figure 1 shows the participant flow through the trial. A total of 1050 migraineurs were assessed for eligibility before enrolment into the trial. Of them 750 migraineurs were excluded because of reasons such as nonfulfillment of the inclusion criterial, refusal to participate in a placebo-controlled trial and other reasons. In total, 300 participants were initially enrolled in the trial and were randomly assigned in the ration of 1:2 to either the placebo group or the vitamin- treated group respectively, but seven participants dropped out before the commencement of the trial and 36 participants dropped out at baseline assessment. Two hundred and fifty seven participants received baseline assessment and successfully commenced trial. One hundred and seventy participants were included in the vitamin- treated group and the remaining 87 participants were included in the placebo-treated group. Sixty eight participants were lost to follow-up because of lack of compliance and 189 participants completed the trial (126 Vitamin treated, 63 Placebo treated).

Baseline analysis

Table 1 shows the baseline clinical characteristics of the participant group. The mean folate concentration was 33.7 nmol/l and 35.6 nmol/l for the placebo and the treatment group respectively, which were above the average folate concentration of 13.7 nmol/l in the general Caucasian population. The mean plasma homocysteine concentration was 9.5 μmol/l and 9.4 μmol/l for the placebo and the treatment group respectively, which were slightly above the average plasma homocysteine level of 8.9 μmol/l in the general Caucasian population. The mean B_6 and B_{12} levels at baseline for both the placebo and treatment groups were within the normal range for a general Caucasian population. The percentage of participants with high migraine frequency and high migraine severity did not significantly differ between the placebo and the treatment group at baseline, however the percentage of participants with high migraine disability significantly differed between the placebo and the treatment group (P =0.02). The placebo group had an increased proportion of participants

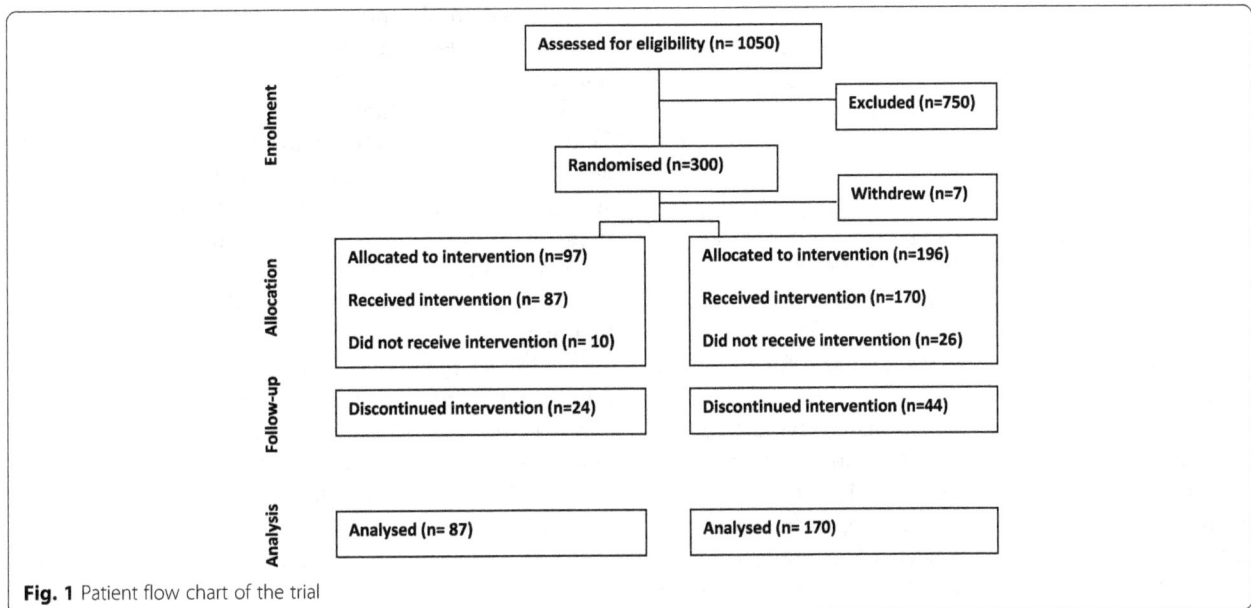

Fig. 1 Patient flow chart of the trial

(91 %) with high migraine disability compared to the treatment group (79 %).

Values are mean (SD) or n (%)

For the blood biochemistries at follow-up (Table 2) - folate, B_6 and B_{12} levels were significantly higher in the treatment group compared to placebo group ($P < 0.0001$) after 6 months of intervention. Plasma homocysteine levels remained at 9.5 μmol/l for the placebo group while in the treatment group, plasma homocysteine levels decreased from 9.4 to 8.5 μmol/l after the 6 months of intervention. However this decrease was not statistically significant ($P = 0.2$). This result is in contrast to our previous results testing the effect of 2 mg of folic acid, which showed a statistically significant reduction in mean homocysteine ($P < 0.001$) in the treatment group. The baseline Hcy plasma levels of the treatment group was lower in the current trial (9.4 μmol/l) compared to the previous trial, this is most likely due to the higher level of baseline folate levels in the current trial (35.6 nmol/l) compared to the previous trial (31.4 nmol/l), which displays a possible floor effect.

For the migraine clinical outcomes at follow-up (Table 3) the treatment group had a lower percentage of participants with high migraine disability, severity and frequency compared to the placebo group at the end of the 6 month intervention. However, these differences were not statistically significant ($P > 0.1$).

When the treatment group was stratified by the MTHFR C677T genotype, an overall decrease in the percentage of high migraine disability, frequency and severity was observed for all three genotype groups after the 6 months of intervention however the decrease was not statistically significant ($P > 0.10$).

Discussion

Migraine is a chronic and debilitating condition that has significant impact on both the sufferer and the society at large [19]. Although there are several migraine therapies and medications currently available to treat migraine, most of them work with differing efficacy and are often associated with adverse effects [20]. Migraine research thus continues to explore new and/or improved migraine

Table 1 Clinical characteristics of patient groups at baseline

Analyte	Placebo ($n = 87$)	1 mg ($n = 170$)
Folate	33.7 (11.6)	35.6 (11.9)
B_6	97.2 (7.3)	132.2 (12.1)
B_{12}	266.1 (94.3)	289.3 (104.4)
Hcy	9.5 (2.6)	9.4 (2.8)
High Disability	79 (91 %)	134 (79 %)
High Frequency	56 (64 %)	109 (64 %)
High Severity	43 (49 %)	73 (43 %)

Table 2 Summary of blood biochemistry measures at follow-up*

Analyte	Placebo ($n = 63$)	1 mg ($n = 126$)	P value*
Folate	34.6 (1.6)	52.6 (0.40)	<0.0001
B6	134.6 (21.5)	490.6 (24.9)	<0.0001
B12	274.1 (11.6)	456.8 (11.6)	<0.0001
Hcy	9.5 (0.32)	8.5 (0.49)	0.2

Values are means (SEM)
Change in folate, B_6, B_{12} and Hcy levels in the treatment and placebo group after 6 months of intervention. Hcy levels did not significantly decrease in the treatment group compared to the placebo group after 6 months of intervention
*P values were determined by t-test

Table 3 Summary of migraine outcomes at follow-up*

Analyte	Placebo (n = 63)	1 mg (n = 126)	P value*
(a) High Disability	34 (52 %)	56 (45 %)	0.4
(b) High Frequency	28 (43 %)	44 (36 %)	0.33
(c) High Severity	12 (19 %)	16 (13 %)	0.31

Values are n (%)
High disability (a) is defined as a MIDAS score >11, High Frequency (b) is defined as a score >10 (median) and High Severity (c) is defined as a score >7 (median). All scores were categorised due to the deviation from non-normal distribution and to improve interpretation
*P value were determined by Chi-square tests

treatments that are both effective and safe for use by all migraineurs [21].

The Genomics Research Centre had previously tested the effects of folate and vitamin B treatment response in migraineurs in two previous studies [13, 14]. The results of these previous studies and have reported the significant decrease in migraine associated symptoms after a 6 month intervention of a vitamin tablet containing 2 mg folic acid, 25 mg of vitamin B_6 and 400 µg of vitamin B_{12}. When the effect of the MTHFRC677T and the MTRR A66G genetic variants on migraine treatment was assessed, it was observed that both these variants exert an independent effect on migraine treatment response [14].

The current trial investigated the effect of 1 mg folic acid, 25 mg of vitamin B_6 and 400 µg of vitamin B_{12} on migraine associated symptoms on adult Caucasian females with MA. The aims of the current study was to investigate the effectiveness of a vitamin supplementation incorporating 1 mg folic acid, 25 mg of vitamin B_6 and 400 µg of vitamin B_{12} in significantly reducing migraine associated symptoms and to investigate the effect of the MTHFRC677T variant on the reduction of homocysteine and migraine associated symptoms in response to the vitamin supplementation.

The results of this trial did not observe a significant reduction in homocysteine levels in the treatment group compared to the placebo group ($P = 0.2$) and there was also no significant decrease observed in migraine disability, frequency or severity in treatment group compared to the placebo group at the end of the treatment period. This result was in contrast to the previous trials which investigated vitamin supplementation of 2 mg folic acid, 25 mg of vitamin B_6 and 400 µg of vitamin B_{12} and reported significant decrease in homocysteine levels as well as migraine associated symptoms compared to the placebo group at the end of treatment period. Similarly while the previous trial reported migraine associated variants, in the MTHFR and MTRR genes to have a significant effect on migraine treatment response, the current trial did not observe any significant effect of the MTHFR C677T gene variant on migraine treatment response. This current study has provided evidence that the folic acid dosage in the proposed vitamin supplementation for migraine treatment plays a pertinent part in reducing homocysteine levels and migraine associated symptoms.

Folate, a water-soluble vitamin, includes endogenous food folate and its synthetic form, folic acid [22]. Folate lacks stability in its naturally occurring form in food storage and preparation; however, folic acid is stable and used for supplements and food fortification [23]. There are many critical cellular pathways dependent on folate as a one-carbon source, including DNA, RNA, and protein methylation, as well as DNA synthesis and maintenance [24]. A number of genetic polymorphisms affect critical components of folate pathways and metabolism, and have been associated with an increased risk for several diseases [25–31]. Mandatory folate fortification of wheat flour was implemented in Australia in 2009. The tolerable upper intake level (UL) (1000 µg/day)of folic acid was established as one-fifth of the lowest observed adverse effect level (5000 µg/day) associated with a potential adverse outcome [32]. Even at dosages of 15,000–100,000 µg of folic acid daily, limited evidence was found of direct toxicity from folic acid [33–38]. However recently the possibility that folic acid intake might lead to changes in epigenetic patterns and thus the plausible hypotheses of how folic acid might affect certain diseases has led to concerns about higher folic acid intake and food fortification programs.

The most important concern has surrounded cancer as the field of epigenetics has been studied largely in the context of tumorogenesis where clear DNA methylation pattern changes in tumors have been reported [39–44]. It has been suggested that early exposure to folic acid might prevent some cancers and in contrast, after the development of tumors, higher intake of folic acid might promote growth of existing tumors [45]. However, a very recent meta-analysis of randomised clinical trials (RCTs) of the effects of B vitamins on 37,485 individuals with existing cardiovascular disease showed no increased risk of cancer incidence. Additionally, since the implementation of mandatory folic acid fortification in the United States in 1998, both incidence and mortality of colorectal cancer have continued to decline [46]. With such varying studies results, extensive research is warranted to fully understand the effect of folic acid on disease risk.

Further research is thus needed to understand the use of vitamin supplementation incorporating various doses of folic acid, vitamin B_6 and B_{12} in regards to not only on the reduction of migraine associated symptoms but also the long term effects of vitamin supplementation on the general well-being of migraineurs.

Conclusion

The recommend dosage of 1 mg folic acid in combination with vitamins vitamin B_6 and B_{12} is less effective in reducing migraine associated symptoms compared to the previously tested dosage of 2 mg folic acid in combination with 25 mg of vitamin B_6 and 400 μg of vitamin B_{12}.

Competing interests
The authors declare that they have no competing interests.

Authors' contributions
LG was involved in the conception and design of the study. SM and was involved in the generation and collection of data. SM and NA were involved in the genotyping of participant samples. MS and SG were involved in the Biochemistry analysis of samples. SM and BN were involved in the assembly of data. RL, SM and BN were involved in the analysis and interpretation of the data. RL, SM and LG were involved in the drafting and revision of the manuscript. LG, RL and CO were involved in approving the final version of the manuscript. All authors have read and approved the final manuscript.

Acknowledgements
The authors acknowledge all the participants of this study who consented and volunteered to participate in the trial.

Funding
This study was supported by funding from a Queensland (Qld) Government Smart State CIF grant. The Genomics Research Centre is a member of the Therapeutic Innovation Australia (TIA), QLD node with funding provided through an ARC EIF Super Science Initiative, TIA NCRIS 2013 and TIA NCRIS 2015.

Author details
[1]Genomics Research Centre, Institute of Health and Biomedical Innovation, Queensland University of Technology, Kelvin Grove, QLD, Australia. [2]Centre for Integrated Preclinical Drug Development Faculty of Medicine and Biomedical Sciences, University of Queensland, Brisbane, QLD, Australia. [3]Blackmores Institute, 20 Jubilee Avenue, Warriewood NSW 2102, Australia.

References
1. de Vries B et al (2009) Molecular genetics of migraine. Hum Genet 126(1): 115–32
2. (1994) Guidelines on the investigation and diagnosis of cobalamin and folate deficiencies. A publication of the British Committee for Standards in Haematology. BCSH General Haematology Test Force. Clin Lab Haematol. 16(2): 101–15
3. Stovner L et al (2007) The global burden of headache: a documentation of headache prevalence and disability worldwide. Cephalalgia 27(3):193–210
4. Goadsby PJ et al (2009) Neurobiology of migraine. Neuroscience 161(2): 327–41
5. Cutrer FM (2010) Pathophysiology of migraine. Semin Neurol 30(2):120–30
6. Pietrobon D, Moskowitz MA (2013) Pathophysiology of migraine. Annu Rev Physiol 75:365–91
7. Kara I et al (2003) Association of the C677T and A1298C polymorphisms in the 5,10 methylenetetrahydrofolate reductase gene in patients with migraine risk. Brain Res Mol Brain Res 111(1–2):84–90
8. Kowa H et al (2000) The homozygous C677T mutation in the methylenetetrahydrofolate reductase gene is a genetic risk factor for migraine. Am J Med Genet 96(6):762–4
9. Lea RA et al (2004) The methylenetetrahydrofolate reductase gene variant C677T influences susceptibility to migraine with aura. BMC Med 2:3
10. Di Rosa G et al (2007) Efficacy of folic acid in children with migraine, hyperhomocysteinemia and MTHFR polymorphisms. Headache 47(9):1342–4
11. Klerk M et al (2002) MTHFR 677C–>T polymorphism and risk of coronary heart disease: a meta-analysis. JAMA 288(16):2023–31
12. Aguilar B, Rojas JC, Collados MT (2004) Metabolism of homocysteine and its relationship with cardiovascular disease. J Thromb Thrombolysis 18(2):75–87
13. Lea R et al (2009) The effects of vitamin supplementation and MTHFR (C677T) genotype on homocysteine-lowering and migraine disability. Pharmacogenet Genomics 19(6):422–8
14. Menon S et al (2012) Genotypes of the MTHFR C677T and MTRR A66G genes act independently to reduce migraine disability in response to vitamin supplementation. Pharmacogenet Genomics 22(10):741–9
15. Stewart WF et al (1999) Validity of an illness severity measure for headache in a population sample of migraine sufferers. Pain 79(2–3):291–301
16. Stewart WF et al (1999) Reliability of the migraine disability assessment score in a population-based sample of headache sufferers. Cephalalgia 19(2):107–14, discussion 74
17. Ghassabian S et al (2014) Fully validated LC-MS/MS method for quantification of homocysteine concentrations in samples of human serum: a new approach. J Chromatogr B Analyt Technol Biomed Life Sci 972:14–21
18. Ghassabian S, Griffiths L, Smith MT (2015) A novel fully validated LC-MS/MS method for quantification of pyridoxal-5'-phosphate concentrations in samples of human whole blood. J Chromatogr B Analyt Technol Biomed Life Sci 1000:77–83
19. Leonardi M et al (2005) The global burden of migraine: measuring disability in headache disorders with WHO's classification of functioning, disability and health (ICF). J Headache Pain 6(6):429–40
20. Rapoport A (2011) New frontiers in headache therapy. Neurol Sci 32(Suppl 1):S105–9
21. Rainero I et al (2013) Genes and primary headaches: discovering new potential therapeutic targets. J Headache Pain 14:61
22. Eitenmiller R, Landen W (1999) Vitamin analysis for the health and food science. Folate, pp 411–465
23. O'Broin JD et al (1975) Nutritional stability of various naturally occurring monoglutamate derivatives of folic acid. Am J Clin Nutr 28(5):438–44
24. Stover PJ (2009) Folate biochemical pathways and their regulation. In: Folate in health and disease. Taylor & Francis Group, Gainesville, pp 49–74
25. Choi SW, Mason JB (2002) Folate status: effects on pathways of colorectal carcinogenesis. J Nutr 132(8 Suppl):2413S–2418S
26. Bjelland I et al (2003) Folate, vitamin B12, homocysteine, and the MTHFR 677C-> T polymorphism in anxiety and depression: the hordaland homocysteine study. Arch Gen Psychiatry 60(6):618–26
27. Perez AB et al (2003) Methylenetetrahydrofolate reductase (MTHFR): incidence of mutations C677T and A1298C in Brazilian population and its correlation with plasma homocysteine levels in spina bifida. Am J Med Genet A 119A(1):20–5
28. Chango A et al (2005) No association between common polymorphisms in genes of folate and homocysteine metabolism and the risk of Down's syndrome among French mothers. Br J Nutr 94(2):166–9
29. Alcasabas P et al (2008) 5,10-methylenetetrahydrofolate reductase (MTHFR) polymorphisms and the risk of acute lymphoblastic leukemia (ALL) in Filipino children. Pediatr Blood Cancer 51(2):178–82
30. Brustolin S, Giugliani R, Felix TM (2010) Genetics of homocysteine metabolism and associated disorders. Braz J Med Biol Res 43(1):1–7
31. Sameer AS et al (2011) Risk of colorectal cancer associated with the methylenetetrahydrofolate reductase (MTHFR) C677T polymorphism in the Kashmiri population. Genet Mol Res 10(2):1200–10
32. Insitute of Medicine, a., Dietary Reference Intakes for Thiamin, Riboflavin, Niacin, Vitamin B6, Folate, Vitamin B12, Patothenic Acid, Biotin and Choline., in Folate. 1998, National Academy Press, Washington, p. 196–305
33. Spies TD, Suarez RM et al (1946) The therapeutic effect of folic acid in tropical sprue. Science 104(2691):75
34. Gibberd FB et al (1970) Toxicity of folic acid. Lancet 1(7642):360–1
35. Hunter R et al (1970) Toxicity of folic acid given in pharmacological doses to healthy volunteers. Lancet 1(7637):61–3
36. Hellstrom L (1971) Lack of toxicity of folic acid given in pharmacological doses to healthy volunteers. Lancet 1(7689):59–61
37. Richens A (1971) Toxicity of folic acid. Lancet 1(7705):912
38. Sheehy TW (1973) Folic acid: lack of toxicity. Lancet 1(7793):37
39. Baylin SB (1997) Tying it all together: epigenetics, genetics, cell cycle, and cancer. Science 277(5334):1948–9
40. Baylin SB, Herman JG (2000) DNA hypermethylation in tumorigenesis: epigenetics joins genetics. Trends Genet 16(4):168–74
41. Momparler RL, Bovenzi V (2000) DNA methylation and cancer. J Cell Physiol 183(2):145–54

42. Feinberg AP (2001) Cancer epigenetics takes center stage. Proc Natl Acad Sci U S A 98(2):392-4
43. Esteller M (2008) Epigenetics in cancer. N Engl J Med 358(11):1148-59
44. Sharma S, Kelly TK, Jones PA (2010) Epigenetics in cancer. Carcinogenesis 31(1):27-36
45. Ciappio E, Mason JB (2009) Folate and carcinogenesis basis mechanisms, in folate in health and disease. Taylor & Francis Group, Boca Raton, pp 235-262
46. Edwards BK et al (2010) Annual report to the nation on the status of cancer, 1975-2006, featuring colorectal cancer trends and impact of interventions (risk factors, screening, and treatment) to reduce future rates. Cancer 116(3):544-73

6

Biofeedback in the prophylactic treatment of medication overuse headache

Marialuisa Rausa[1,2], Daniela Palomba[2,3], Sabina Cevoli[4], Luana Lazzerini[2], Elisa Sancisi[5], Pietro Cortelli[1,4] and Giulia Pierangeli[1,4*] (ORCID)

Abstract

Background: Medication overuse headache (MOH) is a major clinical concern and a common health risk. Recent literature stressed the need to manage chronic headache by using integrated biobehavioral approaches. Few studies evaluated how biofeedback can be useful in MOH.
The aim of the study is to evaluate in a randomized, controlled, single-blind trial the effects of biofeedback associated with traditional pharmacological therapy in the prophylactic treatment of MOH.

Method: Twenty-seven subjects were randomized to frontal electromyographic (EMG) biofeedback associated with prophylactic pharmacological therapy (Bfb Group) or to pharmacological treatment alone (Control Group). The primary outcome was to evaluate the number of patients that return episodic after treatment. Secondly we evaluate the effects of frontal EMG BFB on frequency of headache and analgesic intake. Changes in coping strategies and in EMG frontalis tension were also evaluated. ANOVA was performed on all the variables of interest.

Results: Our results indicate that at the end of treatment the number of patients that returned episodic in the Bfb group was significantly higher than in the Control group. Patients in the Bfb group differed from the Control group in headache frequency, amount of drug intake and active coping with pain. These outcomes were confirmed also after 4 months of follow-up. No significant effects were observed in EMG recordings.

Conclusions: Biofeedback added to traditional pharmacological therapy in the treatment of MOH is a promising approach for reducing headache frequency and analgesic intake. Modification of coping cognitions in the Bfb group, as an adjunct mechanism of self-regulation, needs more evaluations to understand the role of biofeedback in changing maladaptive psychophysiological responses.

Keywords: Biofeedback, Coping strategies, Psychological treatment, Chronic migraine, Medication overuse headache, Preventive therapy

Background

Chronic headache comprise individuals with chronic tension-type headache (CTTH) and chronic migraine (CM), both of which may be associated with medication overuse and medication overuse headache (MOH) [1].

In particular, MOH is a major clinical concern and a common health risk [2]. It has a prevalence of about 1–2 % in the general population [3]. The International Classification of Headache Disorders 3rd edition (beta version) suggests a double diagnosis of either CM or CTTH and MOH, since MOH is excluded or confirmed by analgesic withdrawal.

The treatment of MOH is often complex and includes patient education, discontinuation of the offending drug, rescue therapy for withdrawal symptoms, and preventive therapy [4]. In particular, the withdrawal of the overused medication is recognized as the treatment

* Correspondence: giulia.pierangeli@unibo.it
[1]Department of Biomedical and Neuromotor Sciences DIBINEM, University of Bologna, Bologna, Italy
[4]Padiglione G, Bellaria Hospital, IRCCS Institute of Neurological Sciences of Bologna, Via Altura 3, 40139 Bologna, Italy

of choice [5–10]. Such a treatment is often compromised by lack of motivation and poor patient's self-awareness [11].

In the literature [12–14] the basic psychological factors that are key contributors to MOH are described as follows: a belief that acute medication is the only treatment option, the presence of cephalalgiaphobia [12] (or pain panic, i.e. anticipatory fear of pain), intolerance or difficulty dealing with pain, soporophilia (seeking sedation), the need to maintain the usual daily activities, presence of outside pressures and of psychiatric comorbidities.

Chronic headaches should be treated with multidimensional approaches that can support patients not only pharmacologically but also giving them behavioral and cognitive strategies to cope with their pain [15]. One of the non-pharmacological treatments that has shown positive results in treating migraine and tension-type headache is biofeedback [16–20]. Electromyographic biofeedback (EMG BFB) has proved to be effective in reducing pain symptoms associated with both tension-type headache and migraine [17, 19]. Moreover, it has been shown that many forms of headache, especially if chronic, eventually end up in a mixed headache type, and may meet the criteria for TTH [21, 22]. Although there is a large amount of scientific evidence on biobehavioral therapies for headache [23], few studies evaluated how psychological treatments could be integrated with pharmacological prophylaxis in order to favor the reduction of acute medication intake [18, 21]. Only one study [24] evaluated the effects of EMG BFB in a combined treatment of transformed migraine with analgesic overuse. Data showed that patients treated with biofeedback and pharmacological therapy, after analgesic withdrawal, improved in headache frequency and analgesic intake similarly to control group, but have better improvement after 3 years of follow-up..

No data are available about the role that biofeedback treatment could have in reducing medication overuse without a structured drug withdrawal. Moreover, it has not yet been investigated if biofeedback, as an active self-regulation intervention, could also help MOH patients by changing their strategies to cope with headache attacks in comparison with pharmacological treatment.

Indeed, the role of coping strategies in managing chronic pain and headache has been previously investigated [25–29]. In particular, some studies explored the role of pain catastrophizing (as a maladaptive coping strategy) in migraine. Catastophizing is associated with impaired quality of life [26], chronicity of headache and poorer treatment response [27, 28]; whereas few studies analyzed the effects of biofeedback treatment on coping skills [16].

In his meta-analysis on efficacy of BFB on migraine, Nestoriuc found that self-efficacy yielded higher effect sizes than the actual pain related outcome measures of biofeedback and recommended studies to directly investigate whether changes in self-efficacy (and subsequent changes in coping strategies) mediate the treatment effects of BFB. Currently, no data are available on modifications in coping skills after biofeedback training in MOH.

The aims of the present study were to evaluate the effects of EMG BFB associated with traditional pharmacological interventions on patients with MOH without previous withdrawal intervention in a tertiary headache center. The primary outcome was to evaluate the number of patients that return episodic after treatment. Secondly we evaluate the effects of frontal EMG BFB on frequency of headache and analgesic intake. Changes in coping strategies and in EMG frontalis tension were also evaluated.

Method

Participants

All consecutive patients attending the Headache Center of IRCCS Institute of Neurological Sciences of Bologna in a range of 2 years (from 2008 to 2010), satisfying inclusion criteria for CM and MOH or CTTH and MOH, and accepting to participate were recruited. Headache and drug overuse were classified according to the International Classification of Headache Disorders 3rd Edition (beta version) [1].

Exclusion criteria were: foreign language as mother tongue, pregnancy, secondary headaches, age < 18, noncompliance. Secondary headaches were ruled out by clinical examination, biochemical tests, and neuroimaging studies, when indicated.

Participants gave written informed consent and the study was carried out in accordance with the Declaration of Helsinki; the study protocol was approved by the Ethic Committee of the Local Health Service of Bologna, Italy (protocol number: 07044).

Protocol

During the first visit (T0) patients who gave informed consent and satisfied the inclusion criteria received a headache diary, self-administered questionnaires (see Additional file 1: Measures paragraph), and pharmacological therapy prescription. The pharmacological prophylaxis was chosen by the neurologist according to the prophylactic therapy best suited to each patient, considering efficacy and side effects of previous treatments, comorbidity, and patient's preferences. The neurologist also informed patients about the risks of medication overuse, asking to stop or reduce analgesic intake.

After 1 month (T1) psychophysiological measures were recorded at rest. Headache diary and questionnaires were administered again. At the end of the assessment patients were randomly assigned to the treatment group (Bfb group) or to the control group (Control group). Randomization codes were generated through computer and inserted in numerical sequence into sealed envelopes. Subjects were allocated in 1:1 ratio. The psychologist knew patients' allocation, while neurologists were blinded to it.

Patients in the Bfb group underwent 9 weekly sessions of EMG biofeedback, whereas patients in the Control group underwent 9 weekly sessions with a psychologist in which they were interviewed about their previous week's headaches, their mood, and their analgesic intake. In both groups patients were encouraged to stop or reduce analgesic overuse. Neurologists were blinded to which group the patients belonged.

At the end of the treatment (T2) patients were evaluated from the neurologist and from the psychologist (by psychophysiological assessment). Headache diary and questionnaires were re-administered. The same procedure was followed after 4 months from the end of the treatment (T3). At 1 year from the end of the treatment (T4) patients were visited and evaluated by a neurologist.

Measures

Each time (T0, T1, T2, T3) patients were evaluated by the following measures.

The *Headache Diary* is a monthly diary in which frequency (number of days), intensity (from 1 to 3), and duration (number of hours in a day) of headache attacks were recorded along with the type and the amount of analgesic intake.

PRSS (Pain Related Self Statements Scale) and PRCS (Pain Related Control Scale) [30, 31] are two self-administered questionnaires. The PRSS is an 18-item questionnaire that assesses situation-specific aspects of patients' cognitive coping strategies for pain. Patients have to choose on a Likert scale (0 to 5) how many times they have thoughts such as "If I stay calm and relax I feel better" or "I cannot tolerate this pain anymore". PRSS has two subscales: "Catastrophizing" and "Active Coping". The PRCS is a 15-item questionnaire that measures general attitudes towards pain with statements like "I myself can do something against my pain" and it is divided into 2 subscales: 'Helplessness' and 'Resourcefulness'. Both questionnaires were demonstrated to be valid and sensitive to change, and they are closely related to pain intensity and interference from pain experiences.

At T4 the neurologist evaluated the current headache diagnosis and adherence to pharmacological treatment.

Physiological measures

The frontalis muscle electromyographic activity as a measure of tension was recorded in baseline condition and during the training. The EMG was recorded and fed back to the subject by means of a Biofeedback Modular System (Modulab series 800, SATEM, Rome, Italy).

Treatment

The EMG BFB treatment was carried out by a psychologist at Centro Gruber (Bologna), a service for the diagnosis and treatment of eating disorders and of anxiety and psychosomatic disorders. The initial psychophysiological assessment consisted of 2 sessions in which both clinical data and psychophysiological recordings were collected to assess the state of the patient before treatment at baseline and under stress conditions. The 9 weekly sessions of frontalis muscle EMG BFB aimed to reduce muscle tension. The treatment was divided into three phases: a first acquisition phase, in which the feedback was always present (3 sessions), a second maintenance phase, in which trials with and without feedback were alternated (3 sessions), and a third exposure phase, in which patients attempted to use the technique in imagined situations subjectively perceived as stressful (3 sessions). In all phases patients did not were trained in any relaxation technique, they were encouraged to find muscle tension reduction strategies by themselves. The treatment ended with a reassessment session. The procedure of the entire treatment (12 one hour weekly sessions in all)was standardized and was the same for all patients. The psychologist had to fill a checklist of the status of adherence with the protocol.

Data analysis

The assumptions for the calculation of the sample needed to test the primary end point were: a beta error of 20 %, an alpha error of 5, 50 % of responders in the experimental group and 10 % of responders in the placebo group. Given these assumptions, at least 24 patients per group had to be recruited.

Descriptive statistics (means ± SD) were conducted on the sample features. The sample was randomized into two groups: Biofeedback group (Bfb Group) and Control group. The normality of parameters distribution was checked using Skewedness-Kurtosis. Chi-squared, Student's *T*-test and ANOVA repeated measures were performed to compare data between groups at T1, T2 and T3. Bonferroni correction for multiple comparisons was used. When appropriate, post-hoc analyses were carried out. Data were analyzed using the statistical software SPSS 19.0 (Statistical Package for Social Science). Significance level was set at two-tailed $p < 0.05$.

Results

Forty-seven of 72 patients with MOH consecutively referred to the Headache Center responded to the inclusion criteria and accepted to participate. Three patients were excluded because at T1 they did not fulfill the MOH diagnosis anymore, 10 participants dropped out between T1 and T2 (6 in the Bfb group, 4 in the Control group).

Analyses were conducted only in the 27 participants who provided headache diary data for all measurement periods and completed the study: 15 belonged to the Bfb group, 12 belonged to Control group (Fig. 1).

Patients who did not complete the study did not differ from other participants in: age ($t = -.500$, $p = .620$), sex ($x^2 = 0.688$, $p = 0.41$) educational level ($x^2 = 0.719$, $p = 0.69$) and type of headache at onset ($x^2 = 1.340$, $p = 0.51$), but they differed in age of chronification ($t = 3.924$, $p < 0.001$): participants who dropped out of the study had suffered from MOH for a longer period of time.

According to the original ICHD 3rd edition (beta version), 24 of 27 subjects had a diagnosis of CM and MOH and 3 of CTTH and MOH.

Table 1 shows patients' demographic and headache characteristics. Participants of the Bfb group and Control group did not differ in age ($t = -1.060$, $p = 0.30$), sex ($x^2 = 0.059$, $p = 0.81$), educational level ($x^2 = 0.617$, $p = 0.73$), type of headache at onset ($x^2 = 1.739$, $p = 0.42$), age of chronification ($t = -1.025$, $p = 0.31$). Drugs used for preventive therapy were: antiepileptics (14 patients: 9 in Bfb group and 5 in Control group), beta-blockers (5 patients: 2 in Bfb group and 3 in Control group), antidepressants (6 patients: 3 in Bfb group and 3 in Control group), Ca-antagonists (2 patients in Control group), pizotifen (1 patient in Bfb group).

At the end of the treatment (T2) patients that returned to episodic headache were respectively 10 (67 %) in the Bfb group and 2 (17 %) in the Control group ($x^2 = 6.750$, $p = 0.009$); after 4 months (T3), 12 (80 %) in the Bfb group and 3 (25 %) in the Control group ($x^2 = 8.168$, $p = 0.004$). After 1 year (T4), 7 patients (47 %) in the Bfb group and 2 (17 %) in the Control group ($x^2 = 2.700$, $p = 0.10$) remained episodic (Table 2).

Intention-to treat-analysis was performed on number of responders in the two groups. Including patients that did not complete the study as non responders, the percentages of patients that return episodic at the end of the treatment (T2) were respectively the 37,5 % in the Bfb group, 10 % in the Control Group ($x^2 = 4.417$, $p = 0.036$), at T3 44,44 % in the Bfb group and 15 % in the Control Group ($x^2 = 4.584$, $p = 0.032$), at T4 25,92 % in the Bfb Group and 10 % in the Control Group ($x^2 = 1,88$, $p = 0.170$).

Diary variables

Analyses were performed on the two groups (15 patients of the Bfb group, 12 patients of the Control group) (Table 3).

ANOVA repeated measures on attack frequency (number of attacks per month) yielded main effects for time ($p = 0.014$) and group ($p = 0.001$) and a Group X Time interaction effect ($p = 0.001$).

Post-hoc Fisher's LSD comparisons showed a significant reduction in frequency from T1 to T2 ($p = 0.002$) and from T1 to T3 ($p < 0.001$) only in the Bfb group, no differences in frequency were found in the Control group from T1 to T2 and from T1 to T3. No differences were found between the groups at T1.

Data about the intensity and duration of headache attacks were not analyzed because they were indicated only in 44 % of the diaries filled in by the patients.

Results about analgesic intake showed a main effect for time ($p < 0.025$) and a Group X Time interaction ($p < 0.012$). Group effect was close to the significance level, even if it did not reach it ($p = 0.051$).

Post-hoc Fisher's LSD comparisons showed a significant reduction in analgesic intake from T1 to T2 ($p = 0.001$) and from T1 to T3 ($p = 0.009$) only in the Bfb group, no differences in frequency were found in the Control group from T1 to T2 and from T1 to T3. No differences were found between the groups at T1.

Psychological measures

PRSS and PRCS results were analyzed in 25 patients (14 in Bfb group, 11 in Control group) because their questionnaires were invalid. In PRSS questionnaire ANOVA repeated measures was performed on the two scales: Catastrophizing and Active Coping. In Catastrophizing, analysis showed a main effect for time ($F_{[1, 23]} = 5.762$; $p = 0.006$) and group ($F_{[1, 23]} = 10.98$; $p = 0.003$), but not for the interaction Group x Time ($F_{[1, 23]} = .312$; $p = 0.73$). On post-hoc comparisons, a significant difference emerged between the groups both in pre ($p = 0.018$) and post-training ($p = 0.006$), at T3 the score decreased in both groups, but only in the Bfb group the decrease was significant ($p = 0.019$).

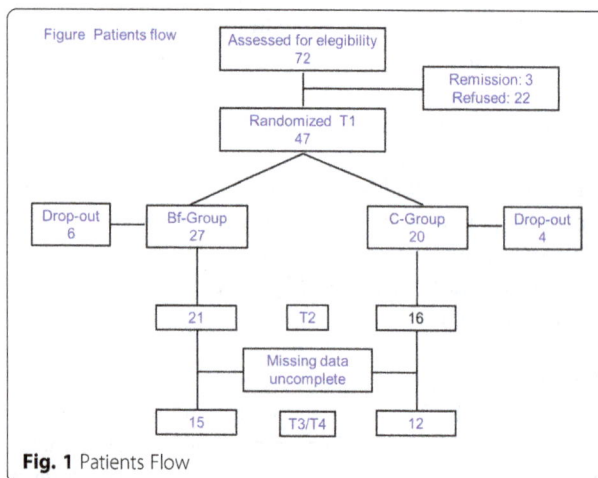

Fig. 1 Patients Flow

Table 1 Patients' demographic and headache characteristics

	Biofeedback Group	Control Group	Total
Gender			
Male	2	2	4
Female	13	10	23
Age (mean ± sd)	40.13 ± 12.41	45.08 ± 11.60	42.33 ± 12.09
Educational Level			
Primary/Secondary	2	3	5
High School	4	3	7
Graduate	9	6	15
Headache at onset			
MWOA	11	10	21
MWA	2	0	2
TTH	2	2	4
Age of chronification (mean ± sd)	28.53 ± 9.96	32.25 ± 8.85	30.18 ± 9.49
Overused drugs			
Triptans	7	5	12
NSAIDs/P	2	0	2
Combination-analgesics	1	2	3
Multiple drug classes	5	5	10
Drug prophylaxis			
Monotherapy	9	7	16
Polytherapy	4	5	9

Abbreviations: *MWOA* migraine without aura, *MWA* migraine with aura, *TTH* tension type headache

In the scale Active Coping a time effect ($F_{[1, 23]}$ = 3.984; $p = 0.044$) and a Group X Time interaction ($F_{[1,23]}$ = 4.499; $p = 0.032$) were detected. Post-hoc Fisher's LSD comparisons showed a significant increase of the scores from T1 to T2 ($p = 0.002$) and from T1 to T3 ($p = 0.047$) only in the Bfb group, no differences in Active Coping were found in the Control group from T1 to T2 ($p = 1.00$) and from T1 to T3 ($p = 1.00$). No differences were found between the groups at T1 ($p = 0.939$).

In PRCS no main interaction effects were detected, only in the subscale Helplessness a group effect was found ($F_{[1,23]} = 8.772$; $p = 0.007$). On post-hoc comparisons, the Bfb group had a lower score than the Control group at T2 ($p = 0.036$) and at T3 ($p = 0.004$). Means and Confidence intervals are available in the Additional files 1, 2 and 3.

EMG data

ANOVA repeated measures performed on frontalis EMG in baseline condition at pre- (T1) and post-treatment (T3) did not yield significant results ($p = 0.52$). No differences were found overall between groups and between the groups at T1 and at T3. No differences were found overall between groups and between the groups at T1 (Bfb Group = 2,47 ± 1,10 µV; Control Group = 2,88 ± 1,25 µV) and at T3 (Bfb Group = 2,28 ± 0,60 µV; Control Group = 2,73 ± 1,17 µV).

Discussion

Our results indicate that at the end of treatment the Bfb group had reduced the headache frequency and the amount of drug intake and showed better active coping with pain, compared with the Control group. These outcomes were confirmed also after 4 months of follow-up.

These results are in line with previous studies, showing that a combined treatment (biofeedback plus pharmacological therapy) for MOH is more effective than pharmacological therapy alone in reducing pain symptoms even

Table 2 Frequencies and percentages of responders (patients that returned episodic) at the end of treatment (T2), after 4 months (T3) and at 1 year (T4)

Responders	Biofeedback group	Control group
T2		
n (%)	10 (67 %)	2 (17 %)
T3		
n (%)	12 (80 %)	3 (25 %)
T4		
n (%)	7 (47 %)	2 (17 %)

Table 3 ANOVA results

Clinical index	Biofeedback group			Control group			Group effect	Time effect	Interaction group X time effect
	T1	T2	T3	T1	T2	T3			
	M(CI95%)	M(CI95%)	M(CI95%)	M(CI95%)	M(CI95%)	M(CI95%)			
Frequency (days/month)	19.93 (17.49; 22.37)	13.93 (10.52; 17.34)	13.00 (9.63; 16.37)	22.08 (19.36; 24.81)	24.25 (20.43;28.06)	22.33 (18.56; 26.10)	**$F_{[1,25]}$ = 14.11; $p = 0.001$	*$F_{[1,25]}$ = 5.44; $p = 0.014$	**$F_{[1,25]}$ = 9.62; $p = 0.001$
Analgesic intake (number tot/ month)	21.27 (13.68; 28.85)	11.93 (4.31; 19.53)	12.40 (2.83; 21.97)	26,62 (18.14; 35.11)	27.04 (18.54; 35.54)	21.17 (16.47; 37.86)	$F_{[1,25]}$ = 4.192; $p = 0.051$	*$F_{[1,25]}$ = 4.52; $p = 0.025$	*$F_{[1,25]}$ = 5.561; $p = 0.012$

Abbreviations: M mean, CI 95 % confidence interval 95 %
*$p<0.05$ **$p<0.01$

in the long run [24]. The combined treatment (biofeedback and pharmacological therapy) was compared with pharmacological treatment after 10 days of drug inpatient withdrawal. Headache frequency and analgesic intake improved even after 3 years of follow-up. Further findings have been obtained from the present study.

First, patients could modify analgesic intake with biofeedback independently of an analgesic-overuse structured withdrawal.

In recent literature the role of drug detoxification has been debated [32–35]. Saper and Lake created a classification system that can be useful in triaging these patients. Type 1 MOH refers to simpler cases of patients who do not have behavioral impairments and do not overuse opioids and barbiturates. Type 2 MOH patients are complex and suffer from behavioral conditions or chronically use opioids or barbiturates [36]. In our study we did not differentiate between simple or complex cases, in future research it could be useful to evaluate such distinction in order to understand which type of patients could benefit from biofeedback treatment. At 1 year of follow-up only 46 % of patients did not return chronic, this result is in line with studies that indicated a high level of relapse in MOH [37, 38] but it would have been better supported if the distinction described above had been used. Moreover, the duration of chronification is one of the characteristics that differed in patients that dropped out of the study. In future research this factor should be taken into account in order to understand if this type of patients need motivational intervention before starting biofeedback treatment or if they could not benefit from this treatment at all.

Second, in our experimental design, patients of the Control and Bfb group were followed up weekly and they were encouraged to stop or reduce analgesic overuse, but our control patients did not benefit from simple advice and support [34], indicating that in order to help patients in reducing drug intake it is necessary to give them different strategies to cope with pain, and biofeedback could help them achieve new self-regulatory strategies.

Third, patients in the Bfb group changed coping cognitions after treatment, they reported using more active coping cognitions than the Control group. Active coping cognitions included thoughts like "If I stay calm and relax, things will be better" or "I can do something about my pain" "I'll manage" "or "I will cope with it". Active coping is opposite to pain catastrophizing, which generally refers to exaggerated negative cognitive and affective reactions to an expected or actual pain experience [39] and it is characterized by magnification of the potential negative aspects of pain, inability to disengage from thoughts about pain, and a feeling of helplessness in coping with pain [40].

It has been stressed that pain catastrophizing may also worsen the experience of pain through physiological and neural pathways by enhancing it via differential patterns of brain activation [41] and by modulating the analgesic effects of medications affecting the endogenous opioid system [42, 43]. Our data allowed us to argue that the acquisition of self-regulation strategies could probably help patients to promote active behaviors and to activate different problem solving strategies. The meta-analysis of Nestoriuc supports this hypothesis, showing that frequency of migraine attacks and perceived self-efficacy had the strongest improvements after the treatment [16].

Nonetheless, modifications of coping cognitions in the biofeedback treatment of MOH needs more evaluations to understand the role of biofeedback in changing coping skills.

Fourth, these results were independent of psychophysiological modification, in fact no differences were found in EMG frontalis muscle level at rest after treatment. It could be hypothesized that if sensors had been placed differently (e.g., on the trapezius muscle or on the site most associated with pain), that would have led to more specific EMG results. Moreover, given the effects of BFB training on patients' coping strategies it could be speculated that BFB acted as a general arousal control strategy [44]. Therefore, in future studies, EMG feedback should be compared with skin conductance or thermal feedback, which more closely reflect the subject's arousal.

The most important limit of this study is the number of participants that concluded it, as the sample size determined by the calculation of the sample had not been reached. It was difficult to recruit patients and, in particular, to obtain all data for two main reasons: the protocol's length and the poor compliance that characterizes this kind of patients [11]. For this reason we considered it a pilot study.

Another limit was that at 1 year of follow-up we could not analyze frequency and intensity of headache attacks due to missing data. Also psychological measures could not be collected. Moreover, at 1 year the number of patients that had returned to episodic headache was reduced in the Bfb group and the difference with the control group did not remain significant.

After 1 year patients generally referred that they were not practicing self-regulatory strategies anymore. In future biofeedback protocols it could be useful to plan "recall sessions" at 4, 6, and 9 months and at 1 year from the end of treatment in order to prevent both relapse and missing data.

The sample of the present study included also patients with CTTH, however it was not possible to evaluate differences in the response to treatment according to diagnosis differences, due to the small number of the CTTH sample.

Conclusions

The results of our study encourage the use of biofeedback in combination with pharmacotherapy in order to stop or reduce analgesic drug overuse. Biofeedback added to traditional pharmacological therapy in the treatment of MOH is a promising approach for reducing the frequency of analgesic intake. Our study also stressed how complex the study of MOH patients is, suggesting that a multicenter randomized control trial could be useful to establish biofeedback efficacy in this kind of patients.

Abbreviations

CM: Chronic migraine; CTTH: Chronic tension-type headache; EMG BFB: Electromyographic biofeedback; MOH: Medication overuse headache

Acknowledgements

We thank Isabella Seràgnoli Foundation that supported this study by a research grant awarded to Dr. Marialuisa Rausa.
We thank Dr. Cecilia Baroncini for help in editing the manuscript.
We thank Dr. Giulia Giannini and Dr. Luca Vignatelli for help in statistical analysis.

Funding

Isabella Seràgnoli Foundation supported this study by a research grant awarded to Dr. Marialuisa Rausa.

Authors' contributions

MR: designed research, performed research, analyzed data, and wrote the paper. DP: designed research, supervised data and paper. SC: performed research, edited paper. LL: analysed data. ES: performed research. PC: designed research and supervised the paper. GP: designed research, performed research and supervised data and paper. All authors read and approved the final manuscript.

Competing interests

The Authors declare that there is no competing interests.

Author details

[1]Department of Biomedical and Neuromotor Sciences DIBINEM, University of Bologna, Bologna, Italy. [2]Service for the Diagnosis and Treatment of Eating Disorders, Service for the Diagnosis and Treatment of Anxiety and Psychosomatic Disorders, Centro Gruber, Bologna, Italy. [3]Department of General Psychology, University of Padova, Padova, Italy. [4]Padiglione G, Bellaria Hospital, IRCCS Institute of Neurological Sciences of Bologna, Via Altura 3, 40139 Bologna, Italy. [5]Neurology, AUSL (Local Health Service) of Ferrara, Ferrara, Italy.

References

1. Headache Classification Committee of the International Headache Society (2013) The International Classification of Headache Disorders, 3rd edition (beta version). Cephalalgia 33(9):629–808. doi:10.1177/0333102413485658
2. Colas R, Muñoz P, Temprano R et al (2004) Chronic daily headache with drug analgesic overuse. Epidemiology and impact on quality of life. Neurology 62:1338–1342. doi:10.1212/01.WNL.0000120545.45443.93
3. Jonsson P, Hedenrud T, Linde M (2011) Epidemiology of medication overuse headache in the general Swedish population. Cephalalgia 31:1015–1022. doi:10.1177/0333102411410082
4. Cheung V, Amoozegar F, Dilli E (2015) Medication overuse headache. Curr Neurol Neurosci Rep Jan 15(1):509. doi:10.1007/s11910-014-0509-x
5. Evers S, Jensen R (2011) Treatment of medication overuse headache-guideline of the EFNS headache panel. Eur J Neurol 18(9):1115–1121. doi:10.1111/j.1468-1331.2011.03497.x
6. Grazzi L, Andrasik F, Usai S et al (2008) In-patient versus day-hospital withdrawal treatment for chronic migraine with medication overuse and disability assessment: results at 1-year follow-up. Neurol Sci 29(Suppl 1): S161–S163. doi:10.1007/s10072-008-0913-6
7. Creac'h C, Frappe P, Cancade M et al (2011) In-patient versus out-patient withdrawal programmes for medication overuse headache: a 2-year randomized trial. Cephalalgia 31:1189–1198. doi:10.1177/0333102411412088
8. Munksgaard S, Bendtsen L, Jensen R (2012) Detoxification of medication-overuse headache by a multidisciplinary treatment programme is highly effective: a comparison of two consecutive treatment methods in an open-label design. Cephalalgia 32:834–844. doi:10.1177/0333102412451363
9. Tassorelli C, Jensen R, Allena M et al (2014) The COMOESTAS Consortium. A consensus protocol for the management of medication-overuse headache: Evaluation in a multicentric, multinational study. Cephalalgia 34(9):645–655. doi:10.1177/0333102414521508
10. Kristoffersen ES, Lundqvist C (2014) Medication-overuse headache: epidemiology, diagnosis and treatment. Ther Adv Drug Saf 5(2):87–99. doi:10.1177/2042098614522683
11. Saper JR, Da Silva AN (2013) Medication overuse headache: history, features, prevention and management strategies. Updated review on MOH including prevention and treatment approach. CNS Drugs 27(11):867–877. doi:10.1007/s40263-013-0081-y
12. Peres MF (2007) Cephalalgiaphobia: a possible specific phobia of illness. J Headache Pain 8:56–59. doi:10.1007/s10194-007-0361-3
13. Saper JR, Hamel RL, Lake AE III (2005) Medication overuse headache (MOH) is a biobehavioural disorder. Cephalalgia 25:545–546. doi:10.1111/j.1468-2982.2005.00879.x
14. Giannini G, Zanigni S, Grimaldi D, et al. (2013) Cephalalgiaphobia as a feature of high-frequency migraine: a pilot study. J Headache Pain 10:14:49. doi: 10.1186/1129-2377-14-49.
15. Andrasik F, Flor H, Turk DC (2005) An expanded view of psychological aspects in head pain: the biopsychosocial model. Neurol Sci 26(Suppl 2): S87–S91. doi:10.1007/s10072-005-0416-7

16. Nestoriuc Y, Martin A (2007) Efficacy of biofeedback for migraine: A meta-analysis. Pain 128:111–127. doi:10.1016/j.pain.2006.09.007

17. Andrasik F (2010) Biofeedback in headache: an overview of approaches and evidence. Cleve Clin J Med 77(Suppl 3):S72–S76. doi:10.3949/ccjm.77.s3.13

18. Pistoia F, Sacco S, Carolei A (2013) Behavioral Therapy for Chronic Migraine. Curr Pain Headache Rep 17:304. doi:10.1007/s11916-012-0304-9

19. Yucha C, Mongomery D. Evidence-Based Practice in Biofeedback and Neurofeedback. Published by AAPB (Association for Applied Psychophysiology and Biofeedback, 2008 edition; http://www.aapb.org)

20. Sherman RA, Herman C. Clinical Efficacy of Psychophysiological Assessments and Biofeedback. Interventions for Chronic Pain Disorders Published by AAPB (Association for Applied Psychophysiology and Biofeedback, accessed 12 April 2004; http://www.aapb.org).

21. Marcus DA, Scharff L, Mercer S, Turk DC (1999) Musculoskeletal abnormalities in chronic headache: a controlled comparison of headache diagnostic groups. Headache 39(1):21–27. doi:10.1046/j.1526-4610.1999.3901021.x

22. Fernández-de-Las-Peñas C (2015) Myofascial Head Pain. Curr Pain Headache Rep 19(7):28. doi:10.1007/s11916-015-0503-2

23. Andrasik F, Buse DC, Grazzi L (2009) Behavioral medicine for migraine and medication overuse headache. Curr Pain Headache Rep 13(3):241–248

24. Grazzi L, Andrasik F, D'Amico D et al (2002) Behavioral and Pharmacologic Treatment of Transformed Migraine With Analgesic Overuse: Outcome at 3 Years. Headache 42:483–490. doi:10.1046/j.1526-4610.2002.02123.x

25. Peres MF, Lucchetti G (2010) Coping strategies in chronic pain. Curr Pain Headache Rep 14(5):331–338. doi:10.1007/s11916-010-0137-3

26. Holroyd KA, Drew JB, Cottrell CK, Romanek KM, Heh V (2007) Impaired functioning and quality of life in severe migraine: The role of catastrophizing and associated symptoms. Cephalalgia 27:1156–1165

27. Radat F, Lanteri-Minet M, Nachit-Ouinekh F et al (2009) The GRIM2005 study of migraine consultation in France. III: Psychological features of subjects with migraine. Cephalalgia 29:338–350

28. Lucas C, Lanteri-Minet M, Massiou H et al (2007) The GRIM2005 study of migraine consultation in France II. Psychological factors associated with treatment response to acute headache therapy and satisfaction in migraine. Cephalalgia 27:1398–1407

29. Radat F, Chanraud S, Di Scala G, Dousset V, Allard M (2013) Psychological and neuropsychological correlates of dependence-related behaviour in medication overuse headaches: a 1 year follow-up study. J Headache Pain 4:14–59. doi:10.1186/1129-2377-14-59

30. Flor H, Behle DJ, Birbaumer N (1993) Assessment of pain-related cognitions in chronic pain patients. Behav Res Ther 31(1):63–73. doi:10.1016/0005-7967(93)90044-U

31. Ferrari R, Fipaldini E, Birbaumer N (2004) La valutazione del controllo percepito sul dolore: la versione italiana del Pain Related Self-Statement Scale e del Pain Related Control Scale. Giornale-Italiano-di-Psicologia 31(1): 187–206. doi:10.1421/13219

32. Olesen J (2012) Detoxification for medication overuse headache is the primary task. Cephalalgia 32:420–422. doi:10.1177/0333102411431309

33. Diener HC (2012) Detoxification for medication overuse headache is not necessary. Cephalalgia 32:423–427. doi:10.1177/0333102411425867

34. Rossi P, Faroni JV, Tassorelli C, Nappi G (2013) Advice alone versus structured detoxification programmes for complicated medication overuse headache (MOH): a prospective, randomized, open-label trial. J Headache Pain 14:10. doi:10.1186/1129-2377-14-10

35. Cheung V, Amoozegar F, Dilli E (2015) Medication Overuse Headache. Curr Neurol Neurosci Rep 15:509. doi:10.1007/s11910-014-0509-x

36. Saper JR, Lake AE III (2006) Medication overuse headache: type I and type II. Cephalalgia 26(10):1262. doi:10.1111/j.1468-2982.2006.01198.x

37. Grazzi L, Andrasik F (2006) Medication-overuse headache: description, treatment, and relapse prevention. Curr Pain Headache Rep 10(1):71–77

38. Katsarava Z, Obermann M (2013) Medication-overuse headache. Broad updated review of MOH. Curr Opin Neurol 26(3):276–281. doi:10.1097/WCO. 0b013e328360d596

39. Sullivan MJL, Thorn B, Haythornthwaite JA et al (2001) Theoretical perspectives on the relation between catastrophizing and pain. Clin J Pain 17:52–64

40. Sullivan MJL, Bishop SR, Pivik J (1995) The Pain Catastrophizing Scale: development and validation. Psychol Assess 7:524–532. doi:10.1037/1040-3590.7.4.524

41. Rhudy JL, Martin SL, Terry EL et al (2011) Pain catastrophizing is related to temporal summation of pain but not temporal summation of the nociceptive flexion reflex. Pain 152:794–801. doi:10.1016/j.pain.2010.12.041

42. King CD, Goodin B, Kindler LL et al (2013) Reduction of conditioned pain modulation in humans by naltrexone: an exploratory study of the effects of pain catastrophizing. J Behav Med 36(3):315–327. doi:10.1007/s10865-012-9424-2

43. Sturgeon JA, Zautra AJ (2013) Psychological resilience, pain catastrophizing, and positive emotions: perspectives on comprehensive modeling of individual pain adaptation. Curr Pain Headache Rep 17(3):317. doi:10.1007/s11916-012-0317-4

44. Rains JC (2008) Change mechanisms in EMG biofeedback training: cognitive changes underlying improvements in tension headache. Headache 48(5): 735–736. doi:10.1111/j.1526-4610.2008.01119_1.x

7

Intravenous ketamine for subacute treatment of refractory chronic migraine

Clinton Lauritsen[1*†] (iD), Santiago Mazuera[1†], Richard B. Lipton[2] and Sait Ashina[3]

Abstract

Background: Refractory migraine is a challenging condition with great impact on health related quality of life. Intravenous (IV) ketamine has been previously used to treat various refractory pain conditions. We present a series of patients with refractory migraine treated with intravenous ketamine in the hospital setting.

Methods: Based on retrospective chart review, we identified six patients with refractory migraine admitted from 2010 through 2014 for treatment with intravenous ketamine. Ketamine was administered using a standard protocol starting with a dose of 0.1 mg/kg/hr and increased by 0.1 mg/kg/hr every 3 to 4 h as tolerated until the target pain score of 3/10 was achieved and maintained for at least 8 h. Visual Analogue Scale (VAS) scores at time of hospital admission were obtained as well as average baseline VAS scores prior to ketamine infusion. A phone interview was conducted for follow-up of migraine response in the 3 to 6 months following ketamine infusion.

Results: The study sample had a median age of 36.5 years (range 29–54) and 83% were women. Pre-treatment pain scores ranged from 9 to 10. All patients achieved a target pain level of 3 or less for 8 h; the average ketamine infusion rate at target was 0.34 mg/kg/hour (range 0.12–0.42 mg/kg/hr). One patient reported a transient out-of-body hallucination following an increase in the infusion rate, which resolved after decreasing the rate. There were no other significant side effects.

Conclusion: IV ketamine was safely administered in the hospital setting to patients with refractory chronic migraine. Treatment was associated with short term improvement in pain severity in 6 of 6 patients with refractory chronic migraine. Prospective placebo-controlled trials are needed to assess short term and long-term efficacy of IV ketamine in refractory chronic migraine.

Background

Chronic migraine and refractory migraine have long challenged clinicians. In the United States, chronic migraine prevalence is nearly 1% and results in enormous impact on headache-related disability, including higher Migraine Disability Assessment Test (MIDAS), reduced health-related quality of life (HRQoL), increased depression and anxiety (PHQ-4 and GAD-7 respectively), compared to episodic migraine [1–6]. Chronic migraine has also been shown to result in greater economic burden and health care resource utilization [1, 3, 7–9]. Annually,

the total economic cost of chronic migraine is over three time that of episodic migraine, when consider direct medical costs and loss from decreased productivity [8].

Refractory migraine is included in ICHD-2 [10] and ICHD-3 beta [11] but criteria for intractable headache have only recently emerged [12]. Silberstein et al. [12] assesses the type and number of treatments the patient failed as well as the clinical setting and the intensity of invention for intractable headache. Multiple treatment options have been proposed for management of refractory migraine including intravenous dihydroergotamine (DHE) and intravenous divalproex sodium [13, 14].

One candidate treatment for intractable migraine is ketamine. Intravenous ketamine has been studied in various refractory pain conditions including complex regional pain [15]. Intranasal ketamine reduced the

---
* Correspondence: Clinton.Lauritsen@jefferson.edu
†Equal contributors
[1]Department of Neurology, Thomas Jefferson University, Jefferson Headache Center, Philadelphia, PA, USA

severity of aura in migraine with prolonged aura in a small randomized trial [16]. The use of intravenous ketamine has only been reported in case series. Krusz et al. [17] demonstrated improvement in pain scores in patients with refractory migraine as well as few side effects associated with treatment.

Ketamine is a dissociative anesthetic that acts on glutamate binding sites at the N-methyl-D-aspartate (NMDA) receptor as well as at opioid, monoaminergic, cholinergic, nicotinic, and muscarinic receptors [18]. There is a theory of functional and electrophysiological dissociation between thalamo-neocortical and limbic systems: sensory inputs may reach cortical receiving areas, but fail to be observed in some of the association areas with the use of ketamine [18]. Analysis of the dose-dependent ketamine effects on pain processing showed a decreasing activation of the secondary somatosensory cortex, insula, and anterior cingulate cortex, which has been linked to the affective pain component that underlines the potency of ketamine in modulating affective pain processing [19]. This theoretical mechanism of action of ketamine has shown to decrease central sensitization and allodynia in pain conditions, which has motived clinicians to use it as treatment for migraine. Ketamine also reduces cortical spreading depression in animal models [20]. Most common known side effects of ketamine may include cardiovascular instability, respiratory changes and psychiatric symptoms including acute psychosis, hallucinations, anxiety but are usually dose-dependent.

Herein, we report the effect of IV ketamine on a series of six patients with intractable migraine treated with escalated doses on an inpatient basis.

Methods

We performed a retrospective chart review study. From 2010 until 2014, a total of six patients were admitted for treatment with continuous intravenous ketamine to Mount Sinai Beth Israel Hospital in New York. Data were collected from charts obtained from the medical record department and electronic medical records (PRISM). The study was approved by the Mount Sinai Institutional Review Board. Prior to admission, a diagnosis of chronic migraine without aura based on ICHD-2 criteria was made by a headache specialist (Sait Ashina). Demographics, number of prior migraine treatments and current use of medications such as opioids, antidepressants, beta blockers, antiepileptic medications and nonsteroidal anti-inflammatory drugs (NSAIDs) were documented, as well as onset age of migraine diagnosis.

All the patients received information regarding side effects and risks associated with the treatment and informed written consent was obtained prior to infusion. Monitoring of the treatment was done according to the

ketamine infusion procedure policy of the Department of Pain Medicine and Palliative Care at Mount Sinai Beth Israel (see Additional file 1 for sources used in protocol development). Following an initial electrocardiogram (EKG) for all patients and a pregnancy test for female patients, ketamine was administered using a standard protocol starting with an initial intravenous infusion of 0.1 mg/kg/hr. The infusion was increased by 0.1 mg/kg/hr every 3 to 4 h as tolerated until the goal pain score of 3/10 was maintained for 8 h. The eighth-hour designation was made based on standard pain assessment intervals in the institution. Thereafter, the infusion was decreased by 0.2 mg/kg/hr every 3to 4 h until the infusion rate reached 0 mg/kg/hr. The dose of ketamine escalated as needed until maximal response or until undesirable side effects including psychomimetic and dysphoric effects.

Visual Analogue scale (VAS) score was used at the moment of admission and follow-up VAS scores at different ketamine infusion rates were assessed from nursing and infusion records. We defined a pain response as a reduction in the initial VAS to a score of three or less. Side effects were identified and reported.

We attempted to contact the patients in this retrospective study for telephone follow-up; however, we were only able to reach two of the six patients. During telephone interview, a questionnaire including MIDAS [21] was administered.

Results

Characteristics of patients admitted for ketamine are summarized in Table 1. Ages ranged from 29 to 54 (median of 36.5) and five out of six were women. VAS scores on admission were nine or ten (see Table 1). All of the patients were Caucasian. The median age of migraine onset was 17 (range 8–29). The median duration of illness was 17 years (range 12–46). The mean number of failed acute migraine treatments was 18 (range 14–26) and failed preventive medications was 25 (range 7–29) (See Table 2). Three patients out of the total six receiving ketamine had a prior psychiatric diagnosis (depression, panic attacks and/or borderline personality disorders). In addition to chronic migraine, concomitant chronic pain disorders were identified in three of six patients, two of whom also had a psychiatric diagnosis. The six patients were on at least one of the following medications: muscle relaxant, NSAID, opioid, antiepileptic, antidepressant, benzodiazepine, triptan, beta blocker or antiemetic (Table 2).

All of the six patients were started on IV ketamine dose of 0.1 mg/kg/hr. All six patients achieved the target endpoint of a pain score of less than three out of ten sustained for at least 8 h. The intravenous ketamine doses are presented in Table 1. We provide the current

Table 1 The demographic and clinical data and intravenous (IV) ketamine infusion rates at which 6 patients achieved a VAS pain score of 3 or less

Patient	Age/sex	Age at migraine onset	Duration of Illness	Psychiatric and Pain Comorbidities	Initial VAS	IV Ketamine Rate VAS < 3	Time to maintain VAS of 3 or less for duration of 8 h
1	42/F	26	16 years	Depression, Panic Attacks, Chronic Back Pain	10	0.42 mg/kg/hr	36 h
2	29/F	15	14 years	Panic Attacks	10	0.38 mg/kg/hr	40 h
3	31/M	19	12 years	Complex Regional Pain Syndrome	9	0.41 mg/kg/hr	20 h
4	54/F	8	46 years	None	9	0.12 mg/kg/hr	12 h
5	30/F	10	20 years	Depression, Borderline Personality Disorder, Chronic Neck Pain	9	0.35 mg/kg/hr	73 h
6	47/F	29	18 years	Depression	9	0.34 mg/kg/hr	82 h

outpatient migraine regimens at the time of admission as well as the number of acute and preventive migraine treatments failed for each patient in Tables 2 and 3. Telephone follow-up was obtained in just two patients, neither of whom reported sustained benefits from intravenous ketamine infusion. One patient reported an out of body hallucination which resolved following decrease in the infusion rate.

Discussion

In this small cases series, all six patients with refractory migraine met the target pain relief endpoint with ketamine over a mean infusion of 44 h (range 12–82). Mean ketamine infusion rate at the time of pain relief endpoint was 0.34 mg/kg/hour (range 0.12–0.42). Patients achieved pain relief without substantial adverse effects. One patient reported a brief dissociative experience, which reversed.

Intravenous ketamine use in treating refractory depression has recently been well established [22, 23]. Studies have also suggested a role for ketamine in the treatment of intractable chronic pain including long-term analgesic effect persisting beyond the duration of

infusion [24]. Long-term ketamine infusion (4–14 days) has been shown to decrease pain for up to 3 months [25]. Allodynia, a marker of chronic pain and central sensitization of nociceptive pathways, has also been shown decrease with intravenous ketamine infusion. Interestingly, this effect was not achieved until 4–5 days of continuous infusion [26].

The existing literature on IV ketamine for the treatment of headache is limited. Though our case series is modest in size, and in the absence of a contemporaneous placebo group, causal inferences are not possible, we demonstrated short-term success in pain relief in intractable migraine patients with one significant but short-lived adverse event. It is biologically plausible that ketamine could be an effective treatment for intractable headache. Ketamine is an antagonist at NMDA receptors, blocking the excitatory action of glutamate (Glu), a neurotransmitter long implicated in the pathophysiology of migraine [27]. Glu has been shown to be implicated in induction of cortical spreading depression (CSD), activation of trigeminal nociceptive neurons as well as play a role in central sensitization. Previous studies have identified variants in the gene for GluA receptors in persons with migraine [28].

To date, there has been a lack of treatments with reliable abortive effect on migraine aura, the phenomenon attributed to CSD. In the rat-model, both ketamine and the non-specific NMDA antagonist, MK-801 have been shown to block CSD, demonstrated electrophysiologically and by fMRI [29]. In a double-blinded, randomized parallel-group controlled study of 18 patients with

Table 2 Outpatient medical regimen in patients with chronic migraine cases at time of scheduled treatment with intravenous ketamine

Patient	1	2	3	4	5	6
Opioid	1		1		1	
Non-steroidal anti-inflammatory	1		2			1
Anti-depressant		1		2	1	2
Muscle relaxant		1			1	1
Benzodiazepine			1	1		
Anti-emetic		1	1		1	1
Neuroleptic					2	1
Anti-epileptic			2			1
Triptan						1
Anti-hypertensive				1	1	1

Table 3 Number of previously failed medications for each patient

Patient	1	2	3	4	5	6
Abortive Medications Failed	19	NA	16	14	18	26
Preventive Medications Failed	25	5	17	28	23	29
OnabotulinumtoxinA Failed	Yes	NA	Yes	Yes	Yes	Yes

NA not available

migraine with aura, Afridi et al. tested the effect of intranasal ketamine compared to midazolam on aura. Ketamine was shown to reduce severity of aura but not duration, whereas midazolam had no effect [16]. Intranasal ketamine has been shown to consistently improve aura symptoms in some patients with familial hemiplegic migraine, although without significant reduction of headache severity [30]. Note: Broadly blocking CSD with long term administration is viewed as a model for preventive treatment [31]. Memantine is a voltage-dependent noncompetitive antagonist at the glutamatergic NMDA receptor, which inhibits the prolonged influx of calcium associated with neuronal excitotoxicity. In order to identify an agent with preventive activity against refractory and chronic migraine, Bigal, et al. administered daily memantine to 28 patients in an unblinded protocol. Compared to baseline, at 3 months, memantine decreased headache frequency severe headaches and MIDAS scores [32]. Ketamine may be a particularly beneficial treatment option for patients that have failed memantine. Because ketamine is the most potent competitive antagonist at the NMDA-type glutamate receptor whereas memantine is a weaker and noncompetitive antagonist, ketamine may have greater impact on central sensitization [33]. Also of interest, in patients concomitantly treated with opioids, ketamine has been shown to increase pain relief.[34] This may suggest a role for ketamine in the treatment of medication overuse headache.

Of the patients that completed follow up questionnaires, none reported lasting benefit from ketamine 3–6 months post infusion. Prior publications have reported lasting effects on chronic non-headache pain reduction following long term infusions of more than 4 days. Of note, none of the patients included in this case series received ketamine infusion for more than 4 days. Thus, we propose that future studies target ketamine infusions for at least this duration. Once placebo controlled studies on acute headache relief are performed, studies assessing long-term benefits should begin. Strategies for maintaining the effect of intravenous ketamine infusion should also be studied, such as the ongoing administration of a daily or as needed NMDA receptor antagonist. Researchers have used similar strategies in prior studies, such as with the use of mexiletine following lidocaine infusion for chronic daily headache. In this fashion, agents including dextromethorphan-quinidine, memantine, oral or intranasal ketamine could be used to maintain the benefit from NDMA receptor antagonism following ketamine infusion [35, 36].

Conclusions

This study highlights the need for further research regarding new treatment options for patients who suffer daily consequences of refractory migraine and have failed many abortive and preventive medications. Our IV ketamine infusion protocol, based on gradually dose escalation, relieves pain without substantial adverse effects. However, future study of this benefit on short-term headache relief needs to be conducted in a placebo-controlled fashion and this publication may serve as the basis for the design of such a trial.

Acknowledgements
Please note a preliminary version of this research was presented as an abstract at the Congress of the International Headache Society in May 2015 [37].

Authors' contributions
CL, SM, SA, and RL were responsible for the conception and design and the study. CL and SM performed chart reviews with analysis of data. CL, SM, SA, and RL were resposible for interpretation of data, drafting of the manuscript and making intellectual contributions to its content. All authors read and approved the final manuscript.

Competing interest
Clinton Lauritsen, Santiago Mazuera and Sait Ashina previously worked at Mount Sinai Beth Israel Hospital. Clinton Lauritsen and Santiago Mazuera have no disclosures. Sait Ashina received honoraria for lecturing from Allergan, Teva Pharmaceuticals, Avanir Pharmaceuticals and served as a consultant for Avanir Pharmaceuticals. Richard Lipton received research support from the NIH [PO1 AG03949 (Program Director), RO1AG025119 (Investigator), RO1AG022374-06A2 (Investigator), RO1AG034119 (Investigator), RO1AG12101 (Investigator), K23AG030857 (Mentor), K23NS05140901A1 (Mentor), and K23NS47256 (Mentor)], the National Headache Foundation, and the Migraine Research Fund; serves on the editorial board of Neurology; has reviewed for the NIA and NINDS; holds stock options in eNeura Therapeutics; and serves as consultant, advisory board member, or has received honoraria from Allergan, American Headache Society, Autonomic Technologies, Boston Scientific, Bristol Myers Squibb, Cognimed, Colucid, Eli Lilly, eNeura Therapeutics, GlaxoSmithKline, MAP, Merck, Nautilus Neuroscience, Novartis, NuPathe, Pfizer, and Vedanta.

Author details
[1]Department of Neurology, Thomas Jefferson University, Jefferson Headache Center, Philadelphia, PA, USA. [2]Department of Neurology, Montefiore Headache Center, Albert Einstein College of Medicine, Bronx, NY, USA. [3]Department of Neurology, New York University School of Medicine, NYU Langone Medical Center, NYU Lutheran Headache Center, New York, NY, USA.

References
1. Blumenfeld AM et al. (2011) Disability, HRQoL and resource use among chronic and episodic migraineurs: results from the International Burden of Migraine Study (IBMS). Cephalalgia 31(3):301–15
2. Buse DC et al. (2012) Chronic migraine prevalence, disability, and sociodemographic factors: results from the American migraine prevalence and prevention study. Headache 52(10):1456–70
3. Lipton RB et al. (2011) OnabotulinumtoxinA improves quality of life and reduces impact of chronic migraine. Neurology 77(15):1465–72
4. Schulman EA et al. (2008) Defining refractory migraine and refractory chronic migraine: proposed criteria from the Refractory Headache Special Interest Section of the American Headache Society. Headache 48(6):778–82
5. Adams AM et al. (2015) The impact of chronic migraine: the chronic migraine epidemiology and outcomes (CaMEO) study methods and baseline results. Cephalalgia 35(7):563–78
6. D'Amico D et al. (2013) Disability and quality of life in headache: where we are now and where we are heading. Neurol Sci 34(Suppl 1):S1–5
7. Lipton RB et al. (2016) OnabotulinumtoxinA improves quality of life and reduces impact of chronic migraine over one year of treatment: pooled results from the PREEMPT randomized clinical trial program. Cephalalgia 36(9):899–908

8. Messali A et al. (2016) Direct and indirect costs of chronic and episodic migraine in the united states: a Web-based survey. Headache 56(2):306–22

9. Wang SJ et al. (2013) Comparisons of disability, quality of life, and resource use between chronic and episodic migraineurs: a clinic-based study in Taiwan. Cephalalgia 33(3):171–81

10. Headache Classification Subcommittee of the International Headache, S (2004) The International Classification of Headache Disorders: 2nd edition. Cephalalgia 24(Suppl 1):9–160

11. Headache Classification Committee of the International Headache, S (2013) The International Classification of Headache Disorders, 3rd edition (beta version). Cephalalgia 33(9):629–808

12. Silberstein SD, Dodick DW, Pearlman S (2010) Defining the pharmacologically intractable headache for clinical trials and clinical practice. Headache 50(9):1499–506

13. Norton J (2000) Use of intravenous valproate sodium in status migraine. Headache 40(9):755–7

14. Peterlin BL et al. (2008) Rational combination therapy in refractory migraine. Headache 48(6):805–19

15. Goldberg ME et al. (2005) Multi-day low dose ketamine infusion for the treatment of complex regional pain syndrome. Pain Physician 8(2):175–9

16. Afridi SK et al. (2013) A randomized controlled trial of intranasal ketamine in migraine with prolonged aura. Neurology 80(7):642–7

17. Krusz J, Cagle J, Hall S (2008) Efficacy of IV ketamine in treating refractory migraines in the clinic. J Pain 9(4):30

18. Corssen G, Domino EF (1966) Dissociative anesthesia: further pharmacologic studies and first clinical experience with the phencyclidine derivative CI-581. Anesth Analg 45(1):29–40

19. Sprenger T et al. (2006) Imaging pain modulation by subanesthetic S-(+)-ketamine. Anesth Analg 103(3):729–37

20. Sanchez-Porras R et al. (2014) The effect of ketamine on optical and electrical characteristics of spreading depolarizations in gyrencephalic swine cortex. Neuropharmacology 84:52–61

21. Stewart WF et al. (1999) An international study to assess reliability of the migraine disability assessment (MIDAS) score. Neurology 53(5):988–94

22. Coyle CM, Laws KR (2015) The use of ketamine as an antidepressant: a systematic review and meta-analysis. Hum Psychopharmacol 30(3):152–63

23. Swiatek KM, K Jordan, J. Coffman (2016) New use for an old drug: oral ketamine for treatment-resistant depression. BMJ Case Rep, 2016

24. Niesters M, Dahan A, van Kleef M (2016) Safety and efficacy of ketamine for pain relief. Ned Tijdschr Geneeskd 160:D58

25. Niesters M, Martini C, Dahan A (2014) Ketamine for chronic pain: risks and benefits. Br J Clin Pharmacol 77(2):357–67

26. Puchalski P, Zyluk A (2016) Results of the treatment of chronic, refractory CRPS with ketamine infusions: a preliminary report. Handchir Mikrochir Plast Chir 48(3):143–147

27. Vikelis M, Mitsikostas DD (2007) The role of glutamate and its receptors in migraine. CNS Neurol Disord Drug Targets 6(4):251–7

28. Ramadan NM (2014) Glutamate and migraine: from Ikeda to the 21st century. Cephalalgia 34(2):86–9

29. Shatillo A et al. (2015) Involvement of NMDA receptor subtypes in cortical spreading depression in rats assessed by fMRI. Neuropharmacology 93:164–70

30. Kaube H et al. (2000) Aura in some patients with familial hemiplegic migraine can be stopped by intranasal ketamine. Neurology 55(1):139–41

31. Ayata C et al. (2006) Suppression of cortical spreading depression in migraine prophylaxis. Ann Neurol 59(4):652–61

32. Bigal M et al. (2008) Memantine in the preventive treatment of refractory migraine. Headache 48(9):1337–42

33. Grande LA et al. (2008) Ultra-low dose ketamine and memantine treatment for pain in an opioid-tolerant oncology patient. Anesth Analg 107(4):1380–3

34. Sveticic G et al. (2003) Combinations of morphine with ketamine for patient-controlled analgesia: a new optimization method. Anesthesiology 98(5):1195–205

35. Taylor CP et al. (2016) Pharmacology of dextromethorphan: relevance to dextromethorphan/quinidine (nuedexta(R)) clinical use. Pharmacol Ther 164:170–82

36. Marmura MJ, Passero FC Jr, Young WB (2008) Mexiletine for refractory chronic daily headache: a report of nine cases. Headache 48(10):1506–10

37. Mazuera S, Ashina S, Lipton RB. (2015) Intravenous Ketamine for the Subacute Treatment of Refractory Chronic Migraine: Case Series: PF24. [Abstract] Headache. 55 Supplement 3:144

8

Network meta-analysis of migraine disorder treatment by NSAIDs and triptans

Haiyang Xu, Wei Han, Jinghua Wang and Mingxian Li[*]

Abstract

Background: Migraine is a neurological disorder resulting in large socioeconomic burden. This network meta-analysis (NMA) is designed to compare the relative efficacy and tolerability of non-steroidal anti-inflammatory agents (NSAIDs) and triptans.

Methods: We conducted systematic searches in database PubMed and Embase. Treatment effectiveness was compared by synthesizing direct and indirect evidences using NMA. The surface under curve ranking area (SUCRA) was created to rank those interventions.

Results: Eletriptan and rizatriptan are superior to sumatriptan, zolmitriptan, almotriptan, ibuprofen and aspirin with respect to pain-relief. When analyzing 2 h-nausea-absence, rizatriptan has a better efficacy than sumatriptan, while other treatments indicate no distinctive difference compared with placebo. Furthermore, sumatriptan demonstrates a higher incidence of all-adverse-event compared with diclofenac-potassium, ibuprofen and almotriptan.

Conclusion: This study suggests that eletriptan may be the most suitable therapy for migraine from a comprehensive point of view. In the meantime ibuprofen may also be a good choice for its excellent tolerability. Multi-component medication also attracts attention and may be a promising avenue for the next generation of migraine treatment.

Keywords: Migraine disorders, Triptans, Non-steroidal anti-inflammatory agents, Network meta-analysis

Background

Migraine is a neurological disorder resulting in large socioeconomic burden affecting approximately 18% of females and 6% of males in the United States [1]. The prevalence of migraine varies with age, females between 35 and 45 years old exhibits the highest prevalence [2]. Apart from the factor of age, the prevalence of migraine in the U.S. also varied with household income and race, and such findings are consistent with studies carried out in other countries [3, 4]. Headache is the primary symptom of migraine and patients may also be afflicted by other symptoms including pulsatile pain, light sensitivity, sound sensitivity, nausea, unilateral pain, blurred vision and emesis. Although a large number of treatments have been developed for migraine over the past decades, several disputes have been encountered by clinicians such as misclassification of migraine, inappropriate selection of treatment and medication overuse. Among them,

medication overuse has become a major issue in chronic migraine patients who may eventually develop a disabling condition called medication-overuse headache [5]. Therefore, awareness and understanding of migraine should be improved and corresponding treatments or medications should be further explored to overcome these issues.

Two types of migraine therapies have been developed: preventive therapies which are used to reduce attack frequency or severity and acute therapies which are used for the sake of aborting attacks. Compared to preventive therapies, acute therapies are able to provide patients with rapid and complete relief with minimal or no adverse events and hence they are recommended for promptly alleviating the symptoms of patients [6]. The selection of acute treatments has been differentiated into two pathways: non-specific medications which include analgesics and non-steroidal anti-inflammatory drugs (NSAIDs); and specific medications which include ergot derivatives and triptans [5]. As suggested by the European Federation of Neurological Societies (EFNS), both oral NSAIDs and

* Correspondence: limingxian_118@163.com; cuilx08@126.com
The First hospital of Jilin University, No. 71 Xinmin Street, Changchun 130021, Jilin, China

triptans are recommended for treating migraine attacks [7]. Moreover, evidence from the American Headache Society (AHS) concluded that the following treatments are deemed to be effective acute therapies for migraine: triptans, NSAIDs, ergotamine derivatives, opioids and other combinational medications [8]. Stratified care is a primary strategy often used in selecting medications for migraine patients and this strategy takes several aspects into account: attack severity, the presence of associated symptoms and the degree of disability resulting from migraine [9]. However, other factors such as dosage may also have significant influence on the overall effectiveness of medications that are used to abort migraine attacks.

Among the common acute treatments that are used for aborting migraine, different levels of evidence have been provided by a wide range of studies. Although the efficacy of some medications have been established, this does not imply that such medications should be considered as the first line treatments for migraine patients since it may cause adverse events that are specifically associated with these medications. Despite the growing popularity of triptans, NSAIDs remain one of the most recommended acute migraine treatments and they are often used as an initial strategy for aborting migraine attacks [9]. On the other hand, triptans are often used as a rescue medication if an initial treatment fails to abort migraine attacks and evidence suggests that about 60% of non-responders to NSAIDs can be treated by triptans [10]. One distinctive advantage of triptans for migraine patients is that they can be effective at any time during a migraine attack and such an advantage may reduce the impact of dosage timing on the overall efficacy. Moreover, some evidence suggests that earlier intervention by using triptans is associated with an enhanced efficacy [11, 12], while some randomized trials do not support such an improved efficacy when patients experienced allodynia in the course of a migraine attack [13, 14].

Despite the fact that both NSAIDs and triptans have been recommended by the EFNS and AHS as acute treatments for migraine, comparing NSAIDs with triptans is a challenging task. Conventional meta-analysis has several limitations due to the lack of evidence as well as lack of indirect evidence.. For this reason, we designed this network meta-analysis (NMA) to compares the relative efficacy and tolerability between NSAIDs and triptans. We hope that the approach of NMA can provide comprehensive evidence with respect to the efficacy and tolerability of these two popular medications.

Methods

Search strategy

We employed search strategies to explore the medical literature for relevant studies in PubMed and EMBASE

systematically, and 2,967 records were identified using the following terms: "migraine disorders", "tryptans", "non-steroidal anti-inflammatory agents", "ergot alkaloids", "opioid analgesics", "sumatriptan", "zolmitriptan", "almotriptan", "rizatriptan", "naratriptan", "ibuprofen", "eletriptan", "diclofenac-potassium" and "aspirin" in PubMed. Reviewers also provided 3 additional references.

As flow chart Fig. 1 illustrates, among the total 2,970 records, 1,263 were identified as duplicates and hence removed after assessment. 1,408 more studies were excluded from the remaining 1,707 records according to the exclusion criteria, leaving 299 remnant studies. Full-text articles were viewed and included if they met the inclusion criteria, or excluded if not. Eventually 88 studies were included in this research [12, 15–101].

Inclusion criteria

Articles were included if they: (1) were randomized clinical trials (RCTs); (2) were categorized as double blind; (3) included relevant clinical outcomes and treatments; (4) contained comparisons between different treatments.

Outcome measures and data extraction

The following data were extracted from eligible studies and shown in Table 1: gender, sample size and diagnostic criteria. Two investigators reviewed the manuscripts of all included studies and extracted data into a database independently. A Jadad scale was generated and is presented in Additional file 1: Table S1. The width of the lines in Fig. 2 is proportional to the number of trials comparing each pair of treatments and the area of circles represents the cumulative number of patients for each intervention.

Statistical analysis

We initially carried out a conventional pair-wise meta-analysis which directly compares each pair of treatments. The corresponding odds ratios (ORs) and 95% confidence intervals (CIs) for each study were pooled in order to obtain the overall effect size. Furthermore, a NMA was performed for each endpoint with a Bayesian framework using R 3.2.3 software. Treatment efficacy was compared through direct and indirect evidence

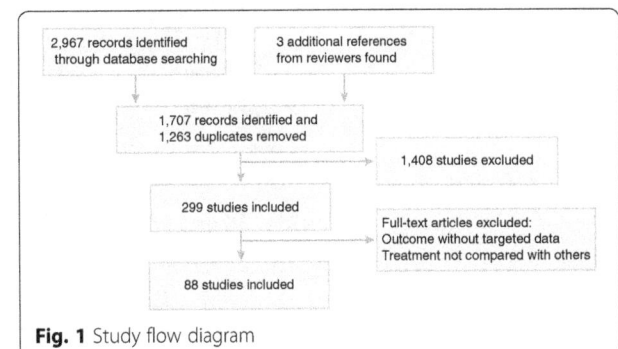

Fig. 1 Study flow diagram

Table 1 Included studies

Study information	Blinding	Number	Female	Diagnostic criteria	Outcomes
Sumatriptan vs Placebo					
Barbanti, 2004, Multinational	Double	432	358	IHS	③
Bigal, 2015, USA	Double	354	386	ICHD-II	③④
Bousser, 1993, France	Double	96	79	IHS	③④⑤⑥⑧
Cady, 1998, USA	Double	132	112	IHS	④⑥⑦⑧
Cady, 2015, USA	Double	212	177	ICHD-II	③④⑤⑥
Diamond, 1998, USA	Double	1077	956	IHS	②④⑤
Diener, 1999, Germany	Double	156	125	IHS	③④⑥⑦⑧⑨
Djupesland, 2010, UK	Double	78	71	IHS	②③④⑥⑧
Fujita, 2014, Japan	Double	144	84	ICHD-II	①②③④⑧⑨
Goldstein, 2005, USA	Double	104	-	IHS	⑥⑦
Gross, 1994, UK	Double	86	69	IHS	②⑥
Henry, 1993, France	Double	76	66	IHS	①②③④⑥⑧
Jelinski, 2006, USA	Double	235	308	IHS	①③⑨
Landy, 2004, UK	Double	449	448	IHS	③⑨
Lipton, 2000, USA	Double	1112	215	IHS	③④
Myllyla, 1998, Finland	Double	94	84	IHS	③④⑤⑥⑦
Nappi, 1994, Italy	Double	244	155	IHS	③④⑤⑥⑦⑧⑨
Peikert, 1999, Multinational	Double	586	408	IHS	②③④⑧
Pini, 1995, Italy	Double	240	-	IHS	④⑥⑦⑧
Rao, 2016, USA	Double	100	54	IHS	③④⑥⑨
Salonen, 1994, Multinational	Double	247	30	IHS	②④
Schulman, 2000, USA	Double	116	105	IHS	⑥⑦⑧
Sheftell, 2005, USA	Double	904	1170	IHS	③⑥⑦⑨
Tfelt-Hansen, 1995, Multinational	Double	248	192	IHS	④⑤⑥⑧⑨
Tfelt-Hansen, 2006, Denmark	Double	100	78	-	③⑧
Wang, 2007, Taipei	Double	56	48	-	①②③④⑦⑧⑨
Wendt, 2006, USA	Double	577	500	-	①②③④⑥⑧⑨
Winner, 2003, USA	Double	354	311	-	①③⑨
Winner, 2006, USA	Double	297	246	-	③④⑥⑨
Zolmitriptan vs Placebo					
Charlesworth, 2003, UK	Double	1372	1138	IHS	⑥⑦⑧
Dahlof, 1998, Multinational	Double	840	701	IHS	③④⑤⑥⑦⑧
Dodick, 2005, USA	Double	1868	1620	IHS	①②③④⑤⑥⑦⑨
Dowson, 2002, Multinational	Double	470	409	IHS	④⑥⑦⑧
Gawel, 2005, Canada	Double	912	798	IHS	①②③④⑥⑧⑨
Klapper, 2004, UK	Double	280	241	IHS	③⑥⑧⑨
Loder, 2005, USA	Double	565	482	IHS	①③⑧⑨
Rothner, 2006, USA	Double	346	410	IHS	①②③④⑧⑨
Ryan Jr, 2000, North America	Double	734	628	IHS	①②③④⑥⑦
Sakai, 2002, Japan	Double	202	150	IHS	②③④⑤⑧
Spierings, 2004, USA	Double	670	580	IHS	①②③④⑤⑧⑨
Tepper, 1999, Multinational	Double	1643	1387	IHS	③⑧
Tuchman, 2006, USA	Double	336	-	-	

Table 1 Included studies *(Continued)*

Study	Blinding	N1	N2	Criteria	Outcomes
Almotriptan vs Placebo					
Diener, 2005, Germany	Double	221	192	IHS	③④⑧
Dowson, 2002, Multinational	Double	470	409	IHS	④⑥⑦⑧
Mathew, 2007, USA	Double	317	275	IHS	①②③④⑧⑨
Pascual, 2000, Multinational	Double	909	788	IHS	①②③④⑤⑦⑧
Rizatriptan vs Placebo					
Ahrens, 1999, USA	Double	555	391	IHS	②③④⑤⑦⑨
Freitag, 2008, USA	Double	82	72	IHS	③④⑤⑨
Mannix, 2007, USA	Double	359	355	IHS	④⑤⑥⑧
Teall, 1998, Multinational	Double	762	653	IHS	②④⑦⑧⑨
Misra, 2007, India	Double	103	76	IHS	③④⑥⑧
Ibuprofen vs Placebo					
Codispoti, 2001, USA	Double	660	556	IHS	③④⑤⑧⑨
Goldstein, 2006, USA	Double	886	722	IHS	④⑨
Kellstein, 2000, USA	Double	729	550	IHS	③④⑤⑥
Misra, 2004, India	Double	105	57	-	④
Sumatriptan-Naproxen vs Placebo					
Mannix, 2009, USA	Double	314	313	-	③⑥⑨
Martin, 2014, USA	Double	623	622	ICHD-II	
Silberstein, 2014, USA	Double	443	331	ICHD-II	①②③⑤⑥⑧⑨
Winner, 2015, USA	Double	349	66	ICHD	③
Eletriptan vs Placebo					
Diener, 2002, Multinational	Double	530	465	IHS	②③④⑨
Diclofenacpotassium vs Placebo					
Comoglu, 2011, Turkey	Double	45	10	IHS	②
Diener, 2006, Germany	Double	590	762	IHS	③④⑥⑦⑨
Lipton, 2010, USA	Double	690	585	IHS	③⑦⑧
Aspirin vs Placebo					
Lange, 2000, Germany	Double	345	-	IHS	③④⑤⑥⑧
Lipton, 2005, USA	Double	401	317	IHS	③④⑥⑦⑧⑨
Sumatriptan vs Zolmitriptan					
Gallagher, 2000, USA	Double	1212	1062	IHS	②④⑥⑦⑧⑨
Gruffyd-Jones, 2001, UK	Double	1522	1299	IHS	①②③④⑥⑦⑧
Sumatriptan vs Almotriptan					
Spierings, 2001, USA	Double	1175	-	IHS	②③④⑤⑥⑦⑧⑨
Sumatriptan vs Naratriptan					
Gobel, 2000, Multinational	Double	247	127	IHS	⑥⑦⑧⑨
Zolmitriptan vs Almotriptan					
Goadsby, 2007, Italy	Double	1062	902	-	③④⑥⑦⑨
Sumatriptan vs Zolmitriptan vs Placebo					
Geraud, 2000, Multinational	Double	558	472	-	①②③④⑥⑦⑧⑨
Sumatriptan vs Almotriptan vs Placebo					
Dodick, 2002, Multinational	Double	292	249	IHS	③⑥
Dowson, 2004, UK	Double	295	-	IHS	③⑧

Table 1 Included studies *(Continued)*

Sumatriptan vs Rizatriptan vs Placebo					
Goldstein, 1998, USA	Double	441	-	IHS	①②③④⑤⑥⑦⑧⑨
Kolodny, 2004, USA	Double	1104	-	IHS	③⑧⑨
Tfelt-Hansen, 1998, Multinational	Double	548	441	IHS	①②③④⑤⑥⑦⑧⑨
Sumatriptan vs Naratriptan vs Placebo					
Dahlof, 1998, Multinational	Double	840	701	IHS	③④⑤⑥⑦⑧
Havanka, 2000, Multinational	Double	189	168	IHS	②④⑤⑥⑦⑧
Sumatriptan vs Sumatriptan-Naproxen vs Placebo					
Brandes, 2007, USA	Double	721	613	-	③④⑤⑥⑦⑨
Smith, 2005, Germany	Double	471	422	IHS	①②③④⑤⑥⑦⑨
Sumatriptan vs Eletriptan vs Placebo					
Mathew, 2003, Multinational	Double	1250	1079	IHS	①②③④⑤⑥⑦⑧
Sumatriptan vs Diclofenacpotassium vs Placebo					
DK/SMSG, 1999, Multinational	Double	220	-	IHS	⑤⑦⑧⑨
Sumatriptan vs Aspirin vs Placebo					
Diener, 2004, Multinational	Double	287	238	IHS	③④⑤⑥⑦⑧
Zolmitriptan vs Rizatriptan vs Placebo					
Pascual, 2000, Multinational	Double	909	788	IHS	①②③④⑤⑦⑧
Zolmitriptan vs Eletriptan vs Placebo					
Steiner, 2003, Multinational	Double	549	460	IHS	①②③④⑤⑦⑧
Rizatriptan vs Naratriptan vs Placebo					
Bomhof, 1999, Multinational	Double	308	262	IHS	①②③④⑤⑥⑦⑧⑨
Rizatriptan vs Ibuprofen vs Placebo					
Misra, 2007, India	Double	103	76	IHS	③④⑥⑧
Sumatriptan vs Ibuprofen vs Aspirin vs Placebo					
Diener, 2004, Multinational	Double	287	238	IHS	③④⑤⑥⑦⑧

① 1 h pain free; ② 1 h pain relief; ③ 2 h pain free; ④ 2 h pain relief; ⑤ 2 h absence of nausea; ⑥ rescue mediaction; ⑦ recurrence; ⑧ all-adverse events; ⑨ nausea

using the ORs and 95% credible intervals (CrIs). Then the surface under curve ranking area (SUCRA) was created to rank those interventions. The ranking probabilities were defined as cumulative probabilities with each intervention being ranked. For each endpoint, an intervention is more desirable than others with a larger SUCRA value.

Results

Trial eligibility

We included double-blind RCTs to investigate the treatment effects of triptans and NASIDs for adults according to the International Classification of Headache Disorders (ICHD), ICHD-II or the International Headache Society (IHS) criteria.

Characteristic of included studies

All studies included were double-blind RCTs involving 1 four-arm trials with 287 participants and 17 three-arm trials with 9,085 participants in all. The remaining 70 studies were two-arm trials that involve 13 comparisons

and a total of 34,850 participants. A detailed list of included studies, patients and diagnostic criteria characteristics is provided in Table 1. All included studies were published between 1993 and 2016.

Pairwise comparisons

We completed pairwise meta-analysis for the 25 comparisons and the weighted ORs for each comparison were calculated. The results of the pair-wise comparisons are shown in Table 2 which illustrates the results of comparison of all 25 direct two-arm trials.

There were a total of 39,004 participants in the placebo controlled trials Direct placebo comparison results suggest all treatments are more effective than placebo with statistical significance in regards to 2 h-pain-free and 2 h-pain-relief (OR > 1, 95% CI excludes 1). All except diclofenac-potassium and almotriptan perform use of rescue medication and most drugs examined show efficacy in 1 h-pain-free and 1 h-pain-relief. Sumatriptan, zolmitriptan, rizatriptan, naratriptan and

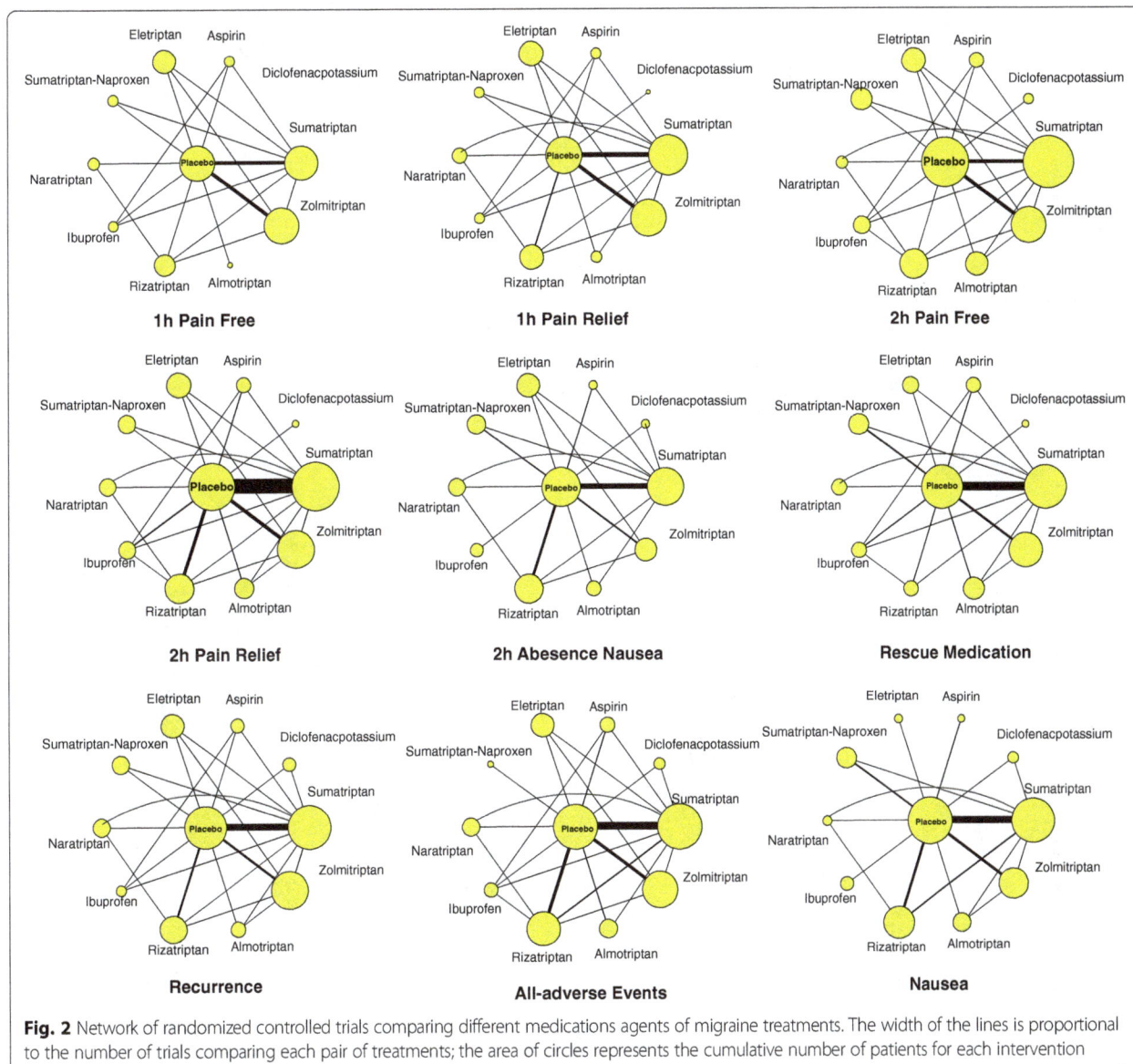

Fig. 2 Network of randomized controlled trials comparing different medications agents of migraine treatments. The width of the lines is proportional to the number of trials comparing each pair of treatments; the area of circles represents the cumulative number of patients for each intervention

aspirin also show an increase in all-adverse events indicating some side effects.

From pairwise meta-analysis between different medications, rizatriptan is more efficacious than naratriptan concerning 1 h-pain-free, 2 h-pain-free and 2 h-pain-relief (OR < 1, 95% CI excludes 1). However, naratriptan manifests a lower recurrence than rizatriptan. Sumatriptan has a worse performance than sumatriptan-naproxen and eletriptan with respect to 2 h-pain-free and use of rescue medication. We can derive that rizatriptan and eletriptan tend to show effective performance with respect to outcomes including 1 h-pain-relief and rescue medication. However, a pairwise meta-analysis provides limited information and does not enable us to synthesize indirect evidence. Therefore we subsequently carried a

NMA for further information so that all treatments could be compared and ranked.

Network meta-analysis

As suggested in Table 3 and Fig. 3, a large number of comparisons were generated by the NMA. As for 1 h-pain-free, all medication except almotriptan and naratriptan show statistical difference over placebo (Additional file 2: Figure S1). Furthermore, zolmitriptan appears to be less effective than rizatriptan and eletriptan, while other comparisons show no significant statistical difference. Likewise, results from NMA with respect to 1 h-pain-relief, only sumatriptan, zolmitriptan, rizatriptan and eletriptan show efficacy when compared with placebo but there were no statistical differences between any two of them.

Table 2 Direct MA comparison of migraine treatments

Comparison	1 h-pain-free	1 h-pain-relief	2 h-pain-free	2 h-pain-relief	2 h-nausea-absence	Rescue medication	Recurrence	All-adverse event	Nausea
Sumatriptan vs Placebo	**2.89 (1.74, 4.81)**	**1.71 (1.34, 2.19)**	**2.93 (2.49, 3.44)**	**1.94 (1.76, 2.14)**	1.08 (0.90, 1.30)	**0.62 (0.54, 0.71)**	**1.34 (1.1, 1.63)**	**1.88 (1.59, 2.23)**	**1.83 (1.45, 2.32)**
Zolmitriptan vs Placebo	**2.45 (2.08, 2.90)**	**1.94 (1.73, 2.18)**	**2.75 (2.06, 3.68)**	**2.17 (1.88, 2.50)**	**1.44 (1.29, 1.62)**	**0.56 (0.51, 0.62)**	1.09 (0.67, 1.76)	**1.94 (1.49, 2.53)**	**2.17 (1.51, 3.12)**
Almotriptan vs Placebo	1.99 (0.99, 3.99)	1.32 (0.89, 1.94)	**1.66 (1.09, 2.53)**	**1.57 (1.29, 1.90)**	1.37 (0.97, 1.93)	0.53 (0.23, 1.21)	1.58 (0.87, 2.84)	1.48 (0.94, 2.33)	0.57 (0.21, 1.53)
Rizatriptan vs Placebo	**3.25 (1.79, 5.90)**	**1.71 (1.21, 2.43)**	**5.36 (4.09, 7.04)**	**2.12 (1.74, 2.58)**	**1.39 (1.24, 1.55)**	**0.60 (0.42, 0.87)**	**1.43 (1.14, 1.8)**	**1.68 (1.44, 1.96)**	1.24 (0.88, 1.76)
Naratriptan vs Placebo	3.50 (0.43, 28.8)	**1.72 (1.16, 2.56)**	**2.75 (1.66, 4.56)**	**1.99 (1.50, 2.62)**	**1.25 (1.00, 1.57)**	**0.52 (0.38, 0.71)**	1.02 (0.61, 1.7)	**1.81 (1.10, 2.98)**	1.00 (0.25, 4.08)
Ibuprofen vs Placebo	**3.14 (1.31, 7.54)**	**2.77 (1.68, 4.55)**	**2.31 (1.70, 3.14)**	**1.83 (1.32, 2.53)**	1.22 (0.97, 1.53)	**0.51 (0.35, 0.74)**	0.82 (0.4, 1.69)	1.01 (0.54, 1.87)	0.77 (0.55, 1.09)
Sumatriptan-Naproxen vs Placebo	3.37 (0.5, 22.48)	1.66 (0.8, 3.41)	**2.81 (2.11, 3.74)**	**2.21 (1.87, 2.61)**	1.09 (0.96, 1.23)	**0.48 (0.42, 0.57)**	**0.55 (0.39, 0.78)**	1.88 (0.82, 4.31)	1.12 (0.62, 2.03)
Eletriptan vs Placebo	**18.4 (4.54, 74.9)**	**3.63 (2.23, 5.92)**	**7.41 (5.16, 10.63)**	**2.70 (2.23, 3.27)**	**1.30 (1.11, 1.53)**	**0.38 (0.30, 0.48)**	**1.52 (1.16, 2)**	0.91 (0.75, 1.11)	**0.19 (0.04, 0.85)**
Diclofenacpotassium vs Placebo	2.00 (0.79, 5.05)	4.00 (0.46, 35.0)	**3.10 (2.02, 4.74)**	**3.68 (2.71, 5.01)**	1.32 (0.91, 1.91)	**1.40 (1.01, 1.94)**	**1.64 (1.25, 2.15)**	1.02 (0.60, 1.74)	0.48 (0.17, 1.41)
Aspirin vs Placebo	–	3.04 (1.87, 4.96)	**2.07 (1.57, 2.72)**	**1.56 (1.29, 1.89)**	1.07 (0.84, 1.37)	**0.66 (0.56, 0.79)**	1.09 (0.81, 1.46)	**2.31 (1.15, 4.64)**	2.99 (0.60, 15.0)
Zolmitriptan vs Sumatriptan	0.86 (0.66, 1.12)	1.01 (0.88, 1.14)	0.97 (0.82, 1.14)	1.00 (0.90, 1.11)	–	0.97 (0.68, 1.40)	1.06 (0.89, 1.26)	1.08 (0.97, 1.21)	1.11 (0.70, 1.76)
Almotriptan vs Sumatriptan	–	0.98 (0.78, 1.22)	0.79 (0.64, 0.97)	1.02 (0.85, 1.24)	1.03 (0.85, 1.25)	1.13 (0.93, 1.37)	1.16 (0.9, 1.5)	0.52 (0.37, 0.73)	0.64 (0.32, 1.30)
Rizatriptan vs Sumatriptan	**1.49 (1.16, 1.91)**	1.11 (0.95, 1.30)	**1.20 (1.08, 1.34)**	1.03 (0.91, 1.16)	1.08 (0.96, 1.23)	0.90 (0.63, 1.28)	1.07 (0.93, 1.24)	0.88 (0.75, 1.04)	0.74 (0.55, 1.00)
Naratriptan vs Sumatriptan	–	0.98 (0.63, 1.50)	0.96 (0.56, 1.62)	0.95 (0.72, 1.27)	1.02 (0.78, 1.33)	1.35 (0.79, 2.31)	0.61 (0.47, 0.79)	0.94 (0.70, 1.26)	0.78 (0.26, 2.28)
Ibuprofen vs Sumatriptan	1.87 (0.90, 3.89)	1.30 (0.87, 1.96)	0.90 (0.62, 1.30)	1.09 (0.80, 1.49)	–	1.01 (0.71, 1.43)	0.84 (0.53, 1.32)	1.07 (0.07, 17.2)	–
Sumatriptan-Naproxen vs Sumatriptan	2.03 (0.91, 4.54)	1.28 (0.86, 1.91)	**1.41 (1.16, 1.72)**	**1.20 (1.04, 1.40)**	1.07 (0.93, 1.24)	**0.66 (0.55, 0.79)**	**0.65 (0.52, 0.81)**	–	1.04 (0.59, 1.84)
Eletriptan vs Sumatriptan	1.42 (0.93, 2.15)	**1.29 (1.05, 1.58)**	**1.35 (1.10, 1.65)**	1.12 (0.96, 1.31)	1.09 (0.94, 1.27)	**0.74 (0.59, 0.93)**	0.94 (0.75, 1.18)	0.83 (0.69, 1.01)	–
Diclofenacpotassium vs Sumatriptan	1.19 (0.54, 2.63)	–	–	–	1.25 (0.87, 1.81)	–	0.88 (0.54, 1.43)	**0.43 (0.26, 0.71)**	0.67 (0.15, 3.03)
Aspirin vs Sumatriptan	–	1.43 (0.97, 2.13)	0.83 (0.59, 1.16)	0.97 (0.76, 1.25)	1.03 (0.71, 1.50)	1.09 (0.83, 1.42)	1.01 (0.73, 1.4)	2.55 (0.11, 61.41)	–
Almotriptan vs Zolmitriptan	–	–	0.90 (0.73, 1.11)	0.93 (0.77, 1.12)	–	0.99 (0.74, 1.32)	1.07 (0.8, 1.42)	–	1.18 (0.52, 2.65)
Rizatriptan vs Zolmitriptan	1.22 (0.73, 2.02)	1.20 (0.88, 1.63)	1.22 (0.90, 1.66)	1.05 (0.81, 1.35)	1.12 (0.87, 1.44)	–	0.96 (0.68, 1.36)	0.89 (0.63, 1.27)	–
Eletriptan vs Zolmitriptan	1.59 (0.96, 2.64)	**1.39 (1.06, 1.81)**	**1.93 (1.50, 2.49)**	1.13 (0.93, 1.38)	1.10 (0.91, 1.34)	–	0.92 (0.68, 1.23)	1.08 (0.85, 1.37)	–

Table 2 Direct MA comparison of migraine treatments *(Continued)*

Naratriptan vs Rizatriptan	**0.35 (0.14, 0.84)**	0.73 (0.49, 1.08)	**0.46 (0.31, 0.69)**	**0.70 (0.51, 0.97)**	0.86 (0.63, 1.18)	-	**0.63 (0.41, 0.96)**	0.70 (0.44, 1.09)	0.47 (0.17, 1.28)
Ibuprofen vs Rizatriptan	-		0.86 (0.40, 1.85)	0.72 (0.39, 1.35)	-	1.75 (0.82, 3.74)	-	0.91 (0.33, 2.53)	-
Aspirin vs Ibuprofen	-	1.10 (0.75, 1.61)	0.81 (0.54, 1.19)	0.87 (0.64, 1.19)	-	1.09 (0.77, 1.53)	1.05 (0.66, 1.68)	1.05 (0.66, 1.68)	-

Values in bold indicate significant difference

Table 3 Network meta-analysis results of migraine treatments

Lower-left triangle: 1 h-Pain-Free; Upper-right triangle: 1 h-Pain-Relief

	A	B	C	D	E	F	G	H	I	J	K
A	**A**	**0.32 (0.20, 0.51)**	**0.33 (0.19, 0.55)**	0.43 (0.11, 1.77)	**0.34 (0.16, 0.70)**	0.45 (0.13, 1.58)	0.25 (0.04, 1.44)	0.43 (0.12, 1.66)	**0.21 (0.07, 0.58)**	0.15 (0.00, 2.63)	0.22 (0.04, 1.28)
B	**0.29 (0.21, 0.38)**	**B**	1.01 (0.53, 1.92)	1.35 (0.33, 5.59)	1.04 (0.48, 2.26)	1.39 (0.39, 5.13)	0.78 (0.13, 4.65)	1.33 (0.36, 5.22)	0.64 (0.21, 1.96)	0.46 (0.01, 8.52)	0.67 (0.11, 4.04)
C	**0.35 (0.26, 0.46)**	1.22 (0.86, 1.75)	**C**	1.34 (0.30, 5.83)	1.03 (0.43, 2.44)	1.39 (0.36, 5.28)	0.77 (0.12, 4.82)	1.32 (0.33, 5.53)	0.63 (0.21, 1.91)	0.46 (0.01, 8.13)	0.66 (0.11, 4.10)
D	0.46 (0.15, 1.23)	1.61 (0.53, 4.62)	1.32 (0.43, 3.68)	**D**	0.77 (0.16, 3.68)	1.04 (0.16, 6.61)	0.58 (0.06, 5.14)	0.99 (0.15, 6.80)	0.47 (0.08, 2.81)	0.34 (0.01, 7.95)	0.51 (0.05, 4.80)
E	**0.20 (0.12, 0.32)**	0.71 (0.46, 1.09)	**0.58 (0.35, 0.93)**	0.44 (0.15, 1.43)	**E**	1.33 (0.35, 5.08)	0.75 (0.11, 4.98)	1.28 (0.29, 5.75)	0.61 (0.17, 2.15)	0.44 (0.01, 8.67)	0.65 (0.10, 4.36)
F	0.56 (0.16, 1.93)	1.98 (0.61, 6.77)	1.61 (0.47, 5.55)	1.24 (0.25, 6.38)	2.80 (0.91, 9.23)	**F**	0.56 (0.07, 4.92)	0.97 (0.16, 5.73)	0.46 (0.09, 2.30)	0.33 (0.01, 7.03)	0.48 (0.06, 4.25)
G	**0.18 (0.07, 0.47)**	0.64 (0.25, 1.68)	0.53 (0.20, 1.41)	0.41 (0.10, 1.67)	0.91 (0.33, 2.58)	0.33 (0.07, 1.47)	**G**	1.76 (0.20, 15.48)	0.82 (0.11, 6.35)	0.57 (0.01, 18.01)	0.87 (0.11, 6.39)
H	**0.28 (0.13, 0.55)**	0.98 (0.46, 2.01)	0.81 (0.37, 1.69)	0.62 (0.17, 2.17)	1.40 (0.59, 3.12)	0.50 (0.12, 1.96)	1.51 (0.46, 4.84)	**H**	0.48 (0.09, 2.46)	0.34 (0.01, 7.70)	0.50 (0.06, 4.55)
I	**0.17 (0.08, 0.30)**	0.59 (0.30, 1.07)	**0.48 (0.25, 0.85)**	0.36 (0.10, 1.25)	0.83 (0.38, 1.71)	0.29 (0.07, 1.10)	0.91 (0.29, 2.62)	0.59 (0.23, 1.50)	**I**	0.73 (0.02, 16.01)	1.04 (0.14, 8.29)
J	–	–	–	–	–	–	–	–	–	**J**	1.50 (0.05, 77.84)
K	**0.31 (0.11, 0.79)**	1.07 (0.40, 2.87)	0.88 (0.31, 2.39)	0.67 (0.16, 2.95)	1.51 (0.53, 4.36)	0.55 (0.11, 2.45)	1.67 (0.58, 4.74)	1.09 (0.33, 3.76)	1.85 (0.60, 5.91)	–	**K**

Lower-left triangle: 2 h-Pain-Free; Upper-right triangle: 2 h-Pain-Relief

	A	B	C	D	E	F	G	H	I	J	K
A	**A**	**0.31 (0.25, 0.41)**	–	**0.22 (0.07, 0.72)**	**0.29 (0.17, 0.39)**	**0.27 (0.18, 0.37)**	**0.23 (0.20, 0.86)**	**0.24 (0.10, 0.30)**	**0.16 (0.12, 0.21)**	**0.03 (0.01, 0.05)**	**0.44 (0.31, 0.50)**
B	**0.21 (0.17, 0.26)**	**B**	–	0.70 (0.26, 1.98)	0.89 (0.47, 1.52)	0.89 (0.44, 1.43)	0.80 (0.67, 2.08)	**0.87 (0.25, 0.99)**	**0.48 (0.39, 0.73)**	**0.08 (0.03, 0.21)**	1.42 (0.75, 2.01)
C	**0.25 (0.18, 0.34)**	1.18 (0.83, 1.68)	**C**	–	–	–	–	–	–	–	–
D	**0.39 (0.25, 0.62)**	1.90 (1.17, 3.04)	1.61 (0.95, 2.68)	**D**	1.28 (0.24, 5.80)	1.01 (0.36, 5.46)	1.52 (0.34, 4.55)	0.71 (0.41, 3.52)	0.69 (0.19, 2.78)	**0.16 (0.01, 0.39)**	1.76 (0.57, 6.84)
E	**0.13 (0.08, 0.19)**	**0.61 (0.40, 0.92)**	**0.51 (0.31, 0.84)**	**0.32 (0.18, 0.58)**	**E**	0.93 (0.68, 1.51)	0.99 (0.51, 3.17)	0.70 (0.38, 1.73)	**0.60 (0.39, 0.81)**	**0.08 (0.06, 0.17)**	**1.40 (1.14, 2.38)**
F	**0.28 (0.12, 0.65)**	1.33 (0.58, 3.17)	1.13 (0.47, 2.80)	0.70 (0.27, 1.83)	2.20 (0.93, 5.29)	**F**	0.84 (0.54, 4.69)	0.76 (0.56, 1.14)	0.52 (0.42, 1.12)	**0.10 (0.04, 0.19)**	**1.63 (1.25, 1.81)**
G	**0.30 (0.16, 0.53)**	1.42 (0.77, 2.63)	1.20 (0.61, 2.35)	0.75 (0.36, 1.58)	**2.33 (1.18, 4.69)**	1.75 (0.96, 3.21)	**G**	1.19 (0.12, 1.22)	**0.56 (0.24, 0.95)**	**0.08 (0.03, 0.25)**	1.98 (0.36, 2.40)
H	**0.22 (0.14, 0.35)**	1.06 (0.65, 1.72)	0.90 (0.51, 1.56)	0.56 (0.29, 1.07)	1.75 (0.96, 3.21)	0.80 (0.30, 2.04)	0.75 (0.36, 1.58)	**H**	0.61 (0.47, 1.98)	**0.15 (0.04, 0.26)**	**1.99 (1.38, 2.99)**
I	**0.10 (0.05, 0.19)**	**0.46 (0.23, 0.95)**	**0.39 (0.19, 0.80)**	**0.24 (0.11, 0.56)**	0.77 (0.35, 1.71)	0.35 (0.12, 1.01)	**0.33 (0.13, 0.80)**	0.44 (0.19, 1.02)	**I**	**0.13 (0.08, 0.44)**	**2.69 (1.51, 4.31)**

Table 3 Network meta-analysis results of migraine treatments (*Continued*)

Upper-right triangle = **Recurrence**; diagonal = treatment (A–K); lower-left triangle = **2 h-Nausea-Absence**

	A	B	C	D	E	F	G	H	I	J	K
	0.23 (0.10, 0.60)	1.12 (0.44, 2.94)	0.95 (0.37, 2.57)	0.59 (0.21, 1.67)	1.86 (0.69, 5.18)	0.84 (0.24, 2.97)	0.79 (0.27, 2.36)	1.05 (0.38, 2.99)	2.40 (0.77, 7.87)	1.48 (0.49, 4.40)	14.32 (9.75, 38.13)
	0.35 (0.19, 0.63)	1.67 (0.89, 3.10)	1.41 (0.72, 2.77)	0.88 (0.41, 1.88)	2.74 (1.34, 5.69)	1.25 (0.43, 3.43)	1.17 (0.53, 2.58)	1.56 (0.75, 3.39)	3.58 (1.43, 9.05)	**J**	**K**
	A	**B**	0.86 (0.57, 1.29)	0.64 (0.29, 1.38)	0.62 (0.39, 0.97)	1.60 (0.85, 3.00)	1.25 (0.49, 3.15)	1.62 (0.84, 3.19)	1.02 (0.44, 2.34)	0.57 (0.27, 1.22)	0.83 (0.41, 1.69)
	0.60 (0.27, 1.29)	0.89 (0.19, 4.11)	**C**	0.75 (0.34, 1.64)	0.89 (0.54, 1.45)	2.30 (1.22, 4.33)	1.80 (0.71, 4.57)	2.34 (1.20, 4.60)	0.83 (0.35, 1.94)	0.82 (0.38, 1.79)	1.20 (0.58, 2.47)
	0.53 (0.14, 2.00)	1.01 (0.09, 10.95)	1.14 (0.08, 18.41)	**D**	0.72 (0.40, 1.29)	1.86 (0.90, 3.85)	1.46 (0.54, 4.00)	1.90 (0.88, 4.12)	1.11 (0.38, 3.33)	0.67 (0.29, 1.57)	0.96 (0.43, 2.21)
	0.61 (0.05, 6.60)	0.27 (0.08, 0.95)	0.31 (0.06, 1.57)	0.27 (0.02, 3.70)	**E**	2.51 (0.94, 6.76)	1.96 (0.58, 6.45)	2.54 (0.96, 6.87)	1.16 (0.46, 2.92)	0.89 (0.31, 2.65)	1.30 (0.47, 3.70)
	0.17 (0.05, 0.49)	0.74 (0.13, 4.34)	0.84 (0.10, 7.13)	0.73 (0.04, 14.17)	2.71 (0.39, 18.41)	2.60 (1.25, 5.32)	2.03 (0.73, 5.64)	2.62 (1.19, 5.87)	0.45 (0.16, 1.23)	0.92 (0.39, 2.23)	1.35 (0.59, 3.10)
	0.44 (0.08, 2.48)	0.98 (0.12, 8.19)	1.11 (0.10, 11.19)	0.97 (0.04, 21.98)	3.57 (0.37, 35.13)	**F**	0.79 (0.26, 2.38)	1.01 (0.41, 2.50)	0.57 (0.17, 1.89)	0.36 (0.13, 0.95)	0.52 (0.21, 1.31)
	0.58 (0.08, 4.22)	0.29 (0.06, 1.48)	0.33 (0.04, 2.64)	0.29 (0.02, 4.94)	1.06 (0.15, 7.12)	1.31 (0.10, 17.60)	**G**	1.30 (0.42, 3.94)	0.44 (0.15, 1.25)	0.46 (0.14, 1.52)	0.66 (0.23, 1.91)
	0.17 (0.03, 0.83)	0.77 (0.09, 7.04)	0.87 (0.09, 8.93)	0.78 (0.03, 17.70)	2.82 (0.28, 29.29)	0.40 (0.04, 3.84)	0.30 (0.02, 3.62)	**H**	**I**	0.35 (0.13, 0.97)	0.51 (0.20, 1.32)
	0.47 (0.06, 3.89)	0.61 (0.03, 11.94)	0.70 (0.03, 17.74)	0.61 (0.01, 27.58)	2.22 (0.10, 54.60)	1.04 (0.07, 15.63)	0.81 (0.04, 14.26)	2.66 (0.21, 37.40)	0.79 (0.02, 28.38)	0.80 (0.27, 2.40)	1.16 (0.40, 3.43)
	0.37 (0.02, 7.04)	1.21 (0.12, 12.49)	1.38 (0.10, 17.99)	1.20 (0.05, 32.12)	4.40 (0.38, 54.35)	0.83 (0.03, 25.26)	0.63 (0.02, 23.22)	2.05 (0.08, 61.86)	1.58 (0.07, 35.45)	**J**	1.44 (0.52, 4.05)
	0.73 (0.08, 6.87)					1.65 (0.10, 29.14)	1.27 (0.06, 25.07)	4.10 (0.29, 65.07)	5.81 (0.99, 35.03)	1.97 (0.05, 76.90)	**K**

Upper-right triangle = **Nausea**; diagonal = treatment (A–G); lower-left triangle = **All Adverse Event**

	A	B	C	D	E	F	G
A	**A**	0.53 (0.42, 0.67)	0.46 (0.32, 0.64)	0.77 (0.41, 1.49)	0.75 (0.52, 1.05)	1.09 (0.45, 2.60)	1.43 (0.76, 2.86)
B	0.31 (0.23, 0.41)	**B**	0.86 (0.60, 1.23)	1.45 (0.77, 2.82)	1.40 (0.99, 1.97)	2.03 (0.85, 4.89)	2.68 (1.40, 5.69)
C	0.37 (0.24, 0.54)	1.17 (0.74, 1.87)	**C**	1.68 (0.86, 3.32)	1.62 (1.04, 2.59)	2.37 (0.93, 5.98)	3.11 (1.52, 6.94)
D	0.64 (0.33, 1.24)	2.04 (1.04, 4.10)	1.74 (0.81, 3.76)	**D**	0.96 (0.46, 1.96)	1.40 (0.47, 4.03)	1.87 (0.74, 4.87)
E	0.41 (0.26, 0.63)	1.31 (0.82, 2.10)	1.11 (0.63, 1.97)	0.64 (0.29, 1.39)	**E**	1.46 (0.60, 3.45)	1.92 (0.92, 4.30)
F	0.26 (0.12, 0.54)	0.84 (0.40, 1.72)	0.71 (0.30, 1.59)	0.41 (0.15, 1.06)	0.64 (0.29, 1.39)	**F**	1.33 (0.45, 4.04)
G	0.89 (0.33, 2.35)	2.84 (1.06, 7.81)	2.42 (0.86, 6.96)	1.39 (0.43, 4.47)	2.17 (0.78, 6.19)	3.39 (1.02, 11.43)	**G**

Table 3 Network meta-analysis results of migraine treatments *(Continued)*

	0.51 (0.10, 2.70)	1.63 (0.31, 9.07)	1.38 (0.25, 7.82)	0.79 (0.13, 4.89)	1.24 (0.22, 6.92)	1.94 (0.32, 12.28)	0.57 (0.09, 3.92)	H	**6.48 (1.06, 39.57)**	1.75 (0.55, 5.65)	0.34 (0.04, 1.79)
	0.64 (0.26, 1.60)	2.05 (0.83, 5.27)	1.76 (0.68, 4.41)	1.00 (0.33, 3.08)	1.57 (0.59, 4.27)	2.45 (0.80, 7.91)	0.72 (0.19, 2.76)	1.27 (0.19, 8.49)	I	0.28 (0.03, 2.14)	**0.05 (0.00, 0.56)**
	0.95 (0.35, 2.54)	**3.04 (1.12, 8.23)**	2.58 (0.90, 7.53)	1.48 (0.45, 4.84)	2.33 (0.79, 6.74)	**3.62 (1.09, 12.42)**	1.07 (0.26, 4.27)	1.85 (0.26, 12.93)	1.48 (0.39, 5.51)	J	**0.18 (0.02, 1.37)**
	0.26 (0.11, 0.58)	0.82 (0.35, 1.91)	0.70 (0.28, 1.73)	0.40 (0.14, 1.13)	0.63 (0.25, 1.57)	0.98 (0.34, 2.92)	**0.29 (0.08, 0.97)**	0.51 (0.08, 3.19)	0.40 (0.12, 1.32)	**0.27 (0.07, 0.97)**	K
Rescue Medication	A	0.43 (0.33, 0.56)	-	-	0.33 (0.17, 0.61)	0.52 (0.25, 1.09)	0.28 (0.14, 0.55)	0.28 (0.17, 0.46)	0.25 (0.08, 0.79)	1.63 (0.43, 6.38)	0.44 (0.24, 0.81)
	2.32 (1.79, 3.05)	B	-	-	0.77 (0.38, 1.50)	1.21 (0.60, 2.56)	0.66 (0.31, 1.32)	0.64 (0.38, 1.10)	0.59 (0.19, 1.83)	3.81 (0.97, 15.25)	1.02 (0.54, 1.95)
	3.03 (1.63, 5.90)	1.30 (0.67, 2.62)	C	-	-	-	-	-	-	-	-
	-	-	-	D	-	-	-	-	-	-	-
	-	-	-	-	E	1.59 (0.61, 4.19)	0.87 (0.36, 2.05)	0.84 (0.38, 1.92)	0.77 (0.21, 2.95)	5.00 (1.18, 22.48)	1.34 (0.57, 3.29)
	1.91 (0.92, 3.97)	0.83 (0.39, 1.68)	-	-	0.63 (0.24, 1.65)	F	0.55 (0.20, 1.46)	0.53 (0.22, 1.27)	0.49 (0.12, 1.85)	3.15 (0.68, 14.14)	0.85 (0.32, 2.13)
	3.52 (1.82, 7.15)	1.52 (0.76, 3.20)	-	-	1.15 (0.49, 2.79)	1.82 (0.69, 5.10)	G	0.97 (0.43, 2.31)	0.90 (0.24, 3.31)	5.77 (1.33, 27.19)	1.55 (0.67, 3.70)
	3.62 (2.16, 6.01)	1.56 (0.91, 2.63)	-	-	1.20 (0.52, 2.61)	1.88 (0.79, 4.48)	1.03 (0.43, 2.34)	H	0.92 (0.27, 3.28)	5.92 (1.48, 25.27)	1.59 (0.72, 3.54)
	3.94 (1.26, 12.29)	1.69 (0.55, 5.32)	-	-	1.30 (0.34, 4.69)	2.05 (0.54, 8.09)	1.11 (0.30, 4.22)	1.09 (0.30, 3.77)	I	6.50 (1.11, 37.90)	1.74 (0.48, 6.35)
	0.61 (0.16, 2.30)	0.26 (0.07, 1.03)	-	-	**0.20 (0.04, 0.84)**	0.32 (0.07, 1.48)	**0.17 (0.04, 0.75)**	**0.17 (0.04, 0.68)**	**0.15 (0.03, 0.90)**	J	0.27 (0.06, 1.13)
	2.27 (1.23, 4.18)	0.98 (0.51, 1.84)	-	-	0.75 (0.30, 1.76)	1.17 (0.47, 3.10)	0.64 (0.27, 1.49)	0.63 (0.28, 1.39)	0.58 (0.16, 2.07)	3.73 (0.89, 16.46)	K

Treatment: A Placebo; B Sumatriptan; C Zolmitriptan; D Almotriptan; E Rizatriptan; F Naratriptan; G Ibuprofen; H Sumatriptan-Naproxen; I Eletriptan; J Diclofenacpotassium; K Aspirin
Values in bold indicate significant difference

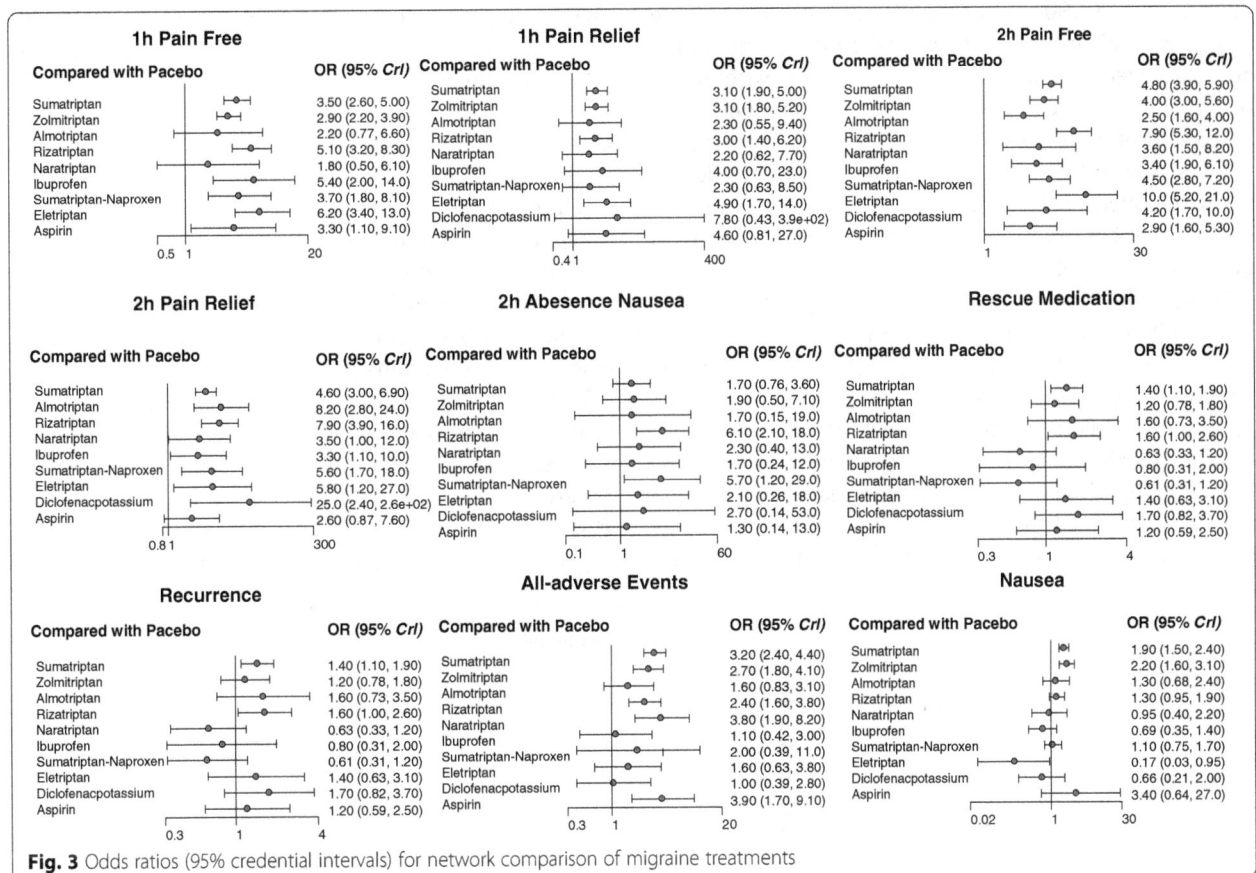

Fig. 3 Odds ratios (95% credential intervals) for network comparison of migraine treatments

For 2 h-pain-free, eletriptan shows efficacy over sumatriptan, zolmitriptan, almotriptan, ibuprofen and aspirin, while rizatriptan is more effective than sumatriptan, zolmitriptan, almotriptan, ibuprofen and aspirin but again there is no statistical evidence to determine the efficacy contrast between rizatriptan and eletriptan (Additional file 3: Figure S2).

Diclofenac-potassium appears to be more effective than any other intervention regarding 2 h-pain-relief. Apart from that, eletriptan also shows promising results compared with sumatriptan, rizatriptan, ibuprofen and aspirin. On the other hand, aspirin is less effective than rizatriptan, naratriptan, sumatriptan-naproxen, eletriptan and diclofenac-potassium. As a traditional treatment, aspirin is regarded as low performance in respect to 2 h-pain-relief, while diclofenac-potassium and eletriptan are outstanding treatments concerning this clinical outcome, and would be promising candidates in acute therapies.

When analyzing 2 h-nausea-absence, rizatriptan has better efficacy than sumatriptan while other treatments except Sumatriptan-Naproxen indicate no distinctive difference even compared with placebo.

Sumatriptan, diclofenac-potassium and rizatriptan present a much higher rate of recurrence figure compared

with naratriptan and sumatriptan-naproxen. Furthermore, solid proof was obtained from the comparison between mono-sumatriptan and sumatriptan-naproxen that naproxen significantly reduces the migraine recurrence rate of sumatriptan while the efficacy of sumatriptan is barely influenced, and further experiments could be designed to investigate this mechanism and to combine treatments with a view to improve their preventive abilities.

Rescue medication data demonstrated that diclofenac-potassium performs the worst compared with rizatriptan, ibuprofen, sumatriptan-naproxen and eletriptan, thus diclofenac-potassium has the most likelihood of all treatments to require a rescue medication. Considering that naproxen has a notable promotion on the tolerability of sumatriptan and that diclofenac-potassium has outstanding behaviors with respect to efficacy, it is desirable to design further experiments to enhance the tolerability of diclofenac-potassium (Additional file 4: Figure S3).

Similarly, sumatriptan demonstrates a high all-adverse-event behavior compared with diclofenac-potassium, ibuprofen and almotriptan. Likewise naratriptan also has a poor all-adverse-event perform when compared with ibuprofen and diclofenac-potassium. In other words, diclofenac-potassium and ibuprofen are milder when compared with naratriptan and sumatriptan, which may indicate that NASIDs offer treatments with less adverse reactions. Aside from this, the combination of sumatriptan and naproxen appears to provide patients with much better tolerance in comparison to sumatriptan alone.

With respect to nausea, zolmitriptan and sumatriptan were significantly inferior to ibuprofen, sumatriptan-naproxen, eletriptan and diclofenac-potassium. Interestingly, eletriptan performs better than several other triptans (Additional file 5: Figure S4).

Finally, Fig. 4 provides the ranking diagrams showing probability of each strategy ranked (1–11) for outcomes and Table 4 provides SUCRA results for further comparison. In general, NASIDs show a more prominent tolerability while some triptans such as rizatriptan and eletriptan exhibit more promising efficacy results. On the other hand, almotriptan has the least effectiveness with respect to 1 h-pain-free and 2 h-pain-free. Similar rankings are displayed in Table 3, which reveals that

diclofenac-potassium and eletriptan has the best efficacy whereas naratriptan and almotriptan are the least efficacious medications.

Discussion

In this NMA, 10 medications were included and the result reveals that eletriptan offers the best efficacy and acceptable tolerability. Besides, our research indicates that ibuprofen exhibited the most desirable tolerability. Furthermore, diclofenac-potassium and sumatriptan-naproxen also showed favorable properties concerning efficacy and tolerability.

Triptans were a group of 5-HT$_{1B/1D}$ agonists [102], three main mechanisms of them were all conduced to anti-migraine function. Firstly, triptans attenuated the release of vasoactive peptides trigeminal system, as well as reduced the migraine vascular inflammation. Moreover, triptans were shown to potentially inhibit the nociceptive

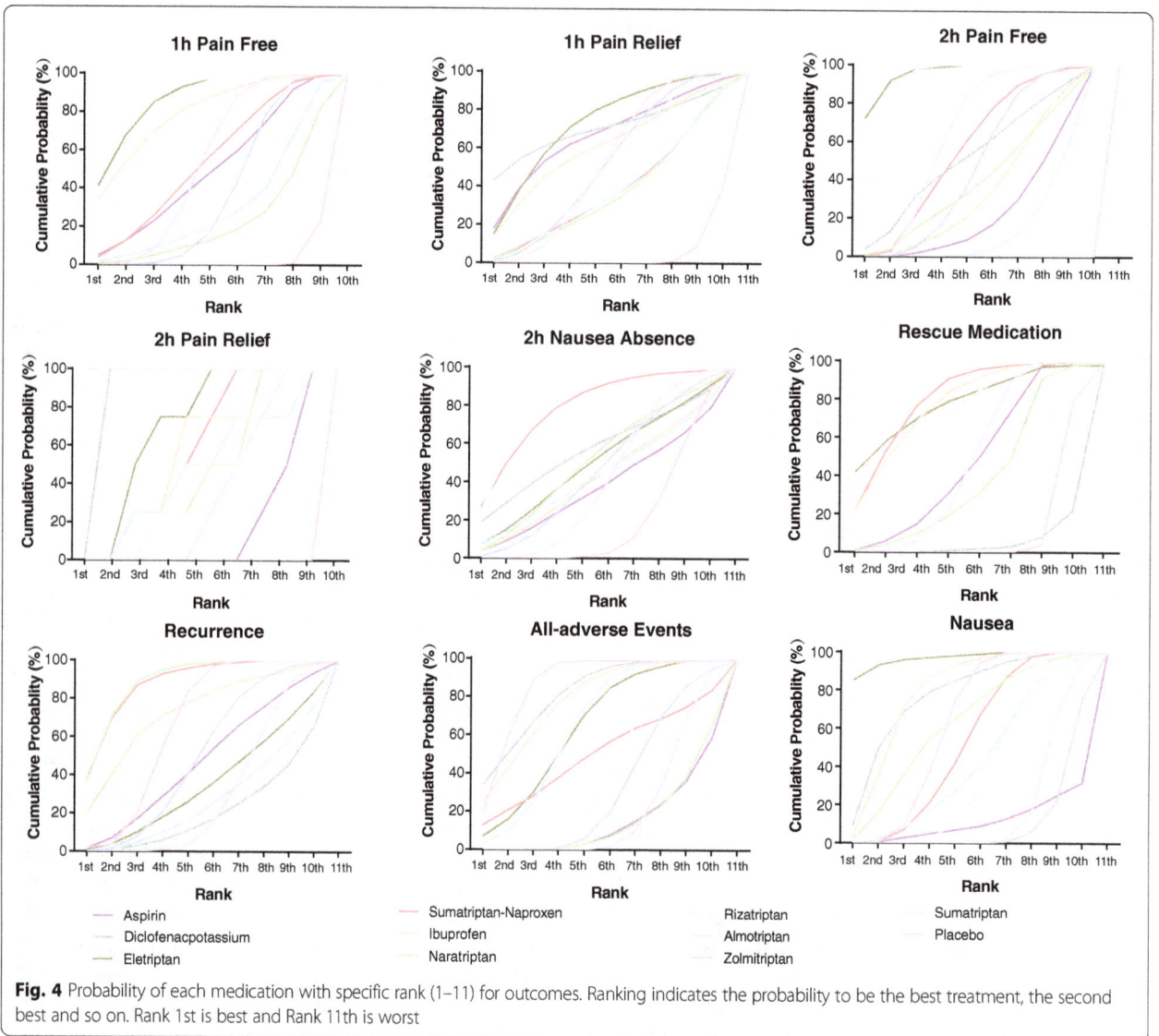

Fig. 4 Probability of each medication with specific rank (1–11) for outcomes. Ranking indicates the probability to be the best treatment, the second best and so on. Rank 1st is best and Rank 11th is worst

Table 4 The SUCRA results of 11 migraine treatments on 9 clinical outcomes

Treatment	1 h-pain-free	1 h-pain-relief	2 h-pain-free	2 h-pain-relief	2 h-nausea-absence	Rescue medication	Recurrence	All-adverse event	Nausea
Placebo	0.024	0.045	0.000	0.000	0.178	0.092	0.602	0.782	0.561
Sumatriptan	0.490	0.483	0.602	0.318	0.376	0.418	0.280	0.189	0.165
Zolmitriptan	0.343	0.476	0.460	0.909	0.418	-	0.457	0.294	0.095
Almotriptan	0.282	0.358	0.186	0.432	0.394	-	0.249	0.589	0.388
Rizatriptan	0.712	0.458	0.824	0.341	0.765	0.602	0.203	0.367	0.358
Naratriptan	0.208	0.344	0.397	0.409	0.467	0.337	0.808	0.137	0.569
Ibuprofen	0.716	0.558	0.356	0.455	0.385	0.678	0.662	0.711	0.715
Sumatriptan-Naproxen	0.493	0.354	0.537	0.523	0.719	0.706	0.801	0.452	0.476
Eletriptan	0.783	0.664	0.874	0.636	0.455	0.689	0.322	0.587	0.880
Diclofenacpotassium	-	0.642	0.504	0.818	0.516	0.040	0.190	0.743	0.705
Aspirin	0.452	0.608	0.262	0.159	0.342	0.417	0.429	0.133	0.103

pathway of central sensitization, thus helped to relieve the pain from migraine [103, 104].

Considering the primary efficacy end-point, triptans perform equally well compared to NSAIDs though eletriptan has the best efficacy, which lends credence to the findings of Chris Cameron et al.'s 2015 study in principle [105]. However, this study did not take adverse events into account. Therefore, we apply 4 adverse-events to characterize this ability in all 10 medications. Additionally we also included a double-component therapy. Here we report this NMA, revealing both the efficacy and the tolerability of present medication against migraine.

At first, we focused on the differences apparent in the primary efficacy end-point between different types of medications. Rizatriptan provides relatively good freedom from pain and nausea though with poor pain relief, the reason for that might be the different criteria for efficacy in each study. When it comes to tolerability, NASIDs seem to be more attractive solutions. Also, it is of significance that this study found naproxen is capable of significantly improving the tolerability of sumatriptan and has no influence on its efficacy.

As suggested by the rank probability of SUCRA, eletriptan exhibited the most considerable efficacy. From the SUCRA data, it is obvious that eletriptan can reduce pain with a better result than any other medication. In the meantime it also performs better than most of others in 1 h pain-free and 2 h pain-free. Eletriptan is a new 5-HT$_{1B/1D/1F}$-selective receptor agonist with a higher affinity to the receptors when compared with other triptans [106]. Besides, more rapid and consistent absorption has been achieved through structural design, and this has made it possible for the drug to pass through the blood-brain barrier [107]. As a result of its enhanced hydrophobility, higher bioavailability and longer plasma half-life have also been reported [108]. When compared with sumatriptan and other triptans, the difference in efficacy

may be explained by the overcoming of the blood-brain barrier, which leads to a faster and more consistent absorption [107].

When we turn attention to the NSAIDs, ibuprofen attracted us by its superior tolerability amongst all observed medications. Though ibuprofen has been available as a non-prescription medication for more than 40 years, the mechanism of how the drug works is still not completely understood. According to a widely accepted theory, it may be related to prostaglandin synthetase inhibition, therefore allowing better tolerability. From the SUCRA data we can observe that ibuprofen ranked top three in all the adverse-event indications.

The results of SUCRA also showed that the diclopenac potassium performs with high efficacy and tolerability, in fact it stood the best option among NSAIDs from a comprehensive point of view. At the mechanism level, NSAIDs inhibit the activity of cyclooxygenase (COX), which is recognized as being composed of two isoforms (COX-1& COX-2). COX acts as a catalyst during the production for prostaglandins, a substance responsible for pain and inflammation. Diclofenac inhibit both COX isoforms, though with a lower activity for COX-2 [109, 110].

Meanwhile we recognized that sumatriptan-naproxen also offered a high-level tolerability, ranking first in rescue medication and recurrence and fourth in the other two indications among the ten medications. The addition of naproxen significantly improved the tolerability of sumatriptan. To understand the reason for this we referred to the mechanism of both the medicines and the migraine.

The pathophysiology mechanism of migraine is quite complex, involving multiple neural pathways that appear to be pivotal during the process [111]. In the early stage of a migraine, vasoactive and substances including calcitonin gene-related peptide and kinins are released by trigeminal nerve endings under the stimulation of cortical spreading depression. At the same time, the central pathways' activation depends on the signals of pain from the periphery. However, in the later stage, central sensitization has no relationship with peripheral neural input [112].

Considering the multiple pathogenic mechanisms, multi-mechanism-targeted therapy may have better effect than monotherapy. Triptans not only decrease transmission of the pain impulses to the trigeminal nucleus caudalis but also release inflammatory mediators from trigeminal nerves, therefore reduce calcitonin gene-related peptide-mediated vasodilation [113]. As for naproxen, it suppressed sensitization of central trigeminovascular neurons in the spinal trigeminal nucleus [20]. In our study, the combination of sumatriptan and naproxen effectively altered peripheral activation of central pathways during early period and development of central sensitization during later periods. As a result, a high-level tolerability was observed, and this possibility was supported by several clinical studies [114–116].

What attracted our attention most is the potentiality to combine different medications together and make use of the advantages of each considering the relevant stage. Applying different medications to intervene at every key point of the multiple pathogenic mechanisms may bring us closer to a better outcome. For instance, we may combine naproxen with eletriptan to attain treatments with both optimal efficacy and tolerability.

As with all analyses, we still cannot avoid several limitations. First, age and gender was not under consideration. Further research is needed in assessing the efficacy for different groups of people. Second, long-term assessment is also important. As we all know, people who suffer from migraine may undergo a long-period treatment and therefore the efficacy and safety of medications are vital. Third, the dosage of medications was not considered and that may cause some deviations.

Conclusions

In conclusion, through this NMA we came to the interpretation that eletriptan may be the most suitable therapy for migraine from a comprehensive point of view. In the meantime ibuprofen may also be a good choice for its excellent tolerability. Multi-component medication also attracted our attention and it may be a promising orientation for the next generation of medication for migraine.

Article highlights

1. Uses NMA to analysis the efficacy and tolerability of NSAIDs and triptans in migraine.

2. Eletriptan may be the most preferable treatment for migraine from a comprehensive point of view.

3. Ibuprofen has the best tolerability among all the medications.

4. Multi-component medication may be a good choice for the migraine medication in the future.

Additional files

Additional file 1: Table S1. Jadad scale table of 88 included studies

Additional file 2: Figure S1. Node splitting of direct and indirect comparisons according to type of interventions for 1 h clinical outcomes.

Additional file 3: Figure S2. Node splitting of direct and indirect comparisons according to type of interventions for 2 h clinical outcomes.

Additional file 4: Figure S3. Node splitting of direct and indirect comparisons according to type of interventions for rescue medication and recurrence.

Additional file 5: Figure S4. Node splitting of direct and indirect comparisons according to type of interventions for all adverse events. Treatment: A Placebo; B Sumatriptan; C Zolmitriptan; D Almotriptan; E Rizatriptan; F Naratriptan; G Ibuprofen; H Sumatriptan-Naproxen; I Eletriptan; J Diclofenacpotassium; K Aspirin. (EPS 2065 kb)

Funding
None.

Authors' contributions
HX and ML were involved in conception and design of the study. WH collected, analyzed, and interpreted the data. The manuscript was drafted by HX and JW. All authors reviewed and approved the final manuscript.

Competing interests
The authors declare that they have no competing interests

References
1. Stewart WF, Lipton RB, Celentano DD, Reed ML (1992) Prevalence of migraine headache in the United States. Relation to age, income, race, and other sociodemographic factors. JAMA 267(1):64–69
2. Lipton RB, Stewart WF, Diamond S, Diamond ML, Reed M (2001) Prevalence and burden of migraine in the United States: data from the American Migraine Study II. Headache 41(7):646–657
3. Gobel H, Petersen-Braun M, Soyka D (1994) The epidemiology of headache in Germany: a nationwide survey of a representative sample on the basis of the headache classification of the International Headache Society. Cephalalgia 14(2):97–106
4. Henry P, Michel P, Brochet B, Dartigues JF, Tison S, Salamon R (1992) A nationwide survey of migraine in France: prevalence and clinical features in adults. GRIM. Cephalalgia 12(4):229–237, discussion 186
5. Antonaci F, Ghiotto N, Wu S, Pucci E, Costa A (2016) Recent advances in migraine therapy. Springerplus 5:637
6. Silberstein SD, Holland S, Freitag F, Dodick DW, Argoff C, Ashman E (2012) Evidence-based guideline update: pharmacologic treatment for episodic migraine prevention in adults: report of the Quality Standards Subcommittee of the American Academy of Neurology and the American Headache Society. Neurology 78(17):1337–1345

7. Evers S, Afra J, Frese A, Goadsby PJ, Linde M, May A et al (2009) EFNS guideline on the drug treatment of migraine–revised report of an EFNS task force. Eur J Neurol 16(9):968–981

8. Marmura MJ, Silberstein SD, Schwedt TJ (2015) The acute treatment of migraine in adults: the american headache society evidence assessment of migraine pharmacotherapies. Headache 55(1):3–20

9. Pringsheim T, Davenport WJ, Marmura MJ, Schwedt TJ, Silberstein S (2016) How to apply the AHS evidence assessment of the acute treatment of migraine in adults to your patient with migraine. Headache 56(7):1194–1200

10. Diamond ML, Hettiarachchi J, Hilliard B, Sands G, Nett R (2004) Effectiveness of eletriptan in acute migraine: primary care for Excedrin nonresponders. Headache 44(3):209–216

11. Pascual J, Cabarrocas X (2002) Within-patient early versus delayed treatment of migraine attacks with almotriptan: the sooner the better. Headache 42(1):28–31

12. Dowson AJ, Massiou H, Lainez JM, Cabarrocas X (2004) Almotriptan improves response rates when treatment is within 1 hour of migraine onset. Headache 44(4):318–322

13. Burstein R, Collins B, Jakubowski M (2004) Defeating migraine pain with triptans: a race against the development of cutaneous allodynia. Ann Neurol 55(1):19–26

14. Linde M, Mellberg A, Dahlof C (2006) Subcutaneous sumatriptan provides symptomatic relief at any pain intensity or time during the migraine attack. Cephalalgia 26(2):113–121

15. (1999) Acute treatment of migraine attacks: efficacy and safety of a nonsteroidal anti-inflammatory drug, diclofenac-potassium, in comparison to oral sumatriptan and placebo. The Diclofenac-K/Sumatriptan Migraine Study Group. Cephalalgia 19(4):232–240

16. Ahrens SP, Farmer MV, Williams DL, Willoughby E, Jiang K, Block GA et al (1999) Efficacy and safety of rizatriptan wafer for the acute treatment of migraine. Cephalalgia 19(5):525–530

17. Barbanti P, Carpay JA, Kwong WJ, Ahmad F, Boswell D (2004) Effects of a fast disintegrating/rapid release oral formulation of sumatriptan on functional ability in patients with migraine. Curr Med Res Opin 20(12):2021–2029

18. Bomhof M, Paz J, Legg N, Allen C, Vandormael K, Patel K (1999) Comparison of rizatriptan 10 mg vs. naratriptan 2.5 mg in migraine. Eur Neurol 42(3):173–179

19. Bousser MG, D'Allens H, Richard A (1993) Efficacy of subcutaneous sumatriptan in the acute treatment of early-morning migraine: a placebo-controlled trial. Early-Morning Migraine Sumatriptan Study Group. J Intern Med 234(2):211–216

20. Brandes JL, Kudrow D, Stark SR, O'Carroll CP, Adelman JU, O'Donnell FJ et al (2007) Sumatriptan-naproxen for acute treatment of migraine: a randomized trial. JAMA 297(13):1443–1454

21. Bussone G, Manzoni GC, Cortelli P, Roncolato M, Fabbri L, Benassuti C (2000) Efficacy and tolerability of sumatriptan in the treatment of multiple migraine attacks. Neurol Sci 21(5):272–278

22. Cady RC, Ryan R, Jhingran P, O'Quinn S, Pait DG (1998) Sumatriptan injection reduces productivity loss during a migraine attack: results of a double-blind, placebo-controlled trial. Arch Intern Med 158(9):1013–1018

23. Carleton SC, Shesser RF, Pietrzak MP, Chudnofsky CR, Starkman S, Morris DL et al (1998) Double-blind, multicenter trial to compare the efficacy of intramuscular dihydroergotamine plus hydroxyzine versus intramuscular meperidine plus hydroxyzine for the emergency department treatment of acute migraine headache. Ann Emerg Med 32(2):129–138

24. Charlesworth BR, Dowson AJ, Purdy A, Becker WJ, Boes-Hansen S, Farkkila M (2003) Speed of onset and efficacy of zolmitriptan nasal spray in the acute treatment of migraine: a randomised, double-blind, placebo-controlled, dose-ranging study versus zolmitriptan tablet. CNS Drugs 17(9):653–667

25. Codispoti JR, Prior MJ, Fu M, Harte CM, Nelson EB (2001) Efficacy of nonprescription doses of ibuprofen for treating migraine headache. A randomized controlled trial. Headache 41(7):665–679

26. Dahlof C, Diener HC, Goadsby PJ, Massiou H, Olesen J, Schoenen J et al (1998) Zolmitriptan, a 5-HT1B/1D receptor agonist for the acute oral treatment of migraine: a multicentre, dose-range finding study. Eur J Neurol 5(6):535–543

27. Dahlof C, Hogenhuis L, Olesen J, Petit H, Ribbat J, Schoenen J et al (1998) Early clinical experience with subcutaneous naratriptan in the acute treatment of migraine: a dose-ranging study. Eur J Neurol 5(5):469–477

28. Diamond S, Elkind A, Jackson RT, Ryan R, DeBussey S, Asgharnejad M (1998) Multiple-attack efficacy and tolerability of sumatriptan nasal spray in the treatment of migraine. Arch Fam Med 7(3):234–240

29. Diener HC (1999) Efficacy and safety of intravenous acetylsalicylic acid lysinate compared to subcutaneous sumatriptan and parenteral placebo in the acute treatment of migraine. A double-blind, double-dummy, randomized, multicenter, parallel group study. The ASASUMAMIG Study Group. Cephalalgia 19(6):581–588, discussion 542

30. Diener HC, Bussone G, De Liano H, Eikermann A, Englert R, Floeter T et al (2004) Placebo-controlled comparison of effervescent acetylsalicylic acid, sumatriptan and ibuprofen in the treatment of migraine attacks. Cephalalgia 24(11):947–954

31. Diener HC, Eikermann A, Gessner U, Gobel H, Haag G, Lange R et al (2004) Efficacy of 1,000 mg effervescent acetylsalicylic acid and sumatriptan in treating associated migraine symptoms. Eur Neurol 52(1):50–56

32. Diener HC, Gendolla A, Gebert I, Beneke M (2005) Almotriptan in migraine patients who respond poorly to oral sumatriptan: a double-blind, randomized trial. Eur Neurol 53(Suppl 1):41–48

33. Diener HC, Jansen JP, Reches A, Pascual J, Pitei D, Steiner TJ (2002) Efficacy, tolerability and safety of oral eletriptan and ergotamine plus caffeine (Cafergot) in the acute treatment of migraine: a multicentre, randomised, double-blind, placebo-controlled comparison. Eur Neurol 47(2):99–107

34. Diener HC, Montagna P, Gács G, Lyczak P, Schumann G, Zöller B et al (2006) Efficacy and tolerability of diclofenac potassium sachets in migraine: a randomized, double-blind, cross-over study in comparison with diclofenac potassium tablets and placebo. Cephalalgia 26(5):537–547

35. Djupesland PG, Docekal P (2010) Intranasal sumatriptan powder delivered by a novel breath-actuated bi-directional device for the acute treatment of migraine: a randomised, placebo-controlled study. Cephalalgia 30(8):933–942

36. Dodick D, Brandes J, Elkind A, Mathew N, Rodichok L (2005) Speed of onset, efficacy and tolerability of zolmitriptan nasal spray in the acute treatment of migraine: a randomised, double-blind, placebo-controlled study. CNS Drugs 19(2):125–136

37. Dodick DW (2002) Almotriptan increases sustained pain-free outcomes in acute migraine: results from three controlled clinical trials. Headache 42(1):21–27

38. Dowson A, Ball K, Haworth D (2000) Comparison of a fixed combination of domperidone and paracetamol (Domperamol) with sumatriptan 50 mg in moderate to severe migraine: a randomised UK primary care study. Curr Med Res Opin 16(3):190–197

39. Dowson AJ, MacGregor EA, Purdy RA, Becker WJ, Green J, Levy SL (2002) Zolmitriptan orally disintegrating tablet is effective in the acute treatment of migraine. Cephalalgia 22(2):101–106

40. Dowson AJ, Massiou H, Lainez JM, Cabarrocas X (2002) Almotriptan is an effective and well-tolerated treatment for migraine pain: results of a randomized, double-blind, placebo-controlled clinical trial. Cephalalgia 22(6):453–461

41. Freitag F, Diamond M, Diamond S, Janssen I, Rodgers A, Skobieranda F (2008) Efficacy and tolerability of coadministration of rizatriptan and acetaminophen vs rizatriptan or acetaminophen alone for acute migraine treatment. Headache 48(6):921–930

42. Gallagher RM, Dennish G, Spierings EL, Chitra R (2000) A comparative trial of zolmitriptan and sumatriptan for the acute oral treatment of migraine. Headache 40(2):119–128

43. Gawel M, Aschoff J, May A, Charlesworth BR (2005) Zolmitriptan 5 mg nasal spray: efficacy and onset of action in the acute treatment of migraine–results from phase 1 of the REALIZE Study. Headache 45(1):7–16

44. Geraud G, Compagnon A, Rossi A (2002) Zolmitriptan versus a combination of acetylsalicylic acid and metoclopramide in the acute oral treatment of migraine: a double-blind, randomised, three-attack study. Eur Neurol 47(2):88–98

45. Geraud G, Olesen J, Pfaffenrath V, Tfelt-Hansen P, Zupping R, Diener HC et al (2000) Comparison of the efficacy of zolmitriptan and sumatriptan: issues in migraine trial design. Cephalalgia 20(1):30–38

46. Goadsby PJ, Massiou H, Pascual J, Diener HC, Dahlof CG, Mateos V et al (2007) Almotriptan and zolmitriptan in the acute treatment of migraine. Acta Neurol Scand 115(1):34–40

47. Gobel H, Winter P, Boswell D, Crisp A, Becker W, Hauge T et al (2000) Comparison of naratriptan and sumatriptan in recurrence-prone migraine patients. Naratriptan International Recurrence Study Group. Clin Ther 22(8):981–989

48. Goldstein J, Ryan R, Jiang K, Getson A, Norman B, Block GA et al (1998) Crossover comparison of rizatriptan 5 mg and 10 mg versus sumatriptan 25 mg and 50 mg in migraine. Rizatriptan Protocol 046 Study Group. Headache 38(10):737–747

49. Goldstein J, Silberstein SD, Saper JR, Elkind AH, Smith TR, Gallagher RM et al (2005) Acetaminophen, aspirin, and caffeine versus sumatriptan succinate in

the early treatment of migraine: results from the ASSET trial. Headache 45(8):973–982

50. Goldstein J, Silberstein SD, Saper JR, Ryan RE Jr, Lipton RB (2006) Acetaminophen, aspirin, and caffeine in combination versus ibuprofen for acute migraine: results from a multicenter, double-blind, randomized, parallel-group, single-dose, placebo-controlled study. Headache 46(3):444–453

51. Gross ML, Kay J, Turner AM, Hallett K, Cleal AL, Hassani H (1994) Sumatriptan in acute migraine using a novel cartridge system self-injector. United Kingdom Study Group. Headache 34(10):559–563

52. Gruffyd-Jones K, Kies B, Middleton A, Mulder LJ, Rosjo O, Millson DS (2001) Zolmitriptan versus sumatriptan for the acute oral treatment of migraine: a randomized, double-blind, international study. Eur J Neurol 8(3):237–245

53. Havanka H, Dahlof C, Pop PH, Diener HC, Winter P, Whitehouse H et al (2000) Efficacy of naratriptan tablets in the acute treatment of migraine: a dose-ranging study. Naratriptan S2WB2004 Study Group. Clin Ther 22(8):970–980

54. Henry P, d'Allens H (1993) Subcutaneous sumatriptan in the acute treatment of migraine in patients using dihydroergotamine as prophylaxis. French Migraine Network Bordeaux-Lyon-Grenoble. Headache 33(8):432–435

55. Jelinski SE, Becker WJ, Christie SN, Ahmad FE, Pryse-Phillips W, Simpson SD (2006) Pain free efficacy of sumatriptan in the early treatment of migraine. Can J Neurol Sci 33(1):73–79

56. Kellstein DE, Lipton RB, Geetha R, Koronkiewicz K, Evans FT, Stewart WF et al (2000) Evaluation of a novel solubilized formulation of ibuprofen in the treatment of migraine headache: a randomized, double-blind, placebo-controlled, dose-ranging study. Cephalalgia 20(4):233–243

57. Klapper J, Lucas C, Rosjo O, Charlesworth B (2004) Benefits of treating highly disabled migraine patients with zolmitriptan while pain is mild. Cephalalgia 24(11):918–924

58. Kolodny A, Polis A, Battisti WP, Johnson-Pratt L, Skobieranda F (2004) Comparison of rizatriptan 5 mg and 10 mg tablets and sumatriptan 25 mg and 50 mg tablets. Cephalalgia 24(7):540–546

59. Lange R, Schwarz JA, Hohn M (2000) Acetylsalicylic acid effervescent 1000 mg (Aspirin) in acute migraine attacks; a multicentre, randomized, double-blind, single-dose, placebo-controlled parallel group study. Cephalalgia 20(7):663–667

60. Le Jeunne C, Gomez JP, Pradalier A, Titus i Albareda F, Joffroy A, Liano H et al (1999) Comparative efficacy and safety of calcium carbasalate plus metoclopramide versus ergotamine tartrate plus caffeine in the treatment of acute migraine attacks. Eur Neurol 41(1):37–43

61. Lewis DW, Kellstein D, Dahl G, Burke B, Frank LM, Toor S et al (2002) Children's ibuprofen suspension for the acute treatment of pediatric migraine. Headache 42(8):780–786

62. Lipton RB, Baggish JS, Stewart WF, Codispoti JR, Fu M (2000) Efficacy and safety of acetaminophen in the treatment of migraine: results of a randomized, double-blind, placebo-controlled, population-based study. Arch Intern Med 160(22):3486–3492

63. Lipton RB, Goldstein J, Baggish JS, Yataco AR, Sorrentino JV, Quiring JN (2005) Aspirin is efficacious for the treatment of acute migraine. Headache 45(4):283–292

64. Lipton RB, Grosberg B, Singer RP, Pearlman SH, Sorrentino JV, Quiring JN et al (2010) Efficacy and tolerability of a new powdered formulation of diclofenac potassium for oral solution for the acute treatment of migraine: results from the International Migraine Pain Assessment Clinical Trial (IMPACT). Cephalalgia 30(11):1336–1345

65. Lipton RB, Stewart WF, Cady R, Hall C, O'Quinn S, Kuhn T et al (2000) Sumatriptan for the range of headaches in migraine sufferers: results of the spectrum study. Headache 40(10):783–791

66. Loder E, Freitag FG, Adelman J, Pearlmand S, Abu-Shakra S (2005) Pain-free rates with zolmitriptan 2.5 mg ODT in the acute treatment of migraine: results of a large double-blind placebo- controlled trial. Curr Med Res Opin 21(3):381–389

67. MacGregor EA, Dowson A, Davies PT (2002) Mouth-dispersible aspirin in the treatment of migraine: a placebo-controlled study. Headache 42(4):249–255

68. Mannix LK, Loder E, Nett R, Mueller L, Rodgers A, Hustad CM et al (2007) Rizatriptan for the acute treatment of ICHD-II proposed menstrual migraine: two prospective, randomized, placebo-controlled, double-blind studies. Cephalalgia 27(5):414–421

69. Mannix LK, Martin VT, Cady RK, Diamond ML, Lener SE, White JD et al (2009) Combination treatment for menstrual migraine and dysmenorrhea using sumatriptan-naproxen: two randomized controlled trials. Obstet Gynecol 114(1):106–113

70. Mathew NT, Finlayson G, Smith TR, Cady RK, Adelman J, Mao L et al (2007) Early intervention with almotriptan: results of the AEGIS trial (AXERT Early Migraine Intervention Study). Headache 47(2):189–198

71. Mathew NT, Schoenen J, Winner P, Muirhead N, Sikes CR (2003) Comparative efficacy of eletriptan 40 mg versus sumatriptan 100 mg. Headache 43(3):214–222

72. Misra UK, Jose M, Kalita J (2004) Rofecoxib versus ibuprofen for acute treatment of migrainne: a randomised placebo controlled trial. Postgrad Med J 80(950):720–723

73. Misra UK, Kalita J, Yadav RK (2007) Rizatriptan vs. ibuprofen in migraine: a randomised placebo-controlled trial. J Headache Pain 8(3):175–179

74. Myllyla VV, Havanka H, Herrala L, Kangasniemi P, Rautakorpi I, Turkka J et al (1998) Tolfenamic acid rapid release versus sumatriptan in the acute treatment of migraine: comparable effect in a double-blind, randomized, controlled, parallel-group study. Headache 38(3):201–207

75. Nappi G, Sicuteri F, Byrne M, Roncolato M, Zerbini O (1994) Oral sumatriptan compared with placebo in the acute treatment of migraine. J Neurol 241(3):138–144

76. Pascual J, Falk RM, Piessens F, Prusinski A, Docekal P, Robert M et al (2000) Consistent efficacy and tolerability of almotriptan in the acute treatment of multiple migraine attacks: results of a large, randomized, double-blind, placebo-controlled study. Cephalalgia 20(6):588–596

77. Pascual J, Vega P, Diener HC, Allen C, Vrijens F, Patel K (2000) Comparison of rizatriptan 10 mg vs. zolmitriptan 2.5 mg in the acute treatment of migraine. Rizatriptan-Zolmitriptan Study Group. Cephalalgia 20(5):455–461

78. Peikert A, Becker WJ, Ashford EA, Dahlof C, Hassani H, Salonen RJ (1999) Sumatriptan nasal spray: a dose-ranging study in the acute treatment of migraine. Eur J Neurol 6(1):43–49

79. Peroutka SJ, Lyon JA, Swarbrick J, Lipton RB, Kolodner K, Goldstein J (2004) Efficacy of diclofenac sodium softgel 100 mg with or without caffeine 100 mg in migraine without aura: a randomized, double-blind, crossover study. Headache 44(2):136–141

80. Pfaffenrath V, Cunin G, Sjonell G, Prendergast S (1998) Efficacy and safety of sumatriptan tablets (25 mg, 50 mg, and 100 mg) in the acute treatment of migraine: defining the optimum doses of oral sumatriptan. Headache 38(3): 184–190

81. Rothner AD, Wasiewski W, Winner P, Lewis D, Stankowski J (2006) Zolmitriptan oral tablet in migraine treatment: high placebo responses in adolescents. Headache 46(1):101–109

82. Ryan RE Jr, Diamond S, Giammarco RAM, Aurora SK, Reed RC, Fletcher PE (2000) Efficacy of Zolmitriptan at early time-points for the acute treatment of migraine and treatment of recurrence: a randomised, placebo-controlled trial. CNS Drugs 13(3):215–226

83. Sakai F, Iwata M, Tashiro K, Itoyama Y, Tsuji S, Fukuuchi Y et al (2002) Zolmitriptan is effective and well tolerated in Japanese patients with migraine: a dose–response study. Cephalalgia 22(5):376–383

84. Salonen R, Ashford E, Dahlof C, Dawson R, Gilhus NE, Luben V et al (1994) Intranasal sumatriptan for the acute treatment of migraine. International Intranasal Sumatriptan Study Group. J Neurol 241(8):463–469

85. Scherl ER, Wilson JF (1995) Comparison of dihydroergotamine with metoclopramide versus meperidine with promethazine in the treatment of acute migraine. Headache 35(5):256–259

86. Schulman EA, Cady RK, Henry D, Batenhorst AS, Putnam DG, Watson CB et al (2000) Effectiveness of sumatriptan in reducing productivity loss due to migraine: results of a randomized, double-blind, placebo-controlled clinical trial. Mayo Clin Proc 75(8):782–789

87. Schulman EA, Dermott KF (2003) Sumatriptan plus metoclopramide in triptan-nonresponsive migraineurs. Headache 43(7):729–733

88. Sheftell FD, Dahlof CG, Brandes JL, Agosti R, Jones MW, Barrett PS (2005) Two replicate randomized, double-blind, placebo-controlled trials of the time to onset of pain relief in the acute treatment of migraine with a fast-disintegrating/rapid-release formulation of sumatriptan tablets. Clin Ther 27(4):407–417

89. Smith TR, Sunshine A, Stark SR, Littlefield DE, Spruill SE, Alexander WJ (2005) Sumatriptan and naproxen sodium for the acute treatment of migraine. Headache 45(8):983–991

90. Spierings EL, Gomez-Mancilla B, Grosz DE, Rowland CR, Whaley FS, Jirgens KJ (2001) Oral almotriptan vs. oral sumatriptan in the abortive treatment of

migraine: a double-blind, randomized, parallel-group, optimum-dose comparison. Arch Neurol 58(6):944–950

91. Spierings EL, Rapoport AM, Dodick DW, Charlesworth B (2004) Acute treatment of migraine with zolmitriptan 5 mg orally disintegrating tablet. CNS Drugs 18(15):1133–1141

92. Steiner TJ, Diener HC, MacGregor EA, Schoenen J, Muirheads N, Sikes CR (2003) Comparative efficacy of eletriptan and zolmitriptan in the acute treatment of migraine. Cephalalgia 23(10):942–952

93. Teall J, Tuchman M, Cutler N, Gross M, Willoughby E, Smith B et al (1998) Rizatriptan (MAXALT) for the acute treatment of migraine and migraine recurrence. A placebo-controlled, outpatient study. Headache 38(4):281–287

94. Tepper SJ, Donnan GA, Dowson AJ, Bomhof MA, Elkind A, Meloche J et al (1999) A long-term study to maximise migraine relief with zolmitriptan. Curr Med Res Opin 15(4):254–271

95. Tfelt-Hansen P, Henry P, Mulder LJ, Scheldewaert RG, Schoenen J, Chazot G (1995) The effectiveness of combined oral lysine acetylsalicylate and metoclopramide compared with oral sumatriptan for migraine. Lancet 346(8980):923–926

96. Tfelt-Hansen P, Teall J, Rodriguez F, Giacovazzo M, Paz J, Malbecq W et al (1998) Oral rizatriptan versus oral sumatriptan: a direct comparative study in the acute treatment of migraine. Rizatriptan 030 Study Group. Headache 38(10):748–755

97. Touchon J, Bertin L, Pilgrim AJ, Ashford E, Bes A (1996) A comparison of subcutaneous sumatriptan and dihydroergotamine nasal spray in the acute treatment of migraine. Neurology 47(2):361–365

98. Tullo V, Allais G, Ferrari MD, Curone M, Mea E, Omboni S et al (2010) Frovatriptan versus zolmitriptan for the acute treatment of migraine: a double-blind, randomized, multicenter, Italian study. Neurol Sci 31 (Suppl 1):S51–S54

99. Wang SJ, Fuh JL, Wu ZA (2007) Intranasal sumatriptan study with high placebo response in Taiwanese patients with migraine. J Chin Med Assoc 70(2):39–46

100. Wendt J, Cady R, Singer R, Peters K, Webster C, Kori S et al (2006) A randomized, double-blind, placebo-controlled trial of the efficacy and tolerability of a 4-mg dose of subcutaneous sumatriptan for the treatment of acute migraine attacks in adults. Clin Ther 28(4):517–526

101. Winner P, Mannix LK, Putnam DG, McNeal S, Kwong J, O'Quinn S et al (2003) Pain-free results with sumatriptan taken at the first sign of migraine pain: 2 randomized, double-blind, placebo-controlled studies. Mayo Clin Proc 78(10):1214–1222

102. Capi M, Curto M, Lionetto L, de Andres F, Gentile G, Negro A et al (2016) Eletriptan in the management of acute migraine: an update on the evidence for efficacy, safety, and consistent response. Ther Adv Neurol Disord 9(5):414–423

103. Lionetto L, Casolla B, Mastropietri F, D'Alonzo L, Negro A, Simmaco M et al (2012) Pharmacokinetic evaluation of zolmitriptan for the treatment of migraines. Expert Opin Drug Metab Toxicol 8(8):1043–1050

104. Napoletano F, Lionetto L, Martelletti P (2014) Sumatriptan in clinical practice: effectiveness in migraine and the problem of psychiatric comorbidity. Expert Opin Pharmacother 15(3):303–305

105. Cameron C, Kelly S, Hsieh SC, Murphy M, Chen L, Kotb A et al (2015) Triptans in the acute treatment of migraine: a systematic review and network meta-analysis. Headache 55(Suppl 4):221–235

106. Napier C, Stewart M, Melrose H, Hopkins B, McHarg A, Wallis R (1999) Characterisation of the 5-HT receptor binding profile of eletriptan and kinetics of [3H]eletriptan binding at human 5-HT1B and 5-HT1D receptors. Eur J Pharmacol 368(2–3):259–268

107. Knyihar-Csillik E, Tajti J, Csillik AE, Chadaide Z, Mihaly A, Vecsei L (2000) Effects of eletriptan on the peptidergic innervation of the cerebral dura mater and trigeminal ganglion, and on the expression of c-fos and c-jun in the trigeminal complex of the rat in an experimental migraine model. Eur J Neurosci 12(11):3991–4002

108. Johnson DE, Rollema H, Schmidt AW, McHarg AD (2001) Serotonergic effects and extracellular brain levels of eletriptan, zolmitriptan and sumatriptan in rat brain. Eur J Pharmacol 425(3):203–210

109. Patrono C, Patrignani P, Garcia Rodriguez LA (2001) Cyclooxygenase-selective inhibition of prostanoid formation: transducing biochemical selectivity into clinical read-outs. J Clin Invest 108(1):7–13

110. Patrono C, Baigent C (2009) Low-dose aspirin, coxibs, and other NSAIDS: a clinical mosaic emerges. Mol Interv 9(1):31–39

111. Goadsby PJ, Lipton RB, Ferrari MD (2002) Migraine–current understanding and treatment. N Engl J Med 346(4):257–270

112. Burstein R, Cutrer MF, Yarnitsky D (2000) The development of cutaneous allodynia during a migraine attack clinical evidence for the sequential recruitment of spinal and supraspinal nociceptive neurons in migraine. Brain 123(Pt 8):1703–1709

113. Burstein R (2001) Deconstructing migraine headache into peripheral and central sensitization. Pain 89(2–3):107–110

114. Loo CY, Tan HJ, Teh HS, Raymond AA (2007) Randomised, open label, controlled trial of celecoxib in the treatment of acute migraine. Singapore Med J 48(9):834–839

115. Krymchantowski AV, Bigal ME (2004) Rizatriptan versus rizatriptan plus rofecoxib versus rizatriptan plus tolfenamic acid in the acute treatment of migraine. BMC Neurol 4:10

116. Krymchantowski AV, Barbosa JS (2002) Rizatriptan combined with rofecoxib vs. rizatriptan for the acute treatment of migraine: an open label pilot study. Cephalalgia 22(4):309–312

9

Volume gain of periaqueductal gray in medication-overuse headache

Zhiye Chen[1,2], Xiaoyan Chen[2], Mengqi Liu[1], Shuangfeng Liu[1], Lin Ma[1*] and Shengyuan Yu[2*]

Abstract

Background: Periaqueductal gray (PAG) is a substantial descending pain modulatory center, and previous voxel-based morphometry study confirmed the clusters with increased volume in PAG region in medication-overuse headache (MOH). The aim of this study is to investigate altered PAG volume in MOH using an automated PAG segment method to measure the true PAG volume.

Methods: High resolution three-dimensional T1-weighted fast spoiled gradient recalled echo MR images were obtained from 22 patients with MOH and 22 normal controls (NC). PAG template was created based on ICBM 152 gray template, and the individual PAG was generated by applying the deformation field from structural image segment to the PAG template, and individual PAG volume was calculated.

Results: There was a significant increased volume of PAG in MOH (0.366 ± 0.005 ml) than that in NC (0.341 ± 0.005 ml)($P < 0.05$). There was no significant correlation between the PAG volume and the clinical variables in MOH patients ($P > 0.05$). The area of receiver operating characteristic (ROC) curve was 0.845, and the cut-off of PAG volume was 0.341 ml with sensitivity 95.5% and specificity 63.6%.

Conclusion: The present study demonstrated that the PAG volume gain was confirmed in MOH patients, and the automated individual PAG volume measure may be considered as a simple and effective imaging biomarker in MOH diagnosis.

Keywords: Medication-overuse headache, Migraine, Periaqueductal gray, Magnetic resonance imaging

Background

Periaqueductal gray (PAG) was an anatomic and functional interface between forebrain and brainstem, and PAG was classified into 4 columns with different cytoarchitecture and included multiple types of neurons (eg. L-glutamate, γ-aminobutyric acid (GABA), opioids (particularly enkephalin), substance P) [1]. The PAG columns had distinct connections with the forebrain, brainstem, and nociceptive neurons of lamina I of the spinal cord and trigeminal nucleus [2–4]. PAG is a critical component of a network that is activated in response to pain, and the different PAG columns receive functionally segregated input from nociceptive pathways [5–7]. Previous studies demonstrated that PAG activation was modulated by expectation of pain [8] and placebo analgesia [9].

PAG is a substantial descending pain modulatory center, which exerts a dual control (including inhibition and facilitation) on nociceptive transmission in the dorsal horn and trigeminal nucleus [10], and the modulatory mechanism was exerted by descending PAG-RVM (rostral ventromedial medulla) pathway contributing to central sensitization and development of secondary hyperalgesia [10, 11]. PAG dysfunction was recognized in migraine [12], and functional MRI studies demonstrated that the PAG dysfunction was associated with increased iron deposition, which may play a role in the genesis or pathophysiology of MOH [13–15].

In the previous studies, the conventional MR imaging demonstrated that specific lesion such as multiple sclerosis and infarction in PAG may produced the migraine-like symptoms [16–21]. and nonspecific lesions without definite clinical diagnosis in PAG region [22]. Voxel-based morphometry (VBM) powerfully demonstrated that the clusters with PAG volume increase in MOH [23] and the clusters

* Correspondence: cjr.malin@vip.163.com; yusy1963@126.com
[1]Department of Radiology, Chinese PLA General Hospital, 28 Fuxing Road, Beijing 100853, China
[2]Department of Neurology, Chinese PLA General Hospital, 28 Fuxing Road, Beijing 100853, China

with PAG volume reducement in MOH with detoxification treatment response [24]. Therefore, PAG volume changes become an important imaging variable in MOH for the diagnosis and the treatment assessment.

VBM methods commonly could compare groups of individuals, and it also could be used to compare single case with control groups although a very high false positive rates presents [25] and non-parametric statistics could addressing the problem of high false positive rate in single case VBM [26]. As these methods were performed over the whole brain level, an automated individual PAG volume measurement was applied to MOH patients in the current study, and the expected cut-off value of PAG volume would be provided for the MOH diagnosis.

Methods

Subjects

Written informed consent was obtained from all participants according to the approval of the ethics committee of the local institutional review board. Twenty-two MOH patients were recruited from the International Headache Center, Department of Neurology, Chinese PLA General Hospital. All the following inclusion criteria should be fulfilled: 1) diagnosis of 8.2 MOH, and 1.1 and 1.2 migraine based on the International Classification of Headache Disorders, third Edition (beta version) (ICHD-III beta) [27]; 2) no migraine preventive medication used in the past 3 months; 3) age between 20 and 60 years; 4) right-handed; 5) patient's willingness to engage in the study. The exclusion criteria were the following: 1) with any chronic disorders, including hypertension, hypercholesterolemia, diabetes mellitus, cardiovascular diseases, cerebrovascular disorders, neoplastic diseases, infectious diseases, connective tissue diseases, other subtypes of headache, chronic pain other than headache, severe anxiety or depression preceding the onset of headache, psychiatric diseases, etc.; 2) with alcohol, nicotine, or other substance abuse; 3) with cranium trauma, illness interfering with central nervous system function, psychotic disorder, and regular use of a psychoactive or hormone medication. Twenty-two normal controls (NCs) were recruited from the hospital's staff and their relatives. Inclusion criteria were similar to those of patients, except for the first two items. NCs should never have had any primary headache disorders or other types of headache in the past year. General demographic and headache information were registered and evaluated in our headache database. Additionally, we evaluated anxiety, depression, and cognitive function of all the participants by using the Hamilton Anxiety Scale (HAMA) [28], the Hamilton Depression Scale (HAMD) [29], and the Montreal Cognitive Assessment (MoCA) Beijing Version (www.mocatest.org). The study protocol was approved by the Ethical Committee of Chinese PLA General Hospital and complied with the Declaration

of Helsinki. Informed consent was obtained from all participants before the study. MRI scans were taken in the interictal stage at least three days after a migraine attack for MOH patients. All the patients were given with the Visual Analogue Scale (VAS). All the subjects were right-handed and underwent conventional MRI examination to exclude the subjects with cerebral infarction, malacia, or occupying lesions. Alcohol, nicotine, caffeine, and other substances were avoided for at least 12 h before MRI examination.

MRI acquisition

Images were acquired on a GE 3.0 T MR system (DISCOVERY MR750, GE Healthcare, Milwaukee, WI, USA) and a conventional eight-channel quadrature head coil was used. All subjects were instructed to lie in a supine position, and formed padding was used to limit head movement. A three-dimensional T1-weighted fast spoiled gradient recalled echo (3D T1-FSPGR) sequence generating 180 contiguous axial slices [TR (repetition time) = 6.3 ms, TE (echo time) = 2.8 ms, flip angle = 15o, FOV (field of view) = 25.6 cm × 25.6 cm, Matrix = 256 × 256, NEX (number of acquisition) = 1] was used to perform the new segment and the individual PAG creation. Conventional T2-weighted imaging (T2WI) and T1 fluid-attenuated inversion recovery (T1-FLAIR) weighted imaging were also acquired. All imaging protocols were identical for all subjects. No obvious structural damage and T2-visible lesion were observed based on the conventional MR images.

MR image processing

All MR structural image data were processed using Statistical Parametric Mapping 12 (SPM 12) (http://www.fil.ion.ucl.ac.uk/spm/) running under MATLAB 7.6 (The Mathworks, Natick, MA, USA) to perform segment [30]. The image processing included following steps: (1) Create PAG template based on mni_icbm152_gm_tal_nlin_asym_09a template by pen tool using MRIcron software (www.mricro.com); (2) Individual PAG segment by apply the deformation field (generated by segment) to the PAG template using the runback strategy; (3) calculate the individual PAG volume using ITK-SNAP (V3.6.0-beta) (http://www.itksnap.org/pmwiki/pmwiki.php) (Fig. 1).

Statistical analysis

The statistical analysis was performed by using PASW Statistics 18.0. The significance differences of PAG volume between MOH group and NC group were computed using general linear model (independent univariate t-test with age and sex as covariates). The Pearson's correlation analysis was applied between PAG volume and the clinical variables in MOH. The age, HAMA, HAMD and MoCA

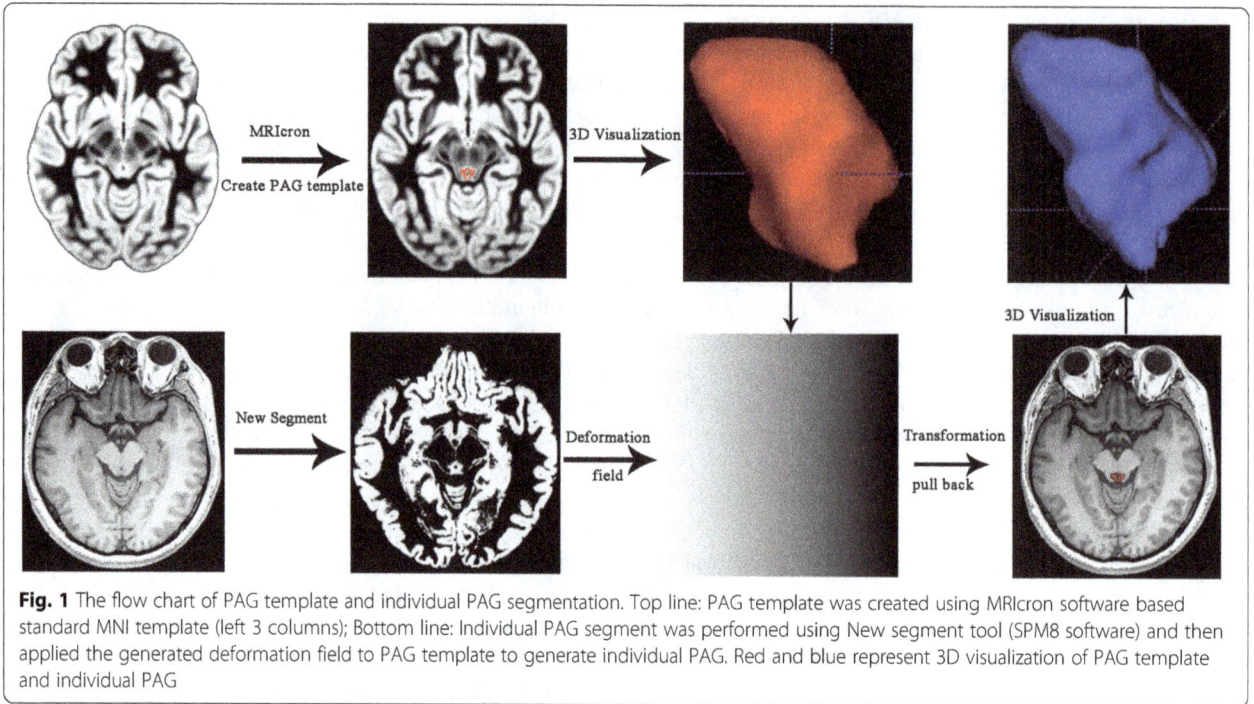

Fig. 1 The flow chart of PAG template and individual PAG segmentation. Top line: PAG template was created using MRIcron software based standard MNI template (left 3 columns); Bottom line: Individual PAG segment was performed using New segment tool (SPM8 software) and then applied the generated deformation field to PAG template to generate individual PAG. Red and blue represent 3D visualization of PAG template and individual PAG

were performed with independent samples T test, and sex was performed with Chi-Square test. Significant difference was set at a P value of < 0.05. Receiver operating characteristic (ROC) curve analysis was performed to identify the diagnostic efficacy and the cut-off value of PAG volume for MOH.

Results
Demography and neuropsychological test
Twenty-two MOH patient (F/M = 14/8) and 22 NCs (F/M = 14/4) were enrolled (Table 1). There was no significant difference for age and sex between MOH (42.55 ± 10.31 years old) and NC (45.09 ± 10.50 years old). There was significant difference for the scores of

HAMA, HAMD and MoCA in MOH compared with that in NC ($P < 0.05$). The disease duration was 6.65 ± 8.00 years, and the scores of VAS were 8.27 ± 1.52. The type of overused medication in MOH patients included:simple analgesics (3/22), simple triptans (1/22), and combination analgesics (18/22).

Comparison of PAG volume between MOH group and NC group
There was a significant increased volume of PAG in MOH (0.366 ± 0.005 ml) than that in NC (0.341 ± 0.005 ml)(F value = 14.41, P value = 0.000) (Fig. 2). There

Table 1 The clinical characteristics of MOH patients and normal controls(NC)

	MOH	NC	T value	P value
Num(F/M)	22(14/8)	22(19/3)	3.03[a]	0.16
Age(yrs)	42.55 ± 10.31	45.09 ± 10.50	0.81	0.42
HAMA	15.82 ± 6.81	9.77 ± 3.15	3.78	0.00
HAMD	17.91 ± 8.88	8.09 ± 4.80	4.54	0.00
MoCA	24.23 ± 3.21	27.50 ± 1.97	4.08	0.00
DD(yrs)	6.65 ± 8.00	NA	NA	NA
VAS	8.27 ± 1.52	NA	NA	NA

NA Not available, *DD* disease duration
[a]Chi-Square test

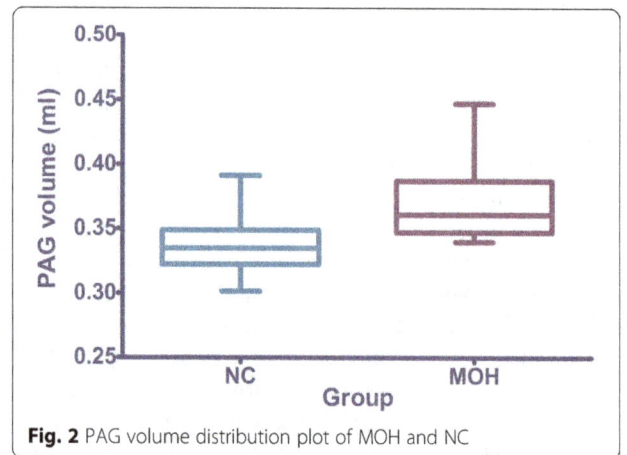

Fig. 2 PAG volume distribution plot of MOH and NC

was no significant correlation between the PAG volume and the clinical variables in MOH patients ($P > 0.05$).

ROC analysis between MOH group and NC group

The area of receiver operating characteristic (ROC) curve was 0.845, and the cut-off of PAG volume was 0.341 ml with sensitivity 95.5% and specificity 63.6% (Fig. 3).

Discussion

PAG dysfunction had been identified in MOH patients, and the investigation methods including resting-state functional MRI [31–33], diffusion kurtosis imaging [34], positron emission tomography [35], and iron deposition study [13]. The altered PAG function [33] may result in the change of PAG volume. The previous VBM study identified clusters in PAG region with volume increase [36], which was based on normalized grey matter. However, the current study provided the true individual PAG volume change firstly in vivo.

The present findings demonstrated the PAG volume gain in MOH compared with NC, which may explain the PAG dysfunction in MOH from the PAG structural pathophysiological change viewpoint. However, the correlation analysis showed that there was no any significant correlation between the PAG volume and the clinical variables in MOH patients. These findings suggested that PAG volume gain may only be associated with the descending pain modulatory network, and the other clinical factor such as anxiety, depress and cognitive function could not influence the PAG structural change in MOH although anxiety scores, depression scores showed significant difference between MOH and NC. The previous study [37] indicated that anxiety and

depression scores was correlated with gray matter volumes of some cerebral regions, therefore, it could assume that anxiety and depression might impair the cerebral regions, and PAG volume gain might be specific change in MOH patients.

Although PAG volume gain was identified in MOH in this study, Fig. 2 present a small overlap between MOH and NC for PAG volume. Further ROC analysis demonstrated PAG volume measurement showed a good level for the diagnosis of MOH from NC. The cut-off value of PAG volume (0.341 ml) could provide a high sensitivity (95.5%), however, the specificity (63.6%) was relative. Therefore, it should be careful to explain the diagnosis of MOH when PAG volume around the cut-off value.

Compared with VBM study, the current study employed an automated PAG volume measurement. VBM study was generally used to compare the difference between groups, and individual PAG volume could not be measured by this method. In this study, the individual PAG segment was generated by applying the deformation filed to the PAG template, which also be recognized as pull back strategy. This automated PAG measurement method could be performed in the routine clinical practice, and had a widespread application for MOH diagnosis, even for the treatment response assessment. However, it should be more prudent when PAG volume was considered as a biomarker for the diagnosis of MOH since MOH is likely to remain a clinical diagnosis.

The limits for this study included as follows: (1) The sample was relative small, and the large sample of MOH and NC should be needed in the future study; (2) The present study was a cross-sectional study, and the longitudinal observation and the treatment response evaluation should further be performed in future study.

Conclusion

In conclusion, PAG volume gain was identified in MOH patients, and PAG volume may be considered as an imaging biomarker for the diagnosis of MOH.

Abbreviations
MOH: Medication-overuse headache; NC: Normal controls; PAG: Periaqueductal gray.

Acknowledgments
This work was supported by the National Natural Sciences Foundation of China (81371514), Special Financial Grant from the China Postdoctoral Science Foundation (2014 T70960) and the Foundation for Medical and health Sci & Tech innovation Project of Sanya (2016YW37).

Authors' contributions
Category 1: (a) Conception and Design: L. M; SY. Y. (b) Acquisition of Data: ZY. C; MQ. L; SF. L; XY. C. (c) Analysis and Interpretation of Data: ZY. C. Category 2: (a) Drafting the Article: ZY. C. (b) Revising It for Intellectual Content: L. M; SY. Y. All authors read and approved the final manuscript.

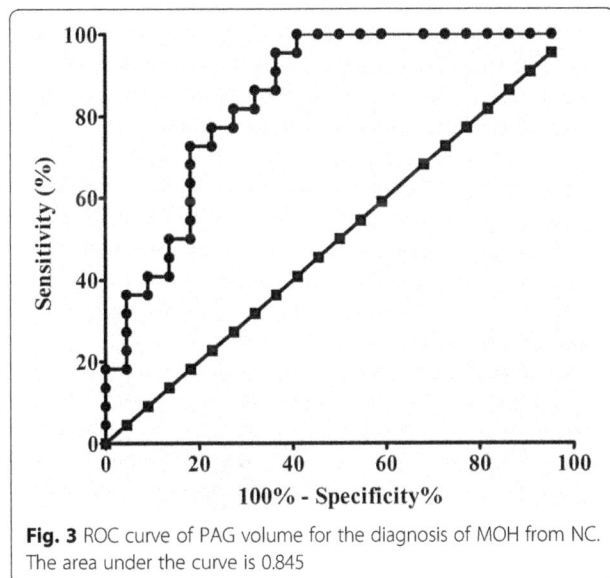

Fig. 3 ROC curve of PAG volume for the diagnosis of MOH from NC. The area under the curve is 0.845

Competing interests

The authors declare that they have no competing interests.

References

1. Benarroch EE (2012) Periaqueductal gray: an interface for behavioral control. Neurology 78:210–7

2. An X, Bandler R, Ongür D, Price JL (1998) Prefrontal cortical projections to longitudinal columns in the midbrain periaqueductal gray in Macaque monkeys. J Comp Neurol 401:455–79

3. Herbert H, Saper CB (1992) Organization of medullary adrenergic and noradrenergic projections to the periaqueductal gray matter in the rat. J Comp Neurol 315:34–52

4. Yezierski RP (1988) Spinomesencephalic tract: projections from the lumbosacral spinal cord of the rat, cat, and monkey. J Comp Neurol 267:131–46

5. Keay KA, Bandler R (2002) Distinct central representations of inescapable and escapable pain: observations and speculation. Exp Physiol 87:275–9

6. Parry DM, Macmillan FM, Koutsikou S, Mcmullan S, Lumb BM (2008) Separation of A- versus C-nociceptive inputs into spinal-brainstem circuits. Neuroscience 152:1076–85

7. Lumb BM (2004) Hypothalamic and midbrain circuitry that distinguishes between escapable and inescapable pain. News Physiol Sci 19:22–6

8. Fairhurst M, Wiech K, Dunckley P, Tracey I (2006) Anticipatory brainstem activity predicts neural processing of pain in humans. Eur J Pain 10:S83b–S

9. Wager TD, Scott DJ, Zubieta JK (2007) Placebo effects on human mu-opioid activity during pain. Proc Natl Acad Sci U S A 104:11056–61

10. Heinricher MM, Tavares I, Leith JL, Lumb BM (2009) Descending control of nociception: specificity, recruitment and plasticity. Brain Res Rev 60:214–25

11. Fields H (2004) State-dependent opioid control of pain. Nat Rev Neurosci 5:565–75

12. Raskin NH, Yoshio H, Sharon L (1987) Headache may arise from perturbation of brain. Headache 27:416–20

13. Welch KM, Nagesh V, Aurora SK, Gelman N (2001) Periaqueductal gray matter dysfunction in migraine: cause or the burden of illness? Headache 41:629–37

14. Kruit MC, Launer LJ, Overbosch J, van Buchem MA, Ferrari MD (2009) Iron accumulation in deep brain nuclei in migraine: a population-based magnetic resonance imaging study. Cephalalgia 29:351–9

15. Tepper SJ, Lowe MJ, Beall E, Phillips MD, Liu K, Stillman MJ et al (2012) Iron deposition in pain-regulatory nuclei in episodic migraine and chronic daily headache by MRI. Headache 52:236–43

16. Gee JR, Chang J, Dublin AB, Vijayan N (2005) The association of brainstem lesions with migraine-like headache: an imaging study of multiple sclerosis. Headache 45:670–7

17. Haas DC, Kent PF, Friedman DI (1993) Headache caused by a single lesion of multiple sclerosis in the periaqueductal gray area. Headache 33:452–5

18. Lin GY, Wang CW, Chiang TT, Peng GS, Yang FC (2013) Multiple sclerosis presenting initially with a worsening of migraine symptoms. J Headache Pain 14:70

19. Tortorella P, Rocca MA, Colombo B, Annovazzi P, Comi G, Filippi M (2006) Assessment of MRI abnormalities of the brainstem from patients with migraine and multiple sclerosis. J Neurol Sci 244:137–41

20. Fragoso YD, Brooks JB (2007) Two cases of lesions in brainstem in multiple sclerosis and refractory migraine. Headache 47:852–4

21. Wang Y, Wang XS (2013) Migraine-like headache from an infarction in the periaqueductal gray area of the midbrain. Pain Med 14:948–9

22. Chen Z, Chen X, Liu M, Liu S, Ma L, Yu S (2016) Nonspecific periaqueductal gray lesions on T2WI in episodic migraine. J Headache Pain 17:101

23. Riederer F, Marti M, Luechinger R, Lanzenberger R, von Meyenburg J, Gantenbein AR et al (2012) Grey matter changes associated with medication-overuse headache: correlations with disease related disability and anxiety. World J Biol Psychiatry 13:517–25

24. Riederer F, Gantenbein AR, Marti M, Luechinger R, Kollias S, Sandor PS (2013) Decrease of gray matter volume in the midbrain is associated with treatment response in medication-overuse headache: possible influence of orbitofrontal cortex. J Neurosci 33:15343–9

25. Scarpazza C, Sartori G, De Simone MS, Mechelli A (2013) When the single matters more than the group: very high false positive rates in single case Voxel Based Morphometry. Neuroimage 70:175–88

26. Scarpazza C, Nichols TE, Seramondi D, Maumet C, Sartori G, Mechelli A (2016) When the Single Matters more than the Group (II): Addressing the Problem of High False Positive Rates in Single Case Voxel Based Morphometry Using Non-parametric Statistics. Front Neurosci 10:6

27. Headache Classification Committee of the International Headache Society (IHS) (2013) The International Classification of Headache Disorders, 3rd edition (beta version). Cephalalgia 33:629–808

28. Maier W, Buller R, Philipp M, Heuser I (1988) The Hamilton Anxiety Scale: reliability, validity and sensitivity to change in anxiety and depressive disorders. J Affect Disord 14:61–8

29. Hamilton M (1967) Development of a rating scale for primary depressive illness. Br J Soc Clin Psychol 6:278–96

30. Ashburner J, Friston KJ (2000) Voxel-based morphometry–the methods. Neuroimage 11:805–21

31. Schwedt TJ, Larson-Prior L, Coalson RS, Nolan T, Mar S, Ances BM et al (2014) Allodynia and descending pain modulation in migraine: a resting state functional connectivity analysis. Pain Med 15:154–65

32. Schwedt TJ, Schlaggar BL, Mar S, Nolan T, Coalson RS, Nardos B et al (2013) Atypical resting-state functional connectivity of affective pain regions in chronic migraine. Headache 53:737–51

33. Mainero C, Boshyan J, Hadjikhani N (2011) Altered functional MRI resting-state connectivity in periaqueductal gray networks in migraine. Ann Neurol 70:838–45

34. Ito K, Kudo M, Sasaki M, Saito A, Yamashita F, Harada T et al (2016) Detection of changes in the periaqueductal gray matter of patients with episodic migraine using quantitative diffusion kurtosis imaging: preliminary findings. Neuroradiology 58:115–20

35. Maniyar FH, Sprenger T, Schankin C, Goadsby PJ (2014) The origin of nausea in migraine-a PET study. J Headache Pain 15:84

36. Rocca MA, Ceccarelli A, Falini A, Colombo B, Tortorella P, Bernasconi L et al (2006) Brain gray matter changes in migraine patients with T2-visible lesions: a 3-T MRI study. Stroke 37:1765–70

37. Chanraud S, Di Scala G, Dilharreguy B, Schoenen J, Allard M, Radat F (2014) Brain functional connectivity and morphology changes in medication-overuse headache: Clue for dependence-related processes? Cephalalgia 34:605–15

10

Randomized, double-blind, crossover study comparing DFN-11 injection (3 mg subcutaneous sumatriptan) with 6 mg subcutaneous sumatriptan for the treatment of rapidly-escalating attacks of episodic migraine

Roger K. Cady[1], Sagar Munjal[2], Ryan J. Cady[1*], Heather R. Manley[1] and Elimor Brand-Schieber[2]

Abstract

Background: A 6-mg dose of SC sumatriptan is the most efficacious and fast-acting acute treatment for migraine, but a 3-mg dose of SC sumatriptan may improve tolerability while maintaining efficacy.

Methods: This randomized, double-blind, crossover study compared the efficacy and tolerability of 3 mg subcutaneous (SC) sumatriptan (DFN-11) with 6 mg SC sumatriptan in 20 adults with rapidly-escalating migraine attacks. Eligible subjects were randomized (1:1) to treat 1 attack with DFN-11 and matching placebo autoinjector consecutively or 2 DFN-11 autoinjectors consecutively and a second attack similarly but with the alternative dose (3 mg or 6 mg).

Results: The proportions of subjects who were pain-free at 60 min postdose, the primary endpoint, were similar following treatment with 3 mg SC sumatriptan and 6 mg SC sumatriptan (50% vs 52.6%, $P = .87$). The proportions of subjects experiencing pain relief ($P \geq .48$); reductions in migraine pain intensity ($P \geq .78$); and relief from nausea, photophobia, or phonophobia ($P \geq .88$) with 3 mg SC sumatriptan and 6 mg SC sumatriptan were similar, as were the mean scores for satisfaction with treatment ($M = 2.6$ vs $M = 2.4$, $P = .81$) and the mean number of rescue medications used ($M = .11$ vs $M = .26$, $P = .32$). The most common adverse events with the 3- and 6-mg doses were triptan sensations — paresthesia, neck pain, flushing, and involuntary muscle contractions of the neck — and the incidence of adverse events with both doses was similar (32 events total: 3 mg, $n = 14$ [44%]; 6 mg, $n = 18$ [56%], $P = .60$). Triptan sensations affected 4 subjects with the 6-mg dose only, 1 subject with the 3-mg dose only, and 7 subjects with both sumatriptan doses. Chest pain affected 2 subjects (10%) treated with the 6-mg dose and no subjects (0%) treated with the 3-mg dose of DFN-11. There were no serious adverse events.

Conclusions: The 3-mg SC dose of sumatriptan in DFN-11 provided relief of migraine pain and associated symptoms comparable to a 6-mg SC dose of sumatriptan. Tolerability was similar with both study medications; DFN-11 treatment was associated with fewer triptan sensations than the 6-mg dose. DFN-11, with its 3-mg dose of sumatriptan, may be a clinically useful alternative to higher-dose autoinjectors.

Keywords: Episodic, Migraine, Rapidly-escalating, Treatment, Sumatriptan, Subcutaneous

* Correspondence: ryancady@clinvest.com
[1]Clinvest/A Division of Banyan Inc., 3805 S Kansas Expy, Springfield, MO 65807, USA
Full list of author information is available at the end of the article

Background

Migraine is a chronic neurologic disease characterized by recurrent episodes of headache associated with a wide array of disruptive symptoms, including photophobia, phonophobia, nausea, and/or vomiting [1, 2]. It is the most common neurological disease for which people seek medical consultation, affecting about 12% of adults in the United States, three quarters of them women [3–5]. Nearly all migraineurs (93%) have some degree of attack-related impairment, and more than half (54%) are severely impaired by their attacks [3]; among women, migraine ranks in the top 10 causes of disability worldwide [6]. Because migraine is heterogeneous and often spans decades of patients' lives, clinical presentations and acute treatment needs can vary considerably over time, and patients often require different formulations of acute medications to optimize treatment outcomes [7]. This is particularly true when attacks are severe, accompanied by nausea and vomiting, or rapid in onset, and parenteral formulations are needed to control symptoms.

Sumatriptan — the first, most widely studied, and most frequently prescribed member of the "triptan" class of medications [2, 8, 9] — is available as a subcutaneous (SC) injection, intranasal spray, oral tablet, and, in some countries, a rectal suppository. The 6 mg SC injection has long been considered optimal for acute therapy of migraine [2]; in large double-blind, randomized, placebo-controlled clinical trials, 70% of subjects with moderate to severe attacks experienced pain relief within 1 h of dosing, and 50% were pain-free [10, 11]. The rapid onset of action of SC sumatriptan is especially important for patients whose attacks become disabling soon after onset [12].

Despite its well-established efficacy and rapid onset of action, sumatriptan 6 mg SC injection has a suboptimal tolerability profile. Many patients (42%) experience triptan sensations [13], such as paresthesia and chest symptoms, that appear to be dose-related [14]. Concerns about drug-related adverse events (AEs), which have caused two thirds of migraine patients to delay or avoid taking a prescription medication, may help to explain why fewer than 10% of eligible migraine patients use the SC formulation of sumatriptan to treat their disease [15]. These concerns can be particularly important in patients with various types of medical conditions (eg, cardiovascular and cerebrovascular disease and some psychiatric illnesses) and/or treated with various medications (eg, monoamine oxidase inhibitors and selective serotonin reuptake inhibitors) [9]. Based on previous research [16], we hypothesized that a formulation using a lower doses of sumatriptan may improve safety and tolerability while maintaining efficacy similar to 6 mg SC sumatriptan, and that a 3-mg dose may be sufficient in many patients. The objective of this exploratory study was to compare the efficacy and tolerability of 3 mg SC sumatriptan (using DFN-11 and matching placebo autoinjectors consecutively) with 6 mg SC sumatriptan (using 2 DFN-11 autoinjectors consecutively) for the acute treatment of episodic migraine attacks.

Methods

This was a double-blind, crossover, pilot study conducted at a single study center (Clinvest; Springfield, MO). The study compared a 3-mg SC dose of sumatriptan with the commonly prescribed 6-mg SC dose in 19 subjects. The protocol was approved by the Sterling Institutional Review Board, and the study was conducted in compliance with good clinical practice and in accordance with the ethical principles set forth in the Declaration of Helsinki. Prior to the initiation of any study-specific procedures, investigators explained the nature of the study to the subjects, and subjects provided informed consent. The first subject was enrolled on 15 September 2015, and the study was completed on 14 April 2016. Additional information about this trial is available online at ClinicalTrials.gov (Identifier: NCT02571049).

Study conduct

To participate, subjects recruited from the clinic and general population had to satisfy a range of inclusion and exclusion criteria (Table 1). The research coordinator and investigator initially evaluated eligibility and obtained informed consent. Final eligibility was determined by the investigator, and the research coordinator completed the enrollment process.

The study consisted of 4 visits: screening, randomization, treatment crossover, and end-of-study. Subjects treated up to 2 attacks within 4 weeks. At the screening visit, subjects provided a detailed medical and headache/migraine history, a physical examination was performed, laboratory assessment samples (ie, hematology, serum chemistry, urine analysis, serology, urine drug screen) were obtained, inclusion/exclusion criteria were verified, and a 12-lead electrocardiogram (ECG) was completed. Eligible subjects returned to the site with 14 days of the screening visit and were trained in the appropriate use of the autoinjector device and given printed instructions to take home that reinforced correct DFN-11 administration.

Subjects were divided into 1 block and randomized (1:1) to receive 3 mg SC sumatriptan (using DFN-11 and matching placebo autoinjectors consecutively) or 6 mg SC sumatriptan (using 2 DFN-11 autoinjectors consecutively) in a crossover design and were dispensed the first treatment in the sequence. The randomization scheme was generated by study personnel with no subject interaction or other monitoring roles using an online tool (http://www.randomization.com); it was provided to the drug packing company, which used it to prepare and pre-label the kits with sequential numbers. The

Table 1 Inclusion and exclusion criteria

Inclusion	Exclusion
ICHD-3-beta episodic migraine[a]	Unable to distinguish migraine from other primary headache conditions
Onset of migraine before age 50	15 or more headache days per month
≥ 3-month history of 2–8 attacks/month; ≥ 75% of attacks progress to moderate or severe pain and/or nausea within 2 h (ie, rapidly-escalating)	Opioid usage > 10 days in the 30 days before screening
Acute headache medication on ≤ 14 days/month in the 3 months prior to enrollment	Use of MAO-A inhibitors within 28 days of randomization
No sumatriptan injections for ≥ 3 months	History of hemiplegic/basilar migraine; epileptogenic conditions; symptoms or signs of ischemic cardiac, cerebrovascular or peripheral vascular syndromes, or uncontrolled hypertension
If taking migraine prophylaxis, stable for 30 days before and throughout the study	Drug or alcohol abuse within the previous 2 years
Females: negative urine pregnancy test at screening, effective birth control, or surgically sterile or postmenopausal for ≥ 1 year before enrollment	Systemic disease or neurological or psychiatric condition[b]
Willing to read and comprehend written instructions and internet access for electronic diary	Investigational medication ≤ 30 days before randomization
Sign informed consent document	Positive urine drug screen for recreational drugs, marijuana, or prescription drugs not explained by stated concomitant medications
	Clinical laboratory or ECG abnormality
	Fridericia's corrected QT interval > 450 msec
	Creatinine > 2 mg/dl; serum total bilirubin > 2.0 mg/dL
	Serum AST, ALT, or alkaline phosphatase > 2.5 times ULN
	Rebound headache from caffeine usage[b]

ICHD International Classification of Headache Disorders, *MAO-A* monoamine oxidase A, *ECG* electrocardiogram, *AST* aspartate aminotransferase, *ALT*, *ULN* upper limit of normal
[a]With or without aura
[b]Contraindicated participation in the opinion of the investigator

research coordinator was instructed to dispense the lowest kit number available.

Diary instruction was provided, and subjects were encouraged to treat an attack within 1 h of onset of headache. They were asked not to use rescue medication until at least 120 min postdose. After subjects treated the first attack, they returned to the clinic for re-evaluation and treatment crossover. Before treating a second attack, subjects had to be pain-free for a minimum of 24 h. The end-of-study visit occurred within 7 days after treatment of the second attack or within 4 weeks of randomization, whichever came first. At the end-of-study visit, the subject's diary information was reviewed, and all end-of-study visit procedures were performed.

Adverse events were monitored from the time subjects gave informed consent until the follow-up visit; physical examinations, vital sign measurements, ECGs, and laboratory assessments were performed at designated visits throughout the study period.

Assessments
Efficacy
The prospectively defined primary efficacy endpoint was the proportion of subjects reporting freedom from pain at 60 min postdose; pain freedom was defined as a headache pain severity rating of 0 (no pain). Secondary endpoints included pain relief, pain freedom, and headache severity at 30, 60, 90, and 120 min postdose, proportion of subjects with relief of associated migraine symptoms (ie, nausea, photophobia, and phonophobia) at 60 min postdose, subject satisfaction with treatment, and use of rescue medication from 2 to 24 h postdose. Pain relief was defined as a 1-point reduction in headache pain intensity, which was rated on a 4-point Likert scale where 0 = no pain, 1 = mild pain, 2 = moderate pain, and 3 = severe pain. Relief of the associated symptoms of nausea, photophobia, and phonophobia was defined as a 1-point reduction in symptom severity where 0 = no symptom, 1 = mild, 2 = moderate, and 3 = severe. Subject satisfaction with treatment was based on a 7-point Likert Scale, with 1 being very satisfied and 7 being very dissatisfied. Use of rescue medication was calculated by totaling the number of rescue medications used from 2 to 24 h postdose.

The primary and most of the secondary endpoint data were derived from an online headache e-diary. Daily diary assessments included onset and duration of headache, severity of pain at the time of onset and at treatment, acute headache pain medication(s) usage, study drug usage, associated symptoms, unusual symptoms, and subject satisfaction with treatment.

Tolerability

Tolerability was assessed by comparing AEs occurring up to 24 h postdose. Safety measures included AEs, physical examinations, vital signs, ECG readings, and laboratory assessments (hematology, serum chemistry, urine analysis). Adverse events were coded with the Medical Dictionary for Regulatory Activities (MedDRA, version 17.0) and classified by date of onset, duration, frequency, severity, and relationship to study medication. The classification of AEs as triptan sensations was determined by principal investigator. Spontaneously reported AEs were recorded for up to 5 days after the last dose of study drug; AEs determined as serious were recorded for up to 30 days.

Statistical analysis

All statistical tests were 2-tailed, and an alpha of .05 was used to determine statistical significance. Descriptive statistics established baseline characteristics and AE frequency. Data for the primary endpoint was analyzed via chi-squared analyses; the secondary outcome measures were analyzed with a 2-tailed Repeated Measures analysis of variance (ANOVA), chi-squared, and/or independent or dependent t-tests, as appropriate. All ANOVAs were followed by univariate post hoc tests, as appropriate, and multiple comparison adjustments were made as needed. A last observation carried forward method was used to impute missing values within a single headache diary attack.

Efficacy analyses were performed on a modified intent-to-treat population, which included all randomized subjects who received at least 1 dose of study drug and obtained at least 1 endpoint measurement (mean change from baseline in the number of hours with headaches) after treatment. The safety population included all randomized subjects.

Results

Twenty-four subjects were screened, 20 subjects were randomized (1 never treated), and 19 subjects treated at least 1 migraine attack (Fig. 1). The study population was 80% female and 95% Caucasian, with a mean age of 39.8 years. At baseline, subjects were experiencing 5 migraine days and 6.8 headache days per month on average (Table 2).

The proportion of subjects who were pain-free at 60 min postdose, the primary efficacy endpoint, was 50.0% for 3 mg SC sumatriptan and 52.6% for 6 mg SC sumatriptan ($P = .87$), as shown in Fig. 2. Pain-free responses to 3 mg SC sumatriptan and 6 mg SC were already apparent at 30 min (22.2% vs 15.8%, respectively; $P = .62$). At 90 min, 66.7% vs 68.4% of subjects were pain-free ($P = .91$), and these responses

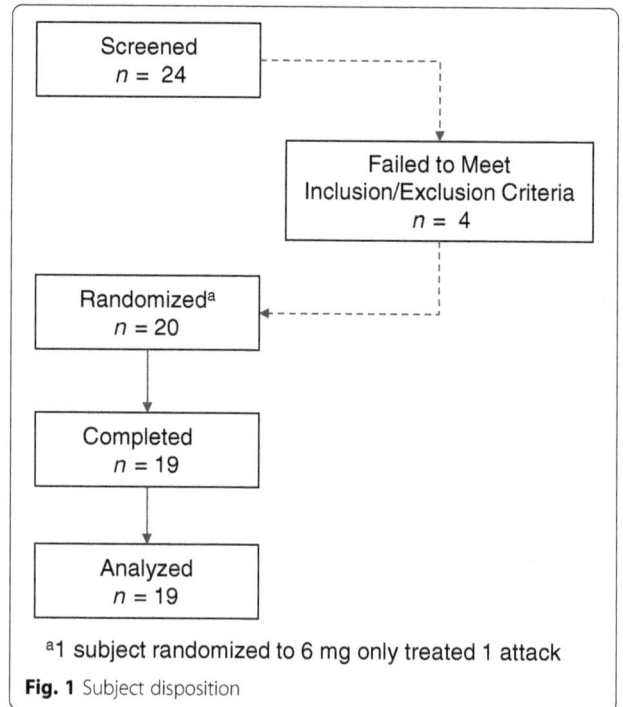

Fig. 1 Subject disposition

Screened
$n = 24$

Failed to Meet Inclusion/Exclusion Criteria
$n = 4$

Randomized[a]
$n = 20$

Completed
$n = 19$

Analyzed
$n = 19$

[a]1 subject randomized to 6 mg only treated 1 attack

were sustained to 120 min postdose (66.7% vs 68.4%; $P = .91$).

Eighty-three percent of subjects experienced pain relief with 3 mg SC sumatriptan at 60, 90, and 120 min postdose; the corresponding pain relief rates with the 6-mg dose, 73.7% ($P = .48$), 79.0% ($P = .73$), and 89.5% ($P = .59$), were not significantly different at any timepoint (Fig. 3). With a mean (SD) predose pain intensity of 2.1 (.6), reductions in migraine pain intensity after treatment with 3 and 6 mg SC sumatriptan were comparable at all time points ($P = .78$) over the 2-h assessment period (Fig. 4).

At 60 min postdose (Fig. 5), there were no significant differences between 3 and 6 mg SC sumatriptan in the proportions of subjects who experienced relief from nausea ($P = .91$), photophobia ($P = .89$), or phonophobia ($P = .88$). The mean number of rescue medication doses used over the course of the study period was not significantly different when subjects treated with 3 mg or 6 mg SC sumatriptan ($M = .11$ vs $M = .26$). Subjects were similarly satisfied with either treatment, with no significant difference in mean scores for 3 and 6 mg SC sumatriptan ($M = 2.6$ vs $M = 2.4$).

Tolerability

In the safety population ($N = 20$), 80% of subjects (16/20) experienced a total of 50 AEs. The overall incidence of AEs with DFN-11 (.72) and 6 mg SC sumatriptan (.74) was comparable ($P = .97$), and the most common AEs were triptan sensations: paresthesia (30%, 6/20), neck pain

Table 2 Baseline demographics

Variable	Value
Gender n (%)	
Male	4 (20)
Female	16 (80)
Age (years)[a]	39.8 (10.4)
Range	19–61
Race n (%)	
Caucasian	19 (95)
Hispanic	1 (5)
Headache Characteristics[a]	
Migraine Days/Month	5.0 (3.7)
Headache Days/Month	6.8 (1.7)

[a]Values are mean (SD)

(20%, 4/20), flushing (10%, 2/20), chest pain (10%, 2/20), involuntary muscle contractions of the neck (10%, 2/20), and vomiting (10%, 2/20). As shown in Table 3, there were no significant differences in the frequency (14 vs 18 events, $P = .60$), duration (27 vs 64 min, $P = .43$), and severity (1.29 vs 1.28 [0–3 scale], $P = .97$) of triptan sensations with DFN-11 and 6 mg SC sumatriptan. Of the 12 subjects who reported triptan sensation AEs, 7 subjects experienced them with DFN-11 and 6 mg SC sumatriptan, 1 subject experienced them only after DFN-11, and 4 subjects experienced them only following 6 mg SC sumatriptan. There were no meaningful changes from baseline in vital signs, ECGs, or laboratory assessments, and no serious AEs were reported.

Discussion

Migraineurs consistently rate rapid onset of pain relief and tolerability of treatment among the most important attributes of acute migraine medication [17, 18]. With an onset of action of approximately 10 min and unparalleled relief of migraine headache and associated symptoms [14], SC sumatriptan has been the most effective acute migraine therapy since its introduction nearly 25 years ago [2]. The primary limitations to its use as an acute therapy are medication-related AEs. Understanding the tolerability of treatment is important as to why migraine patients settle for less effective alternatives [16]. For many, the relatively high likelihood of experiencing triptan sensations is a barrier to effective parenteral migraine-specific therapy. Paradoxically, the characteristics believed to be responsible for the high rate of efficacy seen with the injectable forms — faster bioavailability and greater systemic exposure compared with oral formulations — may also contribute to the relatively high rate of triptan sensations. It has been suggested that novel sumatriptan formulations with pharmacokinetics similar to SC sumatriptan are promising for use in clinical practice [2].

In this study of subjects with rapidly-escalating attacks of episodic migraine, treatment with DFN-11, a 3 mg SC sumatriptan autoinjector, was comparable to SC sumatriptan 6 mg on all clinically relevant efficacy endpoints. The pain-free results at 60 min postdose suggest that DFN-11 may be a fast-acting alternative to commercial formulations of injectable sumatriptan, especially for patients who awaken with full-blown attacks already in progress [19]. In our study, the lower, 3-mg dose of sumatriptan in DFN-11 did not appear to impede the overall therapeutic effect, and DFN-11 maintained an efficacy timecourse similar to SC sumatriptan 6 mg — a finding in accord with a previous report comparing 3 and 6 mg SC sumatriptan [20].

The most common AEs were triptan sensations known to be associated with SC triptan usage; all were mild to

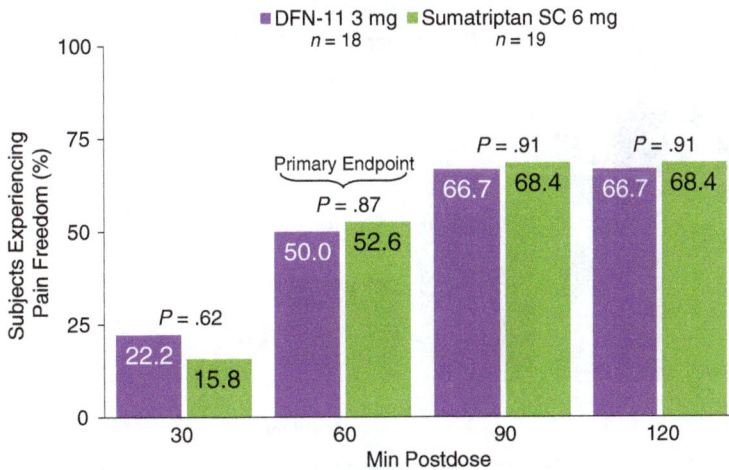

Fig. 2 Pain freedom at 30, 60, 90, and 120 min postdose[a,b]. Legend: SC, subcutaneous. [a]Mean (SD) predose pain intensity average was 2.00 (.58). [b]1 subject randomized to 6 mg only treated 1 attack

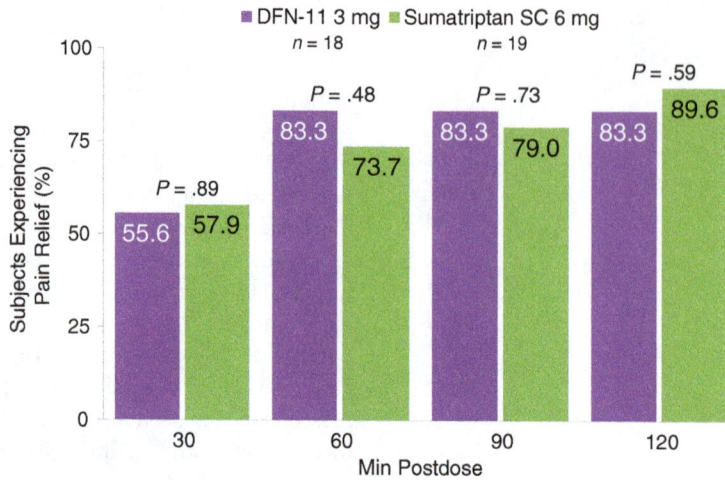

Fig. 3 Pain relief at 30, 60, 90, and 120 min postdose[a]. Legend: SC, subcutaneous. [a]1 subject randomized to 6 mg only treated 1 attack

moderate and similar in frequency and severity to those seen in previous studies of the SC formulation of sumatriptan. Notably, while most subjects experienced symptoms with both sumatriptan doses, fewer subjects had triptan sensations only after treatment with the 3-mg dose than with the 6-mg dose. In addition, the triptan sensation of chest pain, which has been shown to cause up to 10% of sumatriptan-treated patients to discontinue therapy [21] and may lead to substantially increased medical costs for migraine care [22], was not observed after the 3-mg dose of DFN-11 treatment. With the 6 mg SC sumatriptan treatment, 10% of subjects were affected, and the mean duration of the events exceeded 6 h. The implications of these findings deserve to be explored in future research.

While the results with DFN-11 are similar in many aspects to those seen in previous dose-comparing studies of SC sumatriptan, there may be clinically important differences. For example, an open-label trial comparing the 3 and 6 mg SC doses (in which 80% of subjects preferred the 3-mg dose) found, as in the current study, that the proportions of subjects with pain-free responses were similar between the 2 doses at 1 and 2 h after treatment [20]. However, the 1-h pain relief rate for the 3-mg SC dose in this study exceeded previous reports for the 6-mg SC dose at that timepoint (83% vs 70%) [14]. The higher treatment response may reflect the benefits of treating at the first sign of migraine pain, as subjects in the earlier studies [14, 20] waited for pain to reach moderate intensity. AEs were overall slightly more

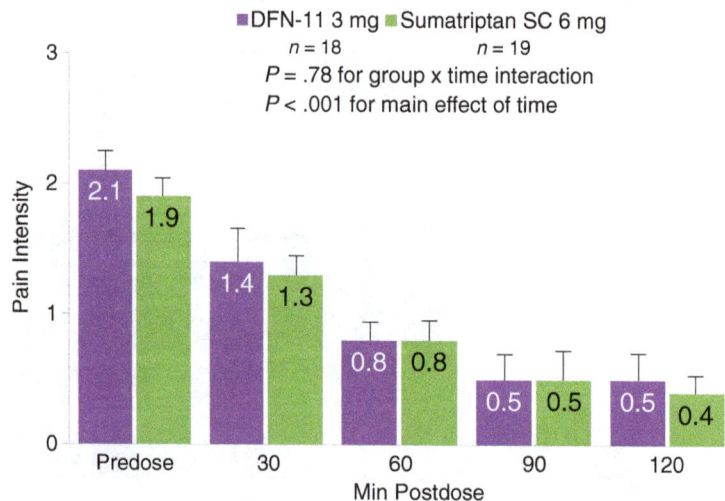

Fig. 4 Pain intensity at predose, 30, 60, 90, and 120 min postdose[a,b,c]. Legend: SC, subcutaneous. [a]1 subject randomized to 6 mg only treated 1 attack. [b]Repeated Measures ANOVA revealed an insignificant group and time interaction: $F_{(2.43, 85.02)} = .61$, $P = .78$. [c]A significant main effect of time was found for pain intensity scores: $F_{(2.43, 85.02)} = .61$, $P < .001$

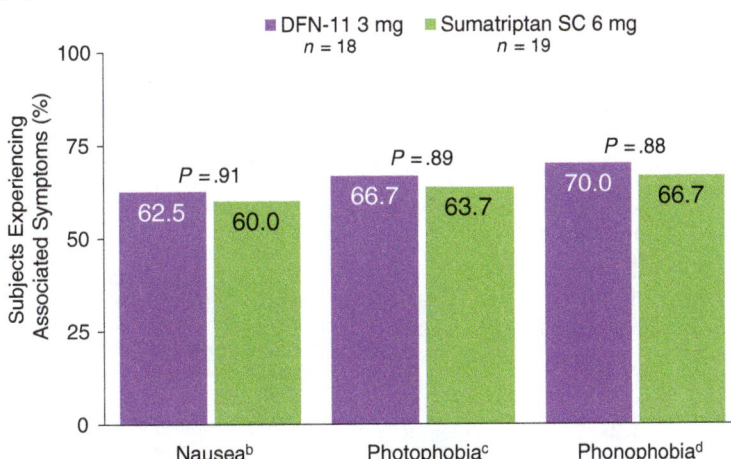

Fig. 5 Proportions of subjects experiencing relief from symptoms associated with migraine at 60 min postdose.[a] Legend: SC, subcutaneous. [a]1 subject randomized to 6 mg only treated 1 attack. [b]3 mg n = 8; 6 mg n = 10. [c]3 mg n = 9; 6 mg n = 11. [d]3 mg n = 10; 6 mg n = 9

frequent with the 6-mg dose than with the 3-mg dose [14, 20].

The current study has strengths and limitations. Its main strength is its originality; this is the first well-controlled study to compare the efficacy and tolerability of 3- and 6-mg SC doses of sumatriptan. Another strength is that because subjects in this study treated at the first sign of migraine, which can prevent the development of central sensitization [23] and optimize pain-free efficacy [24–26], the performance of DFN-

11 was assessed under conditions that simulate actual treatment scenarios. Limitations of the study include the lack of power and sample size calculation, as well as the small sample size, which restrict the validity and generalizability of results. It is also possible that outcomes might have been affected by subjects' using 2 consecutive injections to provide a 6-mg dose of sumatriptan, but there is no evidence that this method of administering study medication influences response to sumatriptan.

Table 3 Triptan sensations after treatment with 3 and 6 mg SC sumatriptan

	3 mg SC sumatriptan			6 mg SC sumatriptan		
	Event frequency n (%)	Duration[a] Min	Severity[a,b] (1–3)	Event frequency n (%)	Duration[a] Min	Severity[a,b] (1–3)
Paresthesia	5 (15.63)	13.0 (.01)	1.20 (.45)	4 (12.50)	20.0 (.01)	1.0 (0.0)
Neck Pain	4 (12.50)	12.0 (.01)	1.25 (.50)	3 (9.38)	11.0 (.00)	1.0 (0.0)
Flushing	2 (6.25)	25.0 (.01)	1.50 (.71)	2 (6.25)	11.0 (.01)	1.50 (.71)
Muscle Contractions (Neck)[c]	1 (3.13)	44 (N/A)	1.0 (N/A)	2 (6.25)	47 (N/A)	1.50 (.71)
Chest Pain	0 (0)	—	—	2 (6.25)	374 (.35)	2.0 (1.41)
Disorientation	0 (0)	—	—	1 (3.13)	19 (N/A)	1.0 (N/A)
Dizziness	0 (0)	—	—	1 (3.13)	20 (N/A)	1.0 (N/A)
Myalgia	0 (0)	—	—	1 (3.13)	44 (N/A)	1.0 (N/A)
Tinnitus	0 (0)	—	—	1 (3.13)	41 (N/A)	1.0 (N/A)
Vomiting	0 (0)	—	—	1 (3.13)	41 (N/A)	1.0 (N/A)
Hyperhidrosis	1 (3.13)	38 (N/A)	1.0 (N/A)	0 (0)	—	—
Malaise	1 (3.13)	130 (N/A)	2.0 (N/A)	0 (0)	—	—
Total	14 (44)[d]	27 (33.12)[e]	1.29 (.47)[f]	18 (56)	64 (167.10)	1.28 (.57)

SC subcutaneous
[a]Mean (SD)
[b]Assessed on a 3-point Likert scale: mild = 1, moderate = 2, and severe = 3
[c]Involuntary
[d]P = .60 vs 6 mg
[e]P = .43 vs 6 mg
[f]P = .97 vs 6 mg

Conclusions

In this randomized, double-blind, crossover pilot study comparing 3 mg SC sumatriptan with 6 mg SC sumatriptan for acute treatment of rapidly-escalating attacks of episodic migraine, both the 3- and 6-mg doses demonstrated comparable efficacy on all efficacy endpoints. The 3-mg and 6-mg SC doses were also similar on safety parameters, but DFN-11 was associated with better tolerability, as shown by a lower incidence of triptan sensation AEs. Of particular interest was the lack of chest pain as an AE with DFN-11. These preliminary results need to be confirmed in larger clinical studies.

Abbreviations

AE: Adverse event; ALT: Alanine aminotransferase; ANOVA: Analysis of variance; AST: Aspartate aminotransferase; ECG: Electrocardiogram; ICHD: International Classification of Headache Disorders; MAO-A: Monoamine oxidase A; SC: Subcutaneous; SD: Standard deviation; ULN: Upper limit of normal

Acknowledgements

The authors wish to thank Carmela Fritz for assistance with the conduct of the study. Medical writing services were provided by Christopher Caiazza. DRL Publication #789.

Funding

This study was sponsored by Dr. Reddy's Laboratories Ltd., which developed DFN-11; its US subsidiary, Promius Pharma, markets DFN-11 as Zembrace™SymTouch™.

Authors' contributions

RKC and SM conceived and designed the study. RJC and HM performed the experiments, and SM, RJC, HM, and EBS analyzed the data and wrote the paper. All authors revised and approved the final manuscript.

Competing interests

This study was supported and funded by Dr. Reddy's Laboratories Ltd, manufacturer of DFN-11. SM is employed by and owns stock in Dr. Reddy's Laboratories Ltd, EBS is an employee of Dr. Reddy's Laboratories Ltd, and RKC, RC, and HM were paid consultants.

Author details

[1]Clinvest/A Division of Banyan Inc., 3805 S Kansas Expy, Springfield, MO 65807, USA. [2]Dr. Reddy's Laboratories Ltd., 107 College Road East, Princeton, NJ 08540, USA.

References

1. Headache Classification Committee of the International Headache Society (IHS) (2013) The International Classification of Headache Disorders, 3rd edition (beta version). Cephalalgia 33:629–808
2. Lionetto L, Negro A, Casolla B et al (2012) Sumatriptan succinate: pharmacokinetics of different formulations in clinical practice. Expert Opin Pharmacother 13:2369–2380
3. Lipton RB, Bigal ME, Diamond M et al (2007) Migraine prevalence, disease burden, and the need for preventive therapy. Neurology 68:343–349
4. Stewart WF, Lipton RB, Celentano DD et al (1992) Prevalence of migraine headache in the United States. Relation to age, income, race, and other sociodemographic factors. JAMA 267:64–69
5. Lipton RB, Stewart WF, Diamond S et al (2001) Prevalence and burden of migraine in the United States: data from the American Migraine Study II. Headache 41:646–657
6. World Health Organization. Global Health Estimates 2014 summary tables. YLD Global 2000–2012, June 2014. Available at: http://www.who.int/entity/healthinfo/global_burden_disease/GHE_YLD_Global_2000_2012.xls?ua=1. http://www.who.int/entity/healthinfo/global_burden_disease/GHE_YLD_Global_2000_2012.xls?ua=1. Accessed 3 Dec 2016.
7. Dowson AJ, Sender J, Lipscombe S et al (2003) Establishing principles for migraine management in primary care. Int J Clin Pract 57:493–507
8. Ferrari MD, Roon KI, Lipton RB et al (2001) Oral triptans (serotonin 5-HT(1B/1D) agonists) in acute migraine treatment: a meta-analysis of 53 trials. Lancet 358:1668–1675
9. Napoletano F, Lionetto L, Martelletti P (2014) Sumatriptan in clinical practice: effectiveness in migraine and the problem of psychiatric comorbidity. Expert Opin Pharmacother 15:303–305
10. Cady RK, Wendt JK, Kirchner JR et al (1991) Treatment of acute migraine with subcutaneous sumatriptan. JAMA 265:2831–2835
11. The Subcutaneous Sumatriptan International Study Group (1991) Treatment of migraine attacks with sumatriptan. N Engl J Med 325:316–321
12. Erlichson K, Waight J (2012) Therapeutic applications for subcutaneous triptans in the acute treatment of migraine. Curr Med Res Opin 28:1231–1238
13. IMITREX (sumatriptan succinate) Injection prescribing information. Available at: https://www.gsksource.com/pharma/content/dam/GlaxoSmithKline/US/en/Prescribing_Information/Imitrex_Injection/pdf/IMITREX-INJECTION-PI-PPI.PDF. Accessed 3 Dec 2016.
14. Mathew NT, Dexter J, Couch J et al (1992) Dose ranging efficacy and safety of subcutaneous sumatriptan in the acute treatment of migraine. US Sumatriptan Research Group. Arch Neurol 49:1271–1276
15. Gallagher RM, Kunkel R (2003) Migraine medication attributes important for patient compliance: concerns about side effects may delay treatment. Headache 43:36–43
16. Goadsby PJ, Lipton RB, Ferrari MD (2002) Migraine–current understanding and treatment. N Engl J Med 346:257–270
17. Gendolla A (2005) Part I: what do patients really need and want from migraine treatment? Curr Med Res Opin 21(Suppl 3):S3–S7
18. Lipton RB, Hamelsky SW, Dayno JM (2002) What do patients with migraine want from acute migraine treatment? Headache 42(Suppl 1):3–9
19. Winner P, Adelman J, Aurora S et al (2006) Efficacy and tolerability of sumatriptan injection for the treatment of morning migraine: two multicenter, prospective, randomized, double-blind, controlled studies in adults. Clin Ther 28:1582–1591
20. Landy SH, Mcginnis JE, Mcdonald SA (2005) Pilot study evaluating preference for 3-mg versus 6-mg subcutaneous sumatriptan. Headache 45:346–349
21. Visser WH, Jaspers NM, De Vriend RH et al (1996) Chest symptoms after sumatriptan: a two-year clinical practice review in 735 consecutive migraine patients. Cephalalgia 16:554–559
22. Wang JT, Barr CE, Goldfarb SD (2002) Impact of chest pain on cost of migraine treatment with almotriptan and sumatriptan. Headache 42(Suppl 1):38–43
23. Burstein R, Jakubowski M (2004) Analgesic triptan action in an animal model of intracranial pain: a race against the development of central sensitization. Ann Neurol 55:27–36
24. Cady RK, Sheftell F, Lipton RB et al (2000) Effect of early intervention with sumatriptan on migraine pain: retrospective analyses of data from three clinical trials. Clin Ther 22:1035–1048
25. Winner P, Mannix LK, Putnam DG et al (2003) Pain-free results with sumatriptan taken at the first sign of migraine pain: 2 randomized, double-blind, placebo-controlled studies. Mayo Clin Proc 78:1214–1222
26. Cady RK, Lipton RB, Hall C et al (2000) Treatment of mild headache in disabled migraine sufferers: results of the Spectrum Study. Headache 40:792–797

11

Unveiling the relative efficacy, safety and tolerability of prophylactic medications for migraine: pairwise and network-meta analysis

Aijie He[1†], Dehua Song[2†], Lei Zhang[3] and Chen Li[4*]

Abstract

Background: A large number patients struggle with migraine which is classified as a chronic disorder. The relative efficacy, safety and tolerability of prophylactic medications for migraine play a key role in managing this disease.

Methods: We conducted an extensive literature search for popular prophylactic medications that are used for migraine patients. Pairwise meta-analysis and network meta-analysis (NMA) were carried out sequentially for determining the relative efficacy, safety and tolerability of prophylactic medications. Summary effect for migraine headache days, headache frequency, at least 50% reduction in headache attacks, all-adverse events, nausea, somnolence, dizziness, withdrawal and withdrawal due to adverse events were produced by synthesizing both direct and indirect evidence.

Results: Patients with three interventions exhibited significantly less average migraine headache days compared with those treated by placebo (topiramate, propranolol, divalproex). Moreover, topiramate and valproate exhibited a significantly increased likelihood of at least 50% reduction in migraine headache attacks compared to placebo. Patients with topiramate and propranolol also exhibited significantly reduced headache frequency compared to those with placebo. On the other hand, patients with divalproex exhibited significantly higher risk of nausea compared to those with placebo, topiramate, propranolol, gabapentin and amitriptyline. Finally, divalproex was associated with an increased risk of withdrawal compared to placebo and propranolol.

Conclusions: Topiramate, propranolol and divalproex may be more efficacious than other prophylactic medications. Besides, the safety and tolerability of divalproex should be further verified by future studies.

Keywords: Migraine, Efficacy, Safety, Tolerability, Network meta-analysis

Background

Migraine is a chronic neurological disorder with high prevalence. Females appeared to have a higher morbidity of migraine than males in developed countries [1]. Although a relatively small number of migraine cases were reported in Asia, the morbidity of migraine attack in this region can reach up to 9.3% [2]. Throbbing headache is usually accompanied with migraine, resulting in both poor productivity

and unstable emotional state [3, 4]. Migraine patients are often managed by medications which are convenient and efficient. However, side effects such as nausea and dizziness resulted from these medications have been observed in patients who exhibited poor level of tolerance [5].

Two types of medications have been introduced to patients: abortive and preventative medications [6]. The above two types of medications differ considerably in their mechanisms: abortive treatments attenuate symptoms arise from acute migraine attacks whereas preventative medications specifically aim at reducing attack severity and frequency. Although several prophylactic medications have been developed for migraine patients,

* Correspondence: dqchangzhigang@126.com
†Equal contributors
⁴Department of Anesthesia, Yantai Hospital of Traditional Chinese Medicine, No. 39 Xingfu Road, Zhifu Disctrict, 264000 Yantai, Shandong, China

no consensus has been reached with respect to their relative efficacy, safety and tolerability [7]. Furthermore, some medications appear to provide inadequate relief since they are not effective to all migraine patients [8]. As a result, some meta-analysis has been designed to compare the relative efficacy between different medications and some conclusions have been obtained in the current literature. For instance, patients treated by sodium valproate were associated with a lower risk of headache compared to the control group [9]. Furthermore, triptans and non-triptans appear to provide patients with different levels of relief [10].

Nevertheless, the current literature does not contain adequate studies that are able to identify the most preferable prophylactic medication for migraine patients and there is an increasing demand for discriminating the available medications with respect to their efficacy, safety and tolerability. For this purpose, we compared several preventative medications for migraine patients by using the approach of network meta-analysis (NMA) and we expect this approach can provide more insights for the selection of prophylactic medications.

Methods
Search strategy
The medical literature for relevant studies in PubMed and EMBASE were systematically searched using electronic search strategies, and 1315 records were identified through searching the following key words, for example "migraine", "topiramate", "propranolol", "gabapentin", "amitriptyline", "divalproex" and "valproate". Two additional references were obtained from reviewers. As flow chart Fig. 1 illustrates, 556 duplicated records were identified and removed. Another 486 irrelevant studies were excluded from the remaining 761 records and a final 32 studies were subject to full-text review (Table 1).

Exclusion criteria
Articles were excluded in our study according to the following criteria: (1) the diagnose of migraine was not firmly confirmed in the study; (2) contain treatments that cannot form a closed network; (3) have no comparisons between different treatments; (4) contain outcomes without proper information; (5) does not have any relevant clinical outcomes or treatments; (6) studies without blinding procedures or studies with sample size less than 30; (7) non-randomized clinical trials such as reviews. A study was not considered to be eligible if any of the above criteria was fulfilled.

Outcome measures, data extraction and comparator network formation
We selected several clinical outcomes in order to measure the relative efficacy, safety and tolerability of prophylactic migraine medications: monthly migraine headache days, headache frequency, the percentages of patients with at least 50% reductions in migraine attacks (efficacy), the number of patients with all adverse events such as nausea, somnolence or dizziness (safety) and the number of patients who withdrew from studies (tolerability). The following data were extracted from eligible studies and shown in Table 1, including country of study, sample size, histology and clinical outcomes. The corresponding data were extracted into a database after two independent investigators reviewed the manuscripts of all the studies. A Jaded scale table was produced for the purpose of study quality assessment (Additional file 1: Table S1). After data extraction was performed for each study, a network plot with respect to each clinical outcome was produced for demonstrating direct and indirect comparisons (Figs. 2, 3 and 4).

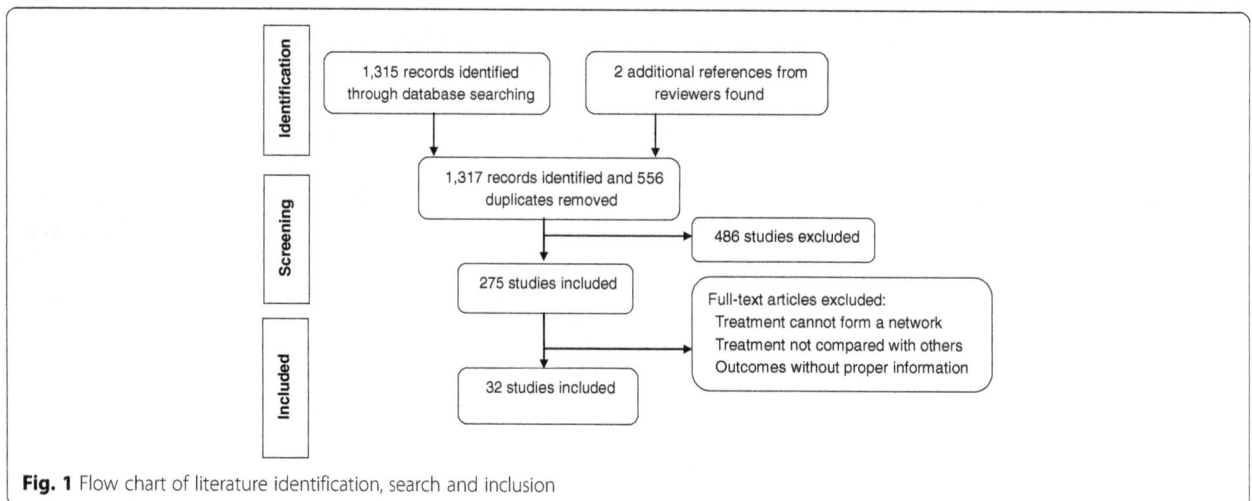

Fig. 1 Flow chart of literature identification, search and inclusion

Unveiling the relative efficacy, safety and tolerability of prophylactic medications for migraine: pairwise...

89

Table 1 Studies identified for the NMA with interventions and outcomes evaluated

Author, Year	Center	Design	Blind	Mechanism of action	Intervention	Size	Male (%)	Follow-up	Age	Clinical outcomes
Silberstein et al., 2013 [42]	Multi	RCT	Double	Anticonvulsants	Gabapentin vs. Placebo	523	21	20w	39.4	①③④⑤⑥⑦⑧⑨
Afshari et al., 2012 [41]	Mono	RCT	Double	Anticonvulsants	Topiramate vs. Valproate	56	21	12w	32.1	②④⑤⑥⑧⑨
Lipton et al., 2011 [40]	Multi	RCT	Double	Anticonvulsants	Topiramate vs. Placebo	330	13	26w	39.6	①④⑤⑥⑦⑧⑨
Holroyd et al., 2010 [39]	Multi	RCT	Double	β blocker	Propranolol vs. Placebo	106	21	16m	38.2	①⑧⑨
Dodick et al., 2009 [38]	Multi	RCT	Double	Anticonvulsants	Topiramate vs. Amitriptyline	346	15	26w	38.8	①④⑤⑥⑦⑧⑨
Ashtari et al., 2008 [37]	Mono	RCT	Double	Anticonvulsants	Topiramate vs. Propranolol	62	21	8w	30.5	②⑥⑦⑧⑨
Silberstein et al., 2007 [36]	Multi	RCT	Double	Anticonvulsants	Topiramate vs. Placebo	306	15	126d	38.2	①④⑤⑥⑦⑧⑨
Gupta et al., 2007 [35]	Mono	Crossover	Double	Anticonvulsants	Topiramate vs. Placebo	60	22	20w	29.4	①④⑧⑨
Diener et al., 2007 [33, 34]	Multi	RCT	Double	Anticonvulsants	Topiramate vs. Placebo	59	26	16w	46.2	①④⑤⑥⑦⑧
Diener et al., 2007 [33, 34]	Multi	RCT	Double	Anticonvulsants	Topiramate vs. Placebo	514	13	6m	39.8	①④⑤⑦⑧
Tommaso et al., 2007 [32]	Mono	RCT	Double	Anticonvulsants	Topiramate vs. Placebo	30	22	1d	37.9	⑨
Silberstein et al., 2006 [31]	Multi	RCT	Double	Anticonvulsants	Topiramate vs. Placebo	211	14	12w	40.5	④
Shaygannejad et al., 2006 [30]	Mono	Crossover	Double	Anticonvulsants	Topiramate vs. Valproate	64	57	24w	34.1	②⑥
Brandes et al., 2006 [29]	Multi	RCT	Double	Anticonvulsants	Topiramate vs. Placebo	468	13	13m	38.8	②⑧⑨
Silberstein et al., 2004 [28]	Multi	RCT	Double	Anticonvulsants	Topiramate vs. Placebo	469	11	26w	40.4	①②③⑤⑥⑧⑨
Mei et al., 2004 [27]	Mono	RCT	Double	Anticonvulsants	Topiramate vs. Placebo	115	46	16w	39.2	②③④⑥⑧⑨
Diener et al., 2004 [26]	Multi	RCT	Double	Anticonvulsants	Topiramate vs. Propranolol	568	20	1y	41.0	①②④⑤⑥⑧⑨
Brandes et al., 2004 [25]	Multi	RCT	Double	Anticonvulsants	Topiramate vs. Placebo	483	13	26w	38.8	③⑧⑨
Freitag et al., 2002 [24]	Multi	RCT	Double	Anticonvulsants	Divalproex vs. Placebo	237	21	12w	40.5	①②③④⑤⑥⑦⑧⑨
Storey et al., 2001 [23]	Mono	RCT	Double	Anticonvulsants	Topiramate vs. Placebo	40	25	12w	38.2	②③⑧⑨
Mathew et al., 2001 [22]	Multi	RCT	Double	Anticonvulsants	Gabapentin vs. Placebo	143	17	16w	39.4	②③④⑥⑦⑧⑨
Klapper, 1997 [21]	Multi	RCT	Single	Anticonvulsants	Divalproex vs. Placebo	176	12	12w	40.5	③④⑤⑥⑧⑨
Kaniecki, 1997 [20]	Mono	RCT	Single	Anticonvulsants	Divalproex vs. Propranolol	37	19	12w	40.1	④⑤⑦⑨
Diener et al., 1996 [19]	Multi	RCT	Double	β blocker	Propranolol vs. Placebo	133	22	12w	39.0	③⑧⑨
Bendtsen et al., 1996 [18]	Mono	Crossover	Double	Antidepressive	Amitriptyline vs. Placebo	40	38	32w	40.0	④⑤⑦⑨
Mathew et al., 1995 [17]	Multi	RCT	Double	Anticonvulsants	Divalproex vs. Placebo	107	20	12w	46.0	①③⑤⑥⑧⑨
Hering and Kuritzky, 1992 [16]	Mono	Crossover	Double	Anticonvulsants	Valproate vs. Placebo	32	21	16w	34.0	⑤⑦⑨
Pradalier et al., 1989 [15]	Multi	RCT	Double	β blocker	Propranolol vs. Placebo	74	24	16w	37.4	②⑤⑦⑧⑨
Mikkelsen et al., 1986 [14]	Mono	Crossover	Double	β blocker	Propranolol vs. Placebo	31	16	12w	38.0	④⑧⑨
Sadeghian andMotiei-Langroudi; 2015 [45]	Mono	RCT	Double	Anticonvulsants	Valproate vs. Placebo	58	27	6m	35.3	③④⑨
Sarchielli et al., 2014 [44]	Multi	RCT	Double	Anticonvulsants	Valproate vs. Placebo	88	21	6m	42.0	④⑤⑥⑦⑧⑨
Nofal et al., 2014 [43]	Moni	RCT	Double	Anticonvulsants	Gabapentin vs. Placebo	86	0	4d	30.9	⑤⑦

Outcomes: ① monthly migraine headache days; ② headache frequency; ③ ≥50% reduction in migraine headache attacks; ④ all-adverse events; ⑤ nausea; ⑥ somnolence; ⑦ dizziness; ⑧ withdrawal; ⑨ withdrawal due to adverse events

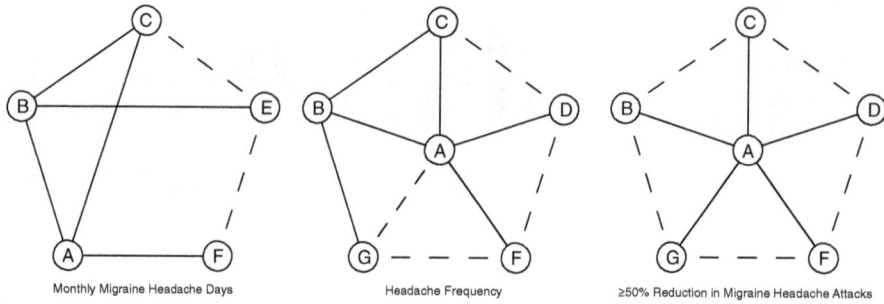

Fig. 2 Network plots of eligible comparisons of migraine intervention (monthly migraine headache days; headache frequency; ≥50% reduction in migraine headache attacks). *A*: Placebo; *B*: Topiramate; *C*: Propranolol; *D*: Gabapentin; *E*: Amitriptyline; *F*: Divalproex; *G*: Valproate. Direct comparisons were connected by solid lines whereas indirect comparisons were connected by dashed lines

Statistical analysis

We implemented a two-step approach in our system review and evidence synthesis. Firstly, a conventional pairwise meta-analysis was carried out in order to pool all direct evidence in the current literature. For continuous outcomes such as monthly migraine headache days and headache frequency, raw mean differences (MD) between two groups were synthesized and a summary effect was produced based on raw mean differences, sample size and sample standard deviation. We selected raw mean differences for evidence synthesis

since all eligible studies reported the above continuous outcomes in the same scale. On the other hand, the statistic of odds ratio (OR) was pooled from each eligible study and a summary OR was produced for each binary outcome. The pairwise meta-analysis was implemented based on the random-effects model because we did not have full knowledge of study participants or implementation for each eligible study [11].

The second step in our study involves conducting a NMA by synthesize both direct and indirect evidence. Similar to the pairwise meta-analysis, summary mean

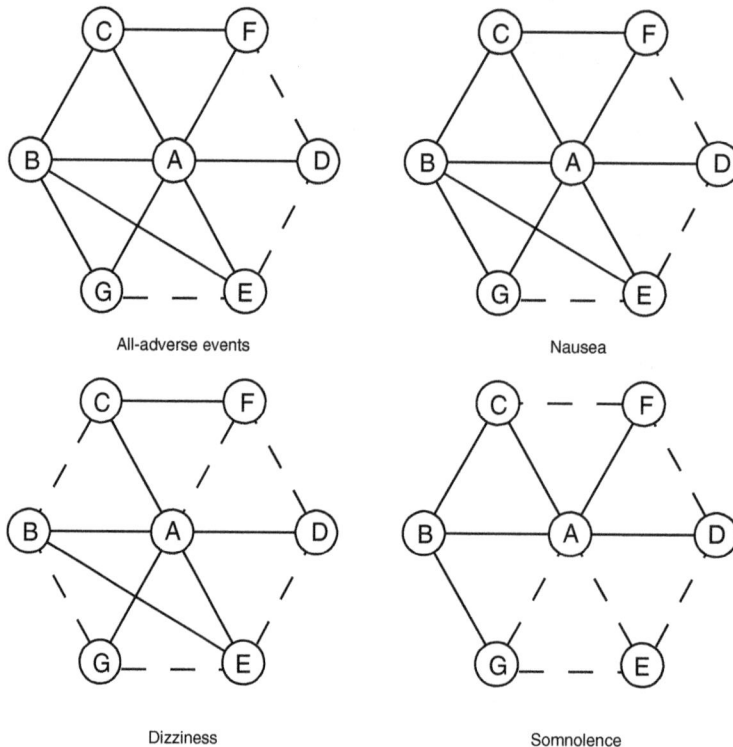

Fig. 3 Network plots of eligible comparisons for adverse events (all adverse events; nausea; somnolence; dizziness) *A*: Placebo; *B*: Topiramate; *C*: Propranolol; *D*: Gabapentin; *E*: Amitriptyline; *F*: Divalproex; *G*: Valproate. Direct comparisons were connected by solid lines whereas indirect comparisons were connected by dashed lines

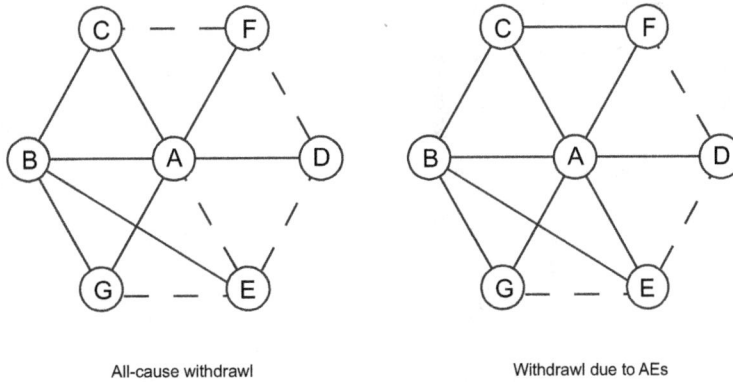

Fig. 4 Network plots of eligible comparisons for discontinued cases (all-cause withdrawal; withdrawal due to AEs). A: Placebo; B: Topiramate; C: Propranolol; D: Gabapentin; E: Amitriptyline; F: Divalproex; G: Valproate. Direct comparisons were connected by solid lines whereas indirect comparisons were connected by dashed lines

differences and summary ORs were produced using the Bayesian framework and the Markov Chain Monte Carlo (MCMC) sampling technique. The corresponding ranking of each intervention was obtained by using the surface under the cumulative ranking curve (SUCRA). If an intervention exhibited a higher SUCRA value compared to other interventions, then it is potentially more preferable than others with respect to an endpoint. After that, the assumption of consistency between direct and indirect evidence was assessed by using the node-splitting method whereas publication bias was visually inspected by using funnel plots [12, 13].

Results

Description of included studies

The prescribed searching strategy and exclusion criteria enabled us to identify and include 32 studies with a total number of 6052 subjects (Table 1) [14–45]. All included studies were carried out by using single or double blinding procedures. These studies were carried out between 1986 and 2015 with a maximum following-up duration of 1 year. The majority of the included studies belonged to typical randomized controlled trials (RCTs), however, we identified and included five crossover RCTs in which participants were randomized to receive a sequence of interventions.

Table 2 Relative treatment efficacy, safety and tolerability produced by pairwise meta-analysis

Comparison	Migraine headache days	Headache frequency	≥50% Reduction	All-adverse events	Nausea	Somnolence	Dizziness	Withdrawal	Withdrawal due to AEs
Placebo vs Topiramate	**−0.28 (−0.53, −0.03)**	**−0.31 (−0.45, −0.17)**	**2.33 (1.58, 3.42)**	**1.35 (1.06, 1.73)**	1.31 (0.97, 1.76)	1.38 (0.70, 2.74)	1.07 (0.54, 2.13)	1.05 (0.91, 1.21)	**2.08 (1.56, 2.78)**
Placebo vs Propranolol	**−0.29 (−0.49, −0.09)**	−1.17 (−2.89, 0.55)	1.37 (0.69, 2.70)	**2.02 (1.05, 4.08)**	1.64 (0.78, 3.47)	**4.33 (1.21, 15.53)**	1.27 (0.20, 8.08)	1.07 (0.76, 1.51)	**1.87 (1.09, 3.19)**
Placebo vs Gabapentin	−0.09 (−0.29, 0.10)	−0.34 (−0.69, 0.01)	1.36 (0.63, 2.95)	1.15 (0.87, 1.51)	0.92 (0.52, 1.64)	**2.23 (1.11, 4.46)**	**3.13 (1.73, 5.66)**	1.21 (0.82, 1.77)	1.57 (0.86, 2.88)
Placebo vs Amitriptyline	-	**−0.36 (−0.62, −0.10)**	**1.81 (1.03, 3.20)**	**2.20 (1.04, 4.66)**	0.33 (0.03, 3.34)	-	1.75 (0.47, 6.45)	-	2.00 (0.17, 22.93)
Placebo vs Divalproex	**−0.40 (−0.61, −0.18)**	-	**4.27 (1.30, 13.99)**	0.98 (0.71, 1.34)	**2.23 (1.21, 4.10)**	1.92 (0.32, 11.63)	-	1.61 (0.92, 2.82)	1.67 (0.70, 3.98)
Placebo vs Valproate	-	-	-	-	3.00 (0.59, 15.37)	-	2.00 (0.36, 11.26)	0.88 (0.29, 2.62)	0.97 (0.26, 3.56)
Topiramate vs Propranolol	−0.12 (−0.32, 0.08)	0.18 (−0.45, 0.81)	-	**0.57 (0.36, 0.90)**	0.81 (0.45, 1.45)	1.42 (0.68, 2.99)	-	**0.66 (0.44, 0.99)**	**0.58 (0.37, 0.91)**
Topiramate vs Amitriptyline	0.01 (−0.20, 0.22)	-	-	1.03 (0.76, 1.41)	0.70 (0.33, 1.49)	1.50 (0.82, 2.72)	1.26 (0.61, 2.57)	1.02 (0.70, 1.50)	1.14 (0.69, 1.88)
Topiramate vs Valproate	-	-	-	1.22 (0.54, 2.76)	1.00 (0.29, 3.48)	1.30 (0.44, 3.84)	-	0.67 (0.24, 1.88)	2000 (0.58, 18.16)
Propranolol vs Divalproex	-	-	-	1.36 (0.58, 3.16)	3.50 (0.67, 18.15)	-	1.00 (0.19, 5.33)	-	4.00 (0.42, 37.78)

Boldface means significance

Table 3 Relative efficacy, safety and tolerability of migraine interventions produced by NMA

Migraine Headache Days

	Placebo	Topiramate	Propranolol	Gabapentin	Amitriptyline	Divalproex	Valproate
Placebo	Placebo	1.20 (0.70, 1.83)	0.98 (0.07, 1.86)	–	1.09 (−0.89, 3.13)	1.28 (0.27, 2.44)	–
Topiramate	−1.20 (−1.83, −0.70)	Topiramate	−0.22 (−1.30, 0.67)	–	−0.10 (−2.03, 1.81)	0.09 (−1.16, 1.31)	–
Propranolol	−0.98 (−1.86, −0.07)	0.22 (−0.67, 1.30)	Propranolol	–	0.13 (−2.02, 2.33)	0.31 (−1.05, 1.83)	–
Gabapentin	–	–	–	Gabapentin	–	–	–
Amitriptyline	−1.09 (−3.13, 0.89)	0.10 (−1.81, 2.03)	−0.13 (−2.33, 2.02)	–	Amitriptyline	0.21 (−2.08, 2.53)	–
Divalproex	−1.28 (−2.44, −0.27)	−0.09 (−1.31, 1.16)	−0.31 (−1.83, 1.05)	–	−0.21 (−2.53, 2.08)	Divalproex	–
Valproate	–	–	–	–	–	–	Valproate

Headache Frequency

≥50% Reduction in Migraine Headache Attacks

	Placebo	Topiramate	Propranolol	Gabapentin	Amitriptyline	Divalproex	Valproate
Placebo	Placebo	1.17 (0.35, 1.98)	1.37 (0.29, 2.49)	1.20 (−0.87, 3.28)	–	0.60 (−1.18, 2.42)	0.84 (−0.81, 2.48)
Topiramate	4.28 (1.35, 14.70)	Topiramate	0.21 (−0.88, 1.33)	0.05 (−2.20, 2.28)	–	−0.56 (−2.53, 1.39)	−0.32 (−1.76, 1.10)
Propranolol	1.65 (0.25, 11.29)	0.38 (0.04, 3.70)	Propranolol	−0.17 (−2.45, 2.15)	–	−0.76 (−2.90, 1.32)	−0.53 (−2.33, 1.23)
Gabapentin	1.59 (0.41, 6.93)	0.37 (0.06, 2.43)	0.96 (0.10, 10.96)	Gabapentin	–	−0.61 (−3.39, 2.12)	−0.36 (−3.01, 2.38)
Amitriptyline	–	–	–	–	Amitriptyline	–	–
Divalproex	2.63 (0.91, 8.79)	0.62 (0.12, 3.11)	1.58 (0.18, 14.74)	1.67 (0.26, 9.65)	–	Divalproex	0.24 (−2.21, 2.67)
Valproate	11.38 (1.31, 111.11)	2.66 (0.22, 32.35)	7.00 (0.37, 128.51)	7.19 (0.51, 94.89)	–	4.30 (0.38, 52.31)	Valproate

All Adverse Events

Nausea

	Placebo	Topiramate	Propranolol	Gabapentin	Amitriptyline	Divalproex	Valproate
Placebo	Placebo				4.66 (1.74, 12.93)	1.13 (0.51, 2.57)	
Topiramate	1.37 (0.99, 1.94)	Topiramate			1.92 (0.72, 5.20)	0.46 (0.19, 1.15)	
Propranolol	1.13 (0.56, 2.24)	0.81 (0.44, 1.59)	Propranolol		4.29 (1.24, 15.39)	1.04 (0.39, 2.75)	
Gabapentin	0.91 (0.47, 1.86)	0.67 (0.32, 1.43)	0.82 (0.32, 2.06)	Gabapentin	2.80 (0.75, 10.80)	0.68 (0.20, 2.19)	
Amitriptyline	0.80 (0.32, 1.84)	0.58 (0.24, 1.37)	0.71 (0.23, 1.89)	0.85 (0.27, 2.50)	Amitriptyline	0.24 (0.07, 0.85)	
Divalproex	3.04 (1.72, 6.47)	2.24 (1.13, 4.93)	2.79 (1.19, 6.48)	3.31 (1.31, 9.25)	3.83 (1.40, 12.81)	Divalproex	
Valproate	2.05 (0.75, 5.65)	1.53 (0.54, 4.07)	1.88 (0.53, 5.59)	2.27 (0.55, 7.43)	2.63 (0.63, 10.29)	0.67 (0.20, 2.32)	Valproate

Somnolence

Dizziness

	Placebo	Topiramate	Propranolol	Gabapentin	Amitriptyline	Divalproex	Valproate
Placebo	Placebo	2.16 (0.25, 17.88)	1.56 (0.24, 10.53)	0.80 (0.04, 10.81)	0.80 (0.05, 11.62)	0.97 (0.05, 15.68)	0.73 (0.06, 10.84)
Topiramate	1.17 (0.48, 2.71)	Topiramate	2.95 (0.55, 13.06)	2.18 (0.31, 13.03)	1.09 (0.07, 10.90)	1.12 (0.10, 8.96)	1.43 (0.07, 20.34)
Propranolol	1.40 (0.11, 17.00)	1.20 (0.09, 17.20)	Propranolol	2.68 (0.55, 14.14)	1.96 (0.32, 14.39)	1.01 (0.07, 12.38)	0.29 (0.01, 15.46)
Gabapentin	3.69 (1.17, 9.63)	3.21 (0.74, 11.22)	2.64 (0.19, 35.35)	Gabapentin	2.20 (0.20, 23.60)	1.58 (0.19, 14.47)	0.81 (0.04, 13.07)
Amitriptyline	1.63 (0.46, 6.07)	1.40 (0.44, 5.06)	1.17 (0.08, 18.83)	0.44 (0.10, 2.67)	Amitriptyline	0.83 (0.04, 12.96)	1.43 (0.07, 20.34)
Divalproex	1.37 (0.05, 34.88)	1.18 (0.04, 35.19)	0.94 (0.11, 9.66)	0.38 (0.01, 11.64)	0.84 (0.02, 27.74)	Divalproex	0.84 (0.02, 27.74)
Valproate	0.44 (0.04, 2.98)	0.37 (0.03, 3.27)	0.30 (0.01, 7.28)	0.12 (0.01, 1.13)	0.26 (0.02, 2.72)	0.29 (0.01, 15.46)	Valproate

Table 3 Relative efficacy, safety and tolerability of migraine interventions produced by NMA (*Continued*)

Withdrawal

Withdrawal due to AEs	Placebo	Topiramate	Propranolol	Gabapentin	Amitriptyline	Divalproex	Valproate
Placebo	**Placebo**	1.10 (0.95, 1.38)	0.81 (0.63, 1.29)	1.17 (0.80, 2.08)	1.19 (0.68, 2.14)	**1.68 (1.14, 3.67)**	1.29 (0.48, 2.68)
Topiramate	**2.33 (1.55, 3.45)**	**Topiramate**	0.71 (0.54, 1.15)	1.04 (0.67, 1.87)	1.09 (0.60, 1.82)	1.48 (0.96, 3.36)	1.14 (0.42, 2.46)
Propranolol	1.51 (0.78, 2.94)	0.64 (0.32, 1.34)	**Propranolol**	1.54 (0.78, 2.63)	1.56 (0.68, 2.56)	**2.09 (1.11, 4.52)**	1.51 (0.49, 3.69)
Gabapentin	1.81 (0.71, 4.58)	0.78 (0.28, 2.18)	1.21 (0.38, 3.72)	**Gabapentin**	1.03 (0.43, 1.95)	1.34 (0.74, 3.37)	1.02 (0.33, 2.38)
Amitriptyline	2.69 (0.93, 7.57)	1.16 (0.43, 3.12)	1.80 (0.51, 5.84)	1.49 (0.35, 5.96)	**Amitriptyline**	1.32 (0.74, 3.73)	1.08 (0.35, 2.33)
Divalproex	**2.25 (1.01, 5.49)**	0.96 (0.41, 2.57)	1.50 (0.57, 4.26)	1.25 (0.38, 4.49)	0.83 (0.24, 3.40)	**Divalproex**	0.68 (0.22, 1.83)
Valproate	2.20 (0.68, 6.92)	0.96 (0.30, 2.97)	1.50 (0.39, 5.28)	1.25 (0.26, 5.38)	0.85 (0.17, 3.58)	0.99 (0.23, 4.28)	**Valproate**

Row treatments were compared to column treatments in the lower diagonal whereas column treatments were compared to row treatments in the upper diagonal

Boldface means significance

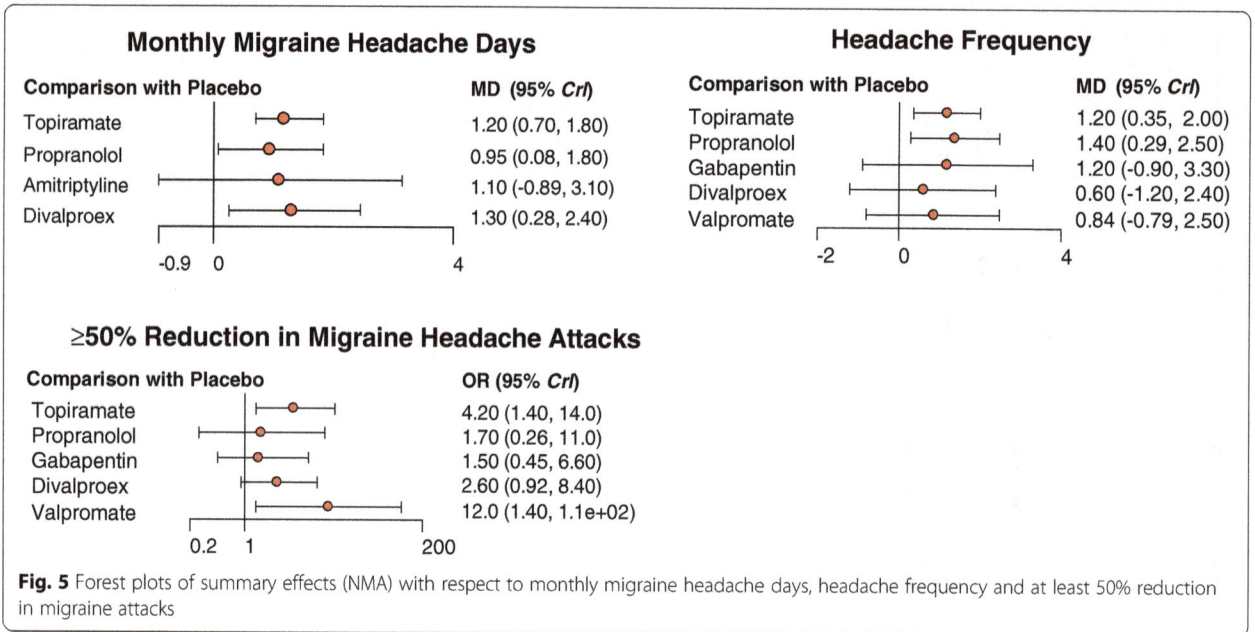

Fig. 5 Forest plots of summary effects (NMA) with respect to monthly migraine headache days, headache frequency and at least 50% reduction in migraine attacks

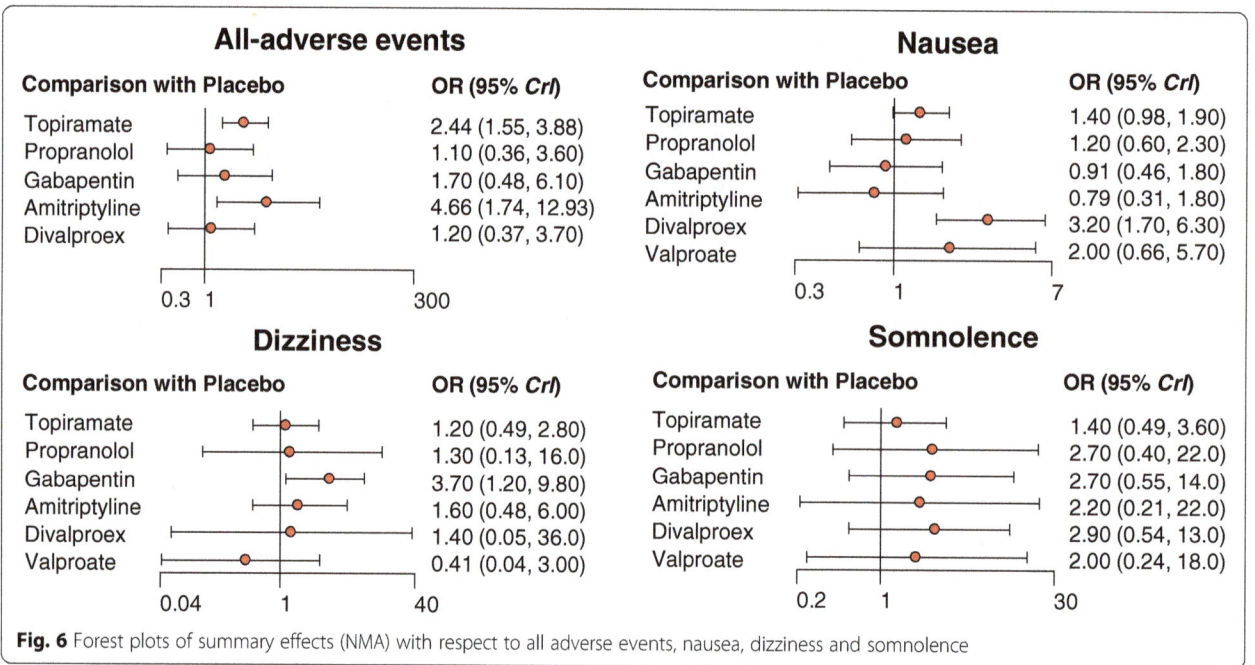

Fig. 6 Forest plots of summary effects (NMA) with respect to all adverse events, nausea, dizziness and somnolence

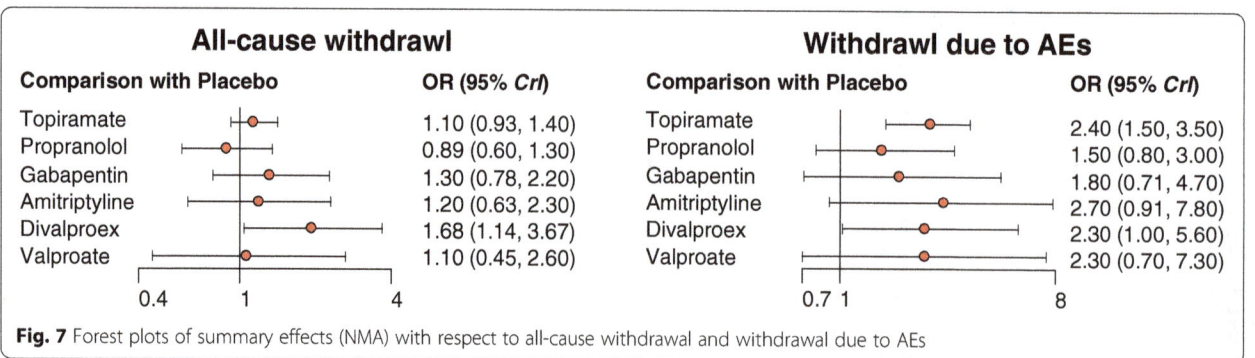

Fig. 7 Forest plots of summary effects (NMA) with respect to all-cause withdrawal and withdrawal due to AEs

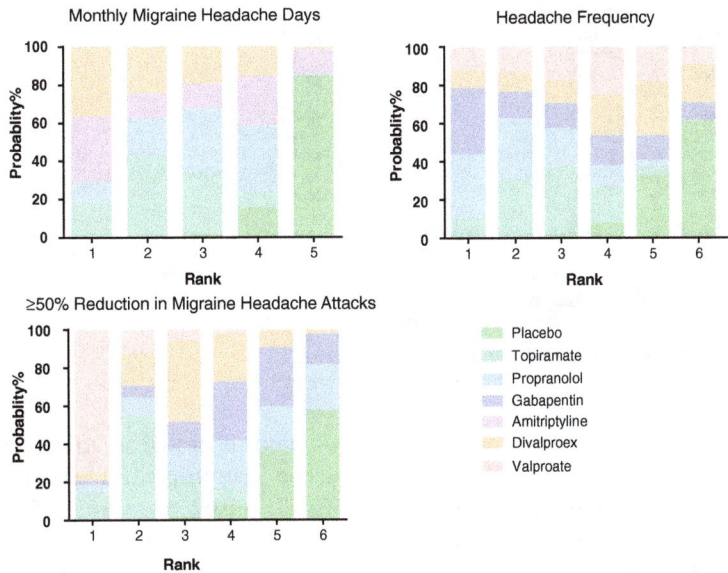

Fig. 8 Probability ranking plot of monthly migraine headache days, headache frequency and at least 50% reduction in migraine attacks

Pairwise comparison using conventional meta-analysis

A total of ten direct comparisons with respect to each endpoint were produced by using pairwise meta-analysis (Table 2). Patients with topiramate exhibited significantly less average headache days, less headache frequency, a higher likelihood of at least 50% reduction compared to those with placebo (migraine headache days: −0.28, 95% CI = −0.53 to −0.03; headache frequency: −0.31, 95% CI = −0.45 to −0.17; ≥ 50% reduction: OR = 2.33, 95% CI = 1.58–3.42). However, patients with topiramate appeared

to have significantly higher risk of all-adverse events and withdrawal due to adverse events compared to those with placebo (all-adverse events: OR = 1.35, 95% CI = 1.06–1.73, withdrawal due to adverse events: OR = 2.08, 95% CI = 1.56–2.78). Patients with propranolol exhibited a significantly less average headache days but higher risk of all-adverse events, somnolence and withdrawal due to adverse events compared to those with placebo (migraine headache days: −0.29, 95% CI = −0.49 to −0.09; all-adverse events: OR = 2.02, 95% CI = 1.05–4.08,

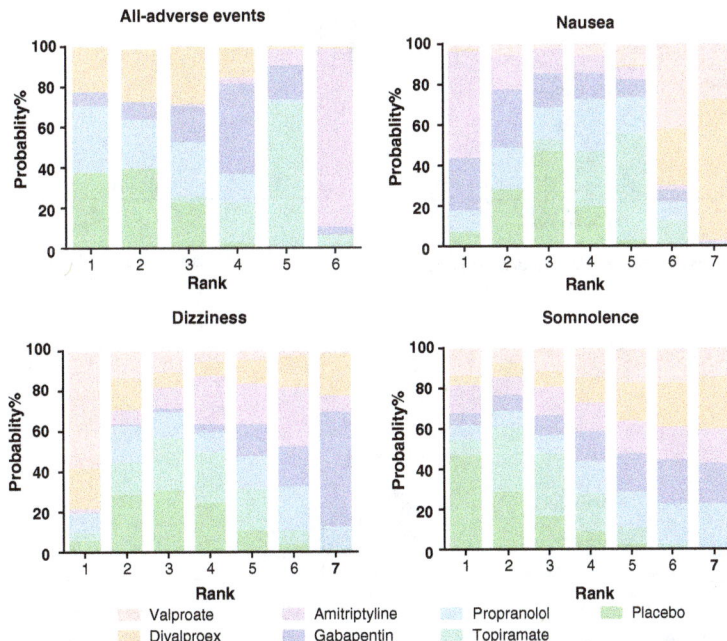

Fig. 9 Probability ranking plot of all adverse events, nausea, dizziness and somnolence

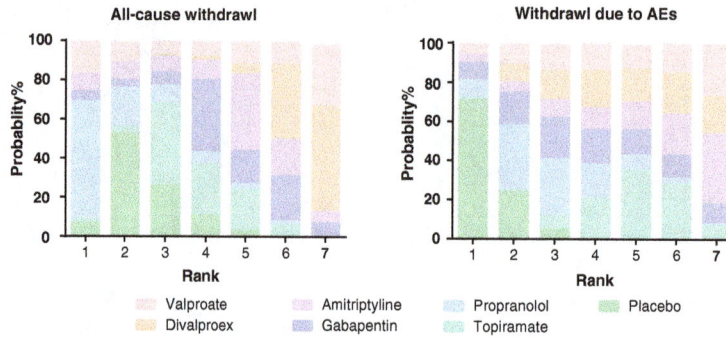

Fig. 10 Probability ranking plot of all-cause withdrawal and withdrawal due to AEs

somnolence: OR = 4.33, 95% CI = 1.21 to 15.53, withdrawal due to adverse events: OR = 1.87, 95% CI = 1.09 to 3.09). Although there is no significant differences in the average migraine days, headache frequency or the likelihood of at least 50% reduction in headache attacks between patients with gabapentin and those with placebo, gabapentin appeared to be associated with an increased risk of somnolence and dizziness (somnolence: OR = 2.23, 95% CI = 1.11 to 4.46; dizziness: OR = 3.13, 95% CI = 1.73 to 5.56). Patients treated with amitriptyline or divalproex exhibited a reduced headache days or headache frequency as well as a better performance in at least 50%

reduction in headache attacks compared to those with placebo (amitriptyline: headache frequency: −0.36, 95% CI = −0.62 to −0.10; ≥ 50% reduction: OR = 1.81, 95% CI = 1.03–3.20; divalproex: migraine headache days: −0.40, 95% CI = −0.61 to −0.18; ≥ 50% reduction: OR = 4.27, 95% CI = 1.30–13.99), however, this was offset by an increased risk of all-adverse events or nausea (amitriptyline: all-adverse events: OR = 2.20, 95% CI = 1.04–4.66; divalproex: nausea: OR = 2.23, 95% CI = 1.21–4.10). Besides that, we were not able to identify any significant results between direct comparisons produced by conventional meta-analysis. Besides, propranolol was safer comparing to topiramate

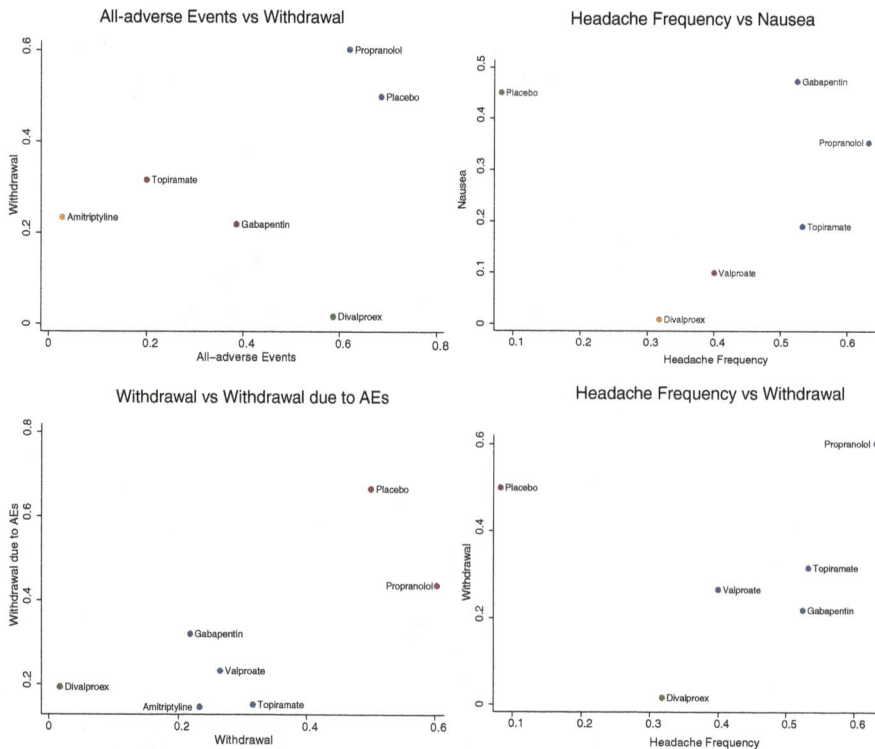

Fig. 11 Clustering of migraine interventions. Interventions with the same level of efficacy, safety or tolerability are shown in the same color. Interventions located in the top right corner were more preferable than those in the lower left corner

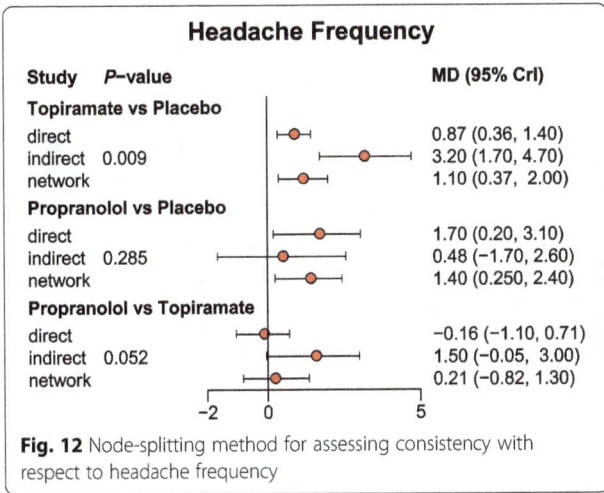

Fig. 12 Node-splitting method for assessing consistency with respect to headache frequency

(all-adverse events: OR = 0.57, 95% CI = 0.36–0.90; withdrawal: OR = 0.66, 95% CI = 0.44–0.99; withdrawal due to adverse events: OR = 0.58, 95% CI = 0.37–0.91).

Including both direct and indirect evidence in the NMA

Results produced by NMA are displayed in Table 3 which determined the relative efficacy, safety and tolerability of prophylactic migraine interventions by using both direct and indirect evidence. Patients with three interventions exhibited significantly less average migraine headache days compared with those treated by placebo (topiramate: −1.20, 95% CrI = −1.83 to −0.70; propranolol: −0.98, 95% CrI = −1.86 to −0.07; divalproex: −1.28, 95% CrI = −2.44 to −0.27; Table 3, Fig. 5). Moreover, patients with topiramate and valproate exhibited a significantly increased likelihood of at least 50% reduction in migraine headache attacks compared to those with placebo (topiramate: OR = 4.28, 95% CrI = 1.35 to 14.70; valproate: 11.38, 95% CrI = 1.31 to 111.11; Table 3, Fig. 5). Patients with topiramate or propranolol also

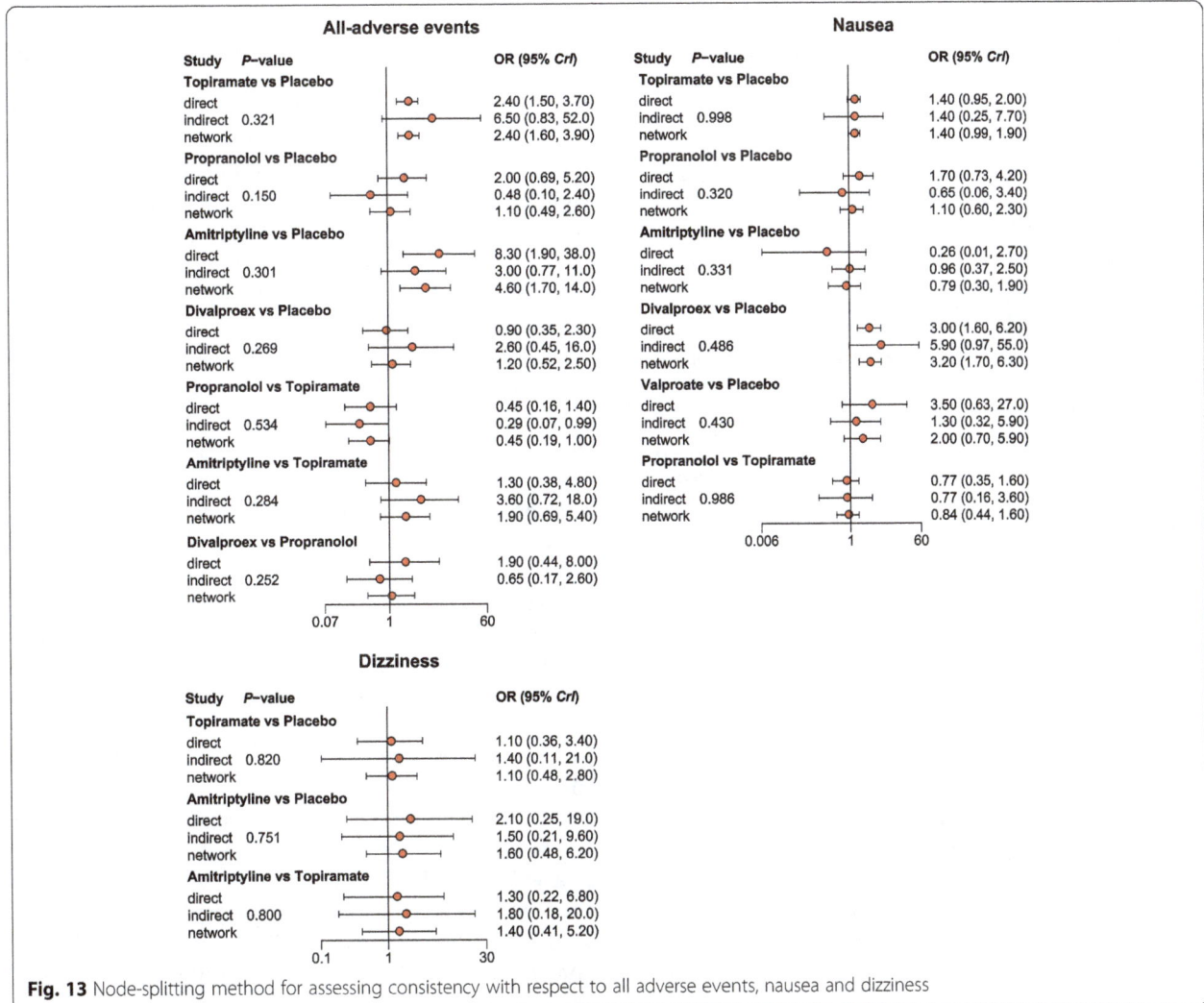

Fig. 13 Node-splitting method for assessing consistency with respect to all adverse events, nausea and dizziness

All-cause withdrawl

Study	P-value	OR (95% CrI)
Topiramate vs Placebo		
direct		1.10 (0.90, 1.30)
indirect	0.165	3.20 (0.70, 15.0)
network		1.10 (0.94, 1.40)
Propranolol vs Placebo		
direct		1.00 (0.71, 1.50)
indirect	0.958	1.20 (0.05, 37.0)
network		0.88 (0.62, 1.30)
Valproate vs Placebo		
direct		2.20 (0.60, 9.30)
indirect	0.142	0.58 (0.18, 2.10)
network		1.10 (0.47, 2.60)
Propranolol vs Topiramate		
direct		0.54 (0.32, 0.88)
indirect	0.066	1.10 (0.64, 2.10)
network		0.77 (0.52, 1.20)
Valproate vs Topiramate		
direct		0.51 (0.16, 1.70)
indirect	0.142	2.00 (0.50, 8.30)
network		0.97 (0.40, 2.30)

0.04   1   40

Withdrawl due to AEs

Study	P-value	OR (95% CrI)
Topiramate vs Placebo		
direct		2.50 (1.60, 3.80)
indirect	0.142	0.73 (0.13, 3.80)
network		2.40 (1.50, 3.60)
Propranolol vs Placebo		
direct		2.10 (1.10, 4.30)
indirect	0.236	0.66 (0.06, 4.00)
network		1.50 (0.79, 2.90)
Amitriptyline vs Placebo		
direct		2.40 (0.16, 97.0)
indirect	0.922	2.80 (0.84, 9.80)
network		2.70 (0.95, 7.60)
Divalproex vs Placebo		
direct		1.90 (0.82, 4.70)
indirect	0.220	10.0 (0.89, 2.8e+02)
network		2.20 (1.00, 5.40)
Valproate vs Placebo		
direct		0.91 (0.23, 4.20)
indirect	0.044	11.0 (1.50, 1.1e+02)
network		2.30 (0.76, 7.40)
Propranolol vs Topiramate		
direct		0.48 (0.19, 1.30)
indirect	0.510	0.75 (0.27, 2.10)
network		0.63 (0.32, 1.40)
Amitriptyline vs Topiramate		
direct		1.20 (0.37, 3.50)
indirect	0.955	1.10 (0.06, 48.0)
network		1.20 (0.42, 3.10)
Valproate vs Topiramate		
direct		4.00 (0.65, 38.0)
indirect	0.050	0.37 (0.08, 1.60)
network		0.96 (0.32, 3.2)
Divalproex vs Propranolol		
direct		6.60 (0.68, 2.2e+02)
indirect	0.219	1.20 (0.37, 3.70)
network		1.50 (0.58, 4.40)

0.06   1   300

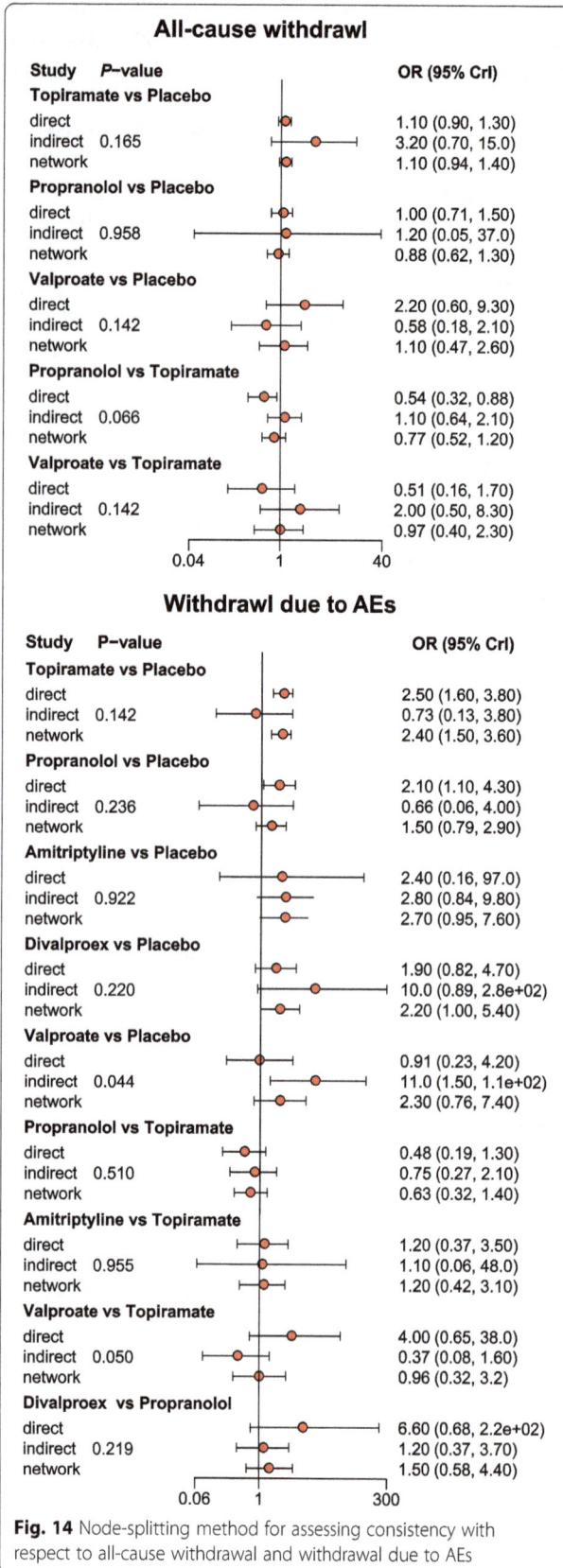

Fig. 14 Node-splitting method for assessing consistency with respect to all-cause withdrawal and withdrawal due to AEs

exhibited significantly reduced headache frequency compared to those with placebo (topiramate: −1.17, 95% CrI = −1.98 to −0.35; propranolol: −1.37, 95% CrI = −2.49 to −0.29; Table 3, Fig. 5).

Our NMA also provides results for the relative safety of migraine interventions. Patients with Divalproex exhibited significantly higher risk of nausea compared to those with placebo, topiramate, propranolol, gabapentin and amitriptyline (all ORs > 1). Furthermore, patients with amitriptyline exhibited a significantly elevated risk of all-adverse events compared to those with propranolol or placebo (all ORs > 1). However, patients with amitriptyline exhibited a significantly reduced risk of all-adverse events compared to those with divalproex (OR = 0.24, 95% CrI = 0.07 to 0.85). Patients with topiramate also exhibited significantly higher risk of all adverse events compared to those with placebo (OR = 2.44, 95% CrI = 1.55 to 3.88; Table 3, Fig. 6). Our NMA also discovered that patients with GABAPENTIN were associated with a significantly increase in the risk of dizziness in comparison to those received placebo (OR = 3.69, 95% CrI = 1.17 to 9.63; Table 3, Fig. 6). The relative tolerability of various migraine interventions were assessed by using the endpoints of all-cause withdrawal and withdrawal due to adverse events. As suggested by Table 3 and Fig. 7, patients with divalproex exhibited a significantly increased risk of all-case withdrawal compared to those with propranolol or placebo (propranolol: OR = 2.09, 95% CrI = 1.11 to 4.52; placebo: OR = 1.68, 95% CrI = 1.14 to 3.67). On the other hand, patients treated with topiramate or divalproex were associated with an increased risk of withdrawals due to adverse events compared to those with placebo (topiramate: OR = 2.33, 95% CrI = 1.55 to 3.45; divalproex: OR = 2.25, 95% CrI = 1.01 to 5.49).

Ranking of migraine interventions using SUCRA values

A ranking plot with respect to each endpoint was produced and a SUCRA table was created in order to differentiate the above migraine interventions (Figs. 8, 9 and 10, Additional file 2: Table S2). Divalproex appeared to have the largest SUCRA value with respect to migraine headache days. Propranolol, topiramate and gabapentin exhibited the largest three SUCRA values with respect to headache frequency. Moreover, valproate, topiramate and divalproex were more preferable than other interventions with respect to the endpoint of at least 50% reduction in migraine attacks. A similar ranking scheme was produced for the above interventions with respect to their safety and tolerability (Additional file 2: Table S2). We also conducted a cluster analysis for grouping the above prophylactic migraine interventions based on the

SUCRA values of two endpoints. Overall, propranolol seemed to be the most desirable intervention when several endpoints were simultaneously considered (Fig. 11).

Assessing consistency between direct and indirect evidence

Since we implemented a consistency model when conducting the NMA, the node-splitting method was used to assess the validity of this assumption (Figs. 12, 13 and 14). Net heat plots were also produced by software in order to visualize the consistency pattern existed in each comparison (Figs. 15, 16 and 17). As suggested by both the node splitting method (*P*-value > 0.05) and net heat plots, there is no significant inconsistency between direct and indirect evidence for the majority of comparisons. Therefore, we concluded that the consistency model is valid in our NMA.

Assessing publication bias using funnel plots

Potential publication bias contained in our NMA was evaluated by using the funnel plots produced by software (Additional file 3: Figures S1, Additional file 4: Figure S2 and Additional file 5: Figure S3). As suggested by the funnel plots, there is no significant asymmetry pattern and most studies were evenly distributed in the funnel plot. Therefore, we concluded that there is no significant publication bias in our study.

Discussion

Migraine is a chronic disabling disease accompanied with recurrent headache. Patients with migraine often suffer from throbbing headache and preventative therapies have been introduced to reduce the risk of migraine onset. Several medications have been applied to migraine patients as prophylaxis and most of these medications are able to reduce the monthly attack frequency by 50% [46]. We conducted an extensive literature review and NMA in order to determine the relative efficacy, safety and tolerability of six popular prophylactic migraine interventions: topiramate, propranolol, gabapentin, amitriptyline, divalproex and valproate.

Results of our NMA indicated that three interventions may be particularly efficacious for reducing the corresponding symptoms of migraine: divalproex, propranolol and valproate. In our study, divalproex ranked the highest with respect to the reduction of monthly headache days whereas propranolol appeared to be the most preferable intervention for reducing headache frequency. Moreover, our study also suggested that valproate exhibited superior performance with respect to at least 50% reduction in headache attacks. Accordingly to the American Academy of Neurology (AAN) and the American Society of Headache (AHS), divalproex is classified as level-A medication and it is offered to patients for migraine prophylaxis [47]. Another study conducted by Kaniecki et al. revealed that both divalproex and propranolol significantly reduced headache frequency and the number of headache days compared to placebo,

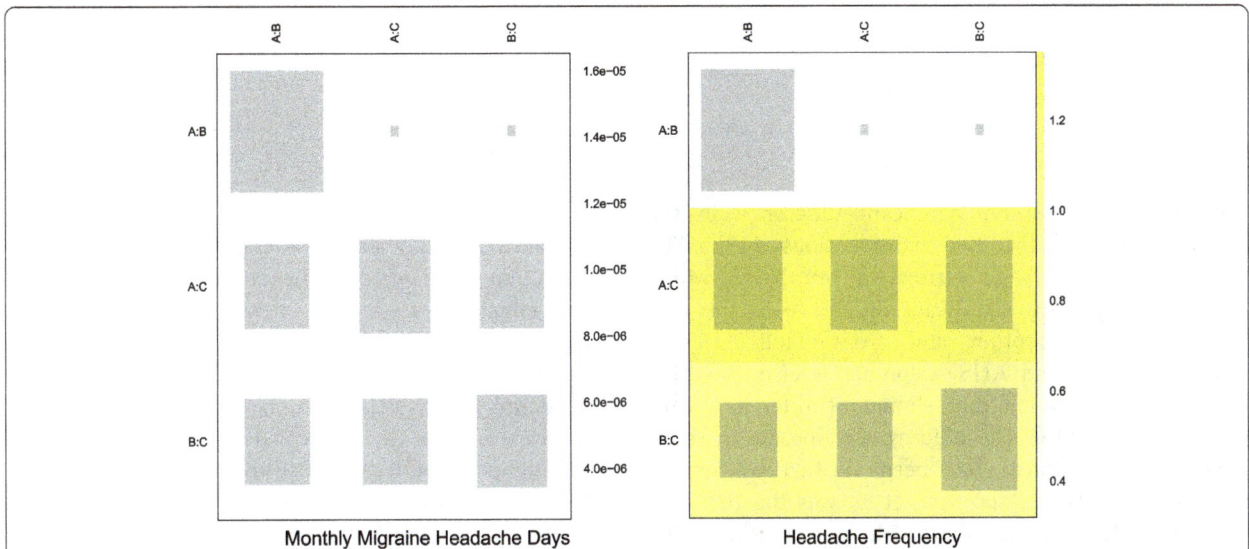

Fig. 15 Net heat plot of study designs with respect to monthly migraine headache days and headache frequency. The area of the gray squares displays the contribution of the direct estimate in design d (shown in the column) to the network estimate in design d (shown in the row). The colors are associated with the change in inconsistency between direct and indirect evidence (shown in the row) after detaching the effect (shown in the column). *Blue colors* indicate an increase and warm colors indicate a decrease (the stronger the intensity of the color, the stronger the change)

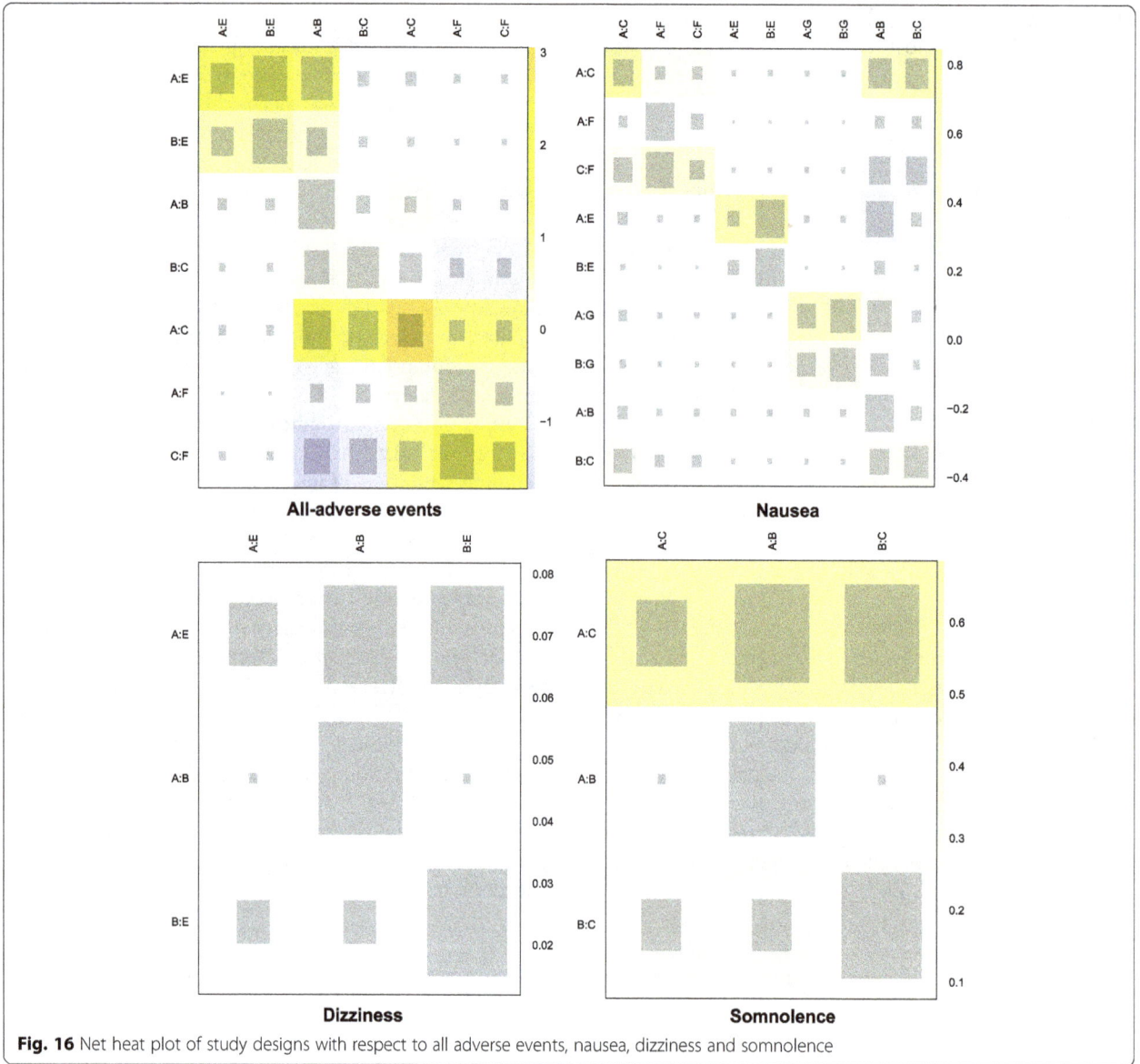

Fig. 16 Net heat plot of study designs with respect to all adverse events, nausea, dizziness and somnolence

however, there was no significant difference in the efficacy between the two interventions [48]. The above conclusions were verified by our NMA which did not suggest any significant difference in the efficacy between divalproex and propranolol. As suggested by AAN and AHS, valproate is also classified as level-A medication that should be offered to migraine patients [49]. The efficacy of valproate in reducing migraine attacks has been verified by several studies, for instance, Sørensen et al. was the first one who suggested that valproate exhibited a noteworthy effect on patients with severe migraine with respect to migraine prophylaxis [50]. Although our study suggested that patients with valproate were more likely to experience at least 50% reduction in migraine attacks than those with placebo, the wide

confidence interval resulted from potential inconsistency or inadequate evidence should be addressed by conducting large-scale studies in order to verify the above conclusions.

Apart from efficacy, the safety of migraine medication is another predominating factor that must be considered by physicians when selecting an appropriate intervention. As suggested by previous studies, migraine patients treated by antiepileptic drugs may experience several side-effects, including nausea, dizziness and paresthesia [51]. One significant result produced by our NMA is that patients with divalproex exhibited a significantly increased risk of nausea compared to those with placebo or other interventions. This result was confirmed by our SUCRA ranking tables in which the SUCRA value of

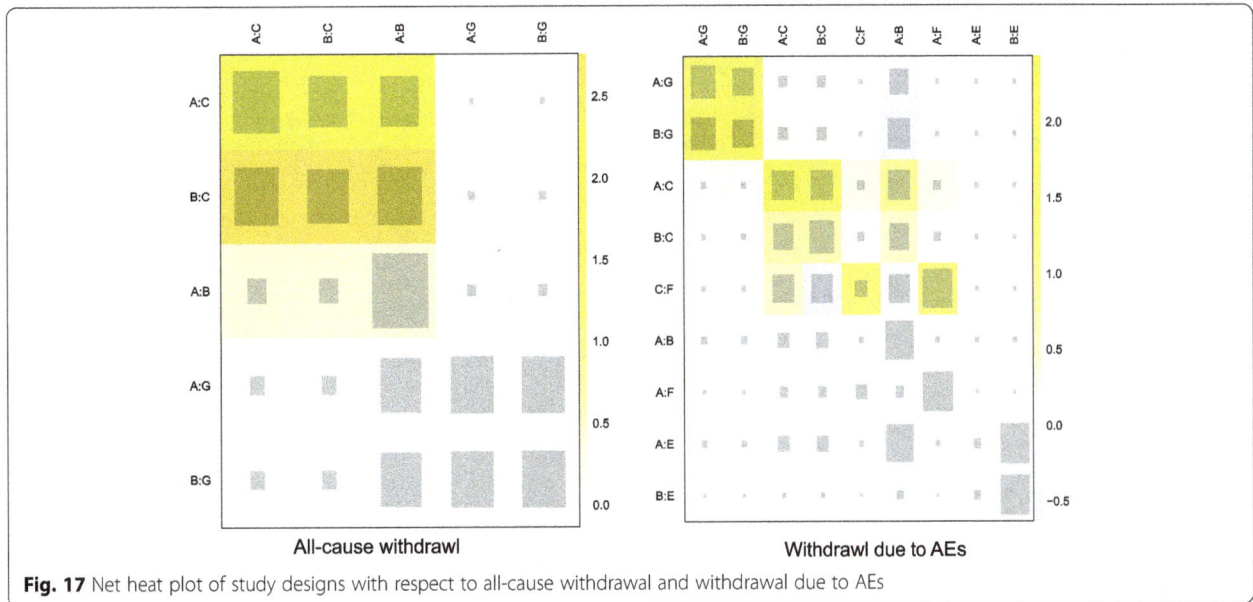

Fig. 17 Net heat plot of study designs with respect to all-cause withdrawal and withdrawal due to AEs

divalproex appeared to be the lowest with respect to the endpoint of nausea. Apart from that, our pairwise meta-analysis discovered that patients with divalproex were associated with a significantly increased risk of nausea compared to those with placebo. Furthermore, our NMA revealed that patients with divalproex may have poor medication compliance since they appeared to have an increased risk of withdrawal. We urged future researchers to design and conducted prospective studies in order to confirm the safety of divalproex.

Despite that some new findings have been suggested by our study, it is essential to discuss several key issues that may have impact on our conclusions. Firstly, we include both RCTs and crossover studies in our NMA; this may significantly increase the heterogeneity resulted from the design and implantation of different studies. For instance, crossover studies involves randomly assigning a sequence of interventions to different groups over the study period, therefore, the randomization technique used in crossover studies was completely different from that in RCTs. However, the inclusion of crossover studies did not enable us to adjust for the corresponding sequences where a serious of treatments was assigned. Furthermore, the inclusion of crossover studies produced some extra confounding factors that were not presented in RCTs. For instance, a wash-out period between interventions is often used in crossover studies and the duration of the wash-out period may have significant impact on medication compliance as well as on the corresponding endpoints. Our NMA did not adjust for the corresponding dose used for each intervention either. The above uncontrolled factors may independently affect our conclusion or interacted with each other, producing significant effect modification. Nevertheless,

the corresponding conclusions and limitations underlying our study provide researchers with key guidelines for designing new trials or prospective studies for migraine patients.

Conclusions

Our NMA suggested that topiramate, propranolol and divalproex may be more efficacious than other prophylactic medications. However, based on the above limitations, our results need to be interpreted with caution. Besides, safety and tolerability of divalproex should be further verified by future studies.

Additional files

Additional file 1:Table S1. Jadad scale of 32 studies included.

Additional file 2: Table S2. Ranking of migraine interventions using SUCRA values.

Additional file 3: Figure S1. Funnel plot of studies assessing the efficacy of migraine interventions.

Additional file 4: Figure S2. Funnel plot of studies assessing the safety of migraine interventions.

Additional file 5: Figure S3. Funnel plot of studies assessing the tolerability of migraine interventions.

Funding
None.

Authors' contributions
AH, DS, and CL initiated the concept and design of the study; collected data; prepared the manuscript; and finalized it according to the recommendations. AH, DS, and LZ initiated the study design, analyzed and interpreted the data. AH, DS, and LZ acquired the data and tested them for accuracy and integrity and interpreted the data. All authors read and approved the final manuscript.

Competing interest
The authors declare that they have no competing interests.

Author details
[1]Department of Neurosurgery, the Affiliated Yantai Yuhuangding Hospital of Qingdao University, 264000 Yantai, Shandong, China. [2]Department of Radiotherapy, the Affiliated Yantai Yuhuangding Hospital of Qingdao University, 264000 Yantai, Shandong, China. [3]Department of Pharmacy, Yantai Hospital of Traditional Chinese Medicine, 264000 Yantai, Shandong, China. [4]Department of Anesthesia, Yantai Hospital of Traditional Chinese Medicine, No. 39 Xingfu Road, Zhifu Disctrict, 264000 Yantai, Shandong, China.

References

1. Eyre HA, Air T, Pradhan A, Johnston J, Lavretsky H, Stuart MJ et al (2016) A meta-analysis of chemokines in major depression. Prog Neuropsychopharmacol Biol Psychiatry 68:1–8

2. Koenig J, Kemp AH, Feeling NR, Thayer JF, Kaess M (2016) Resting state vagal tone in borderline personality disorder: A meta-analysis. Prog Neuropsychopharmacol Biol Psychiatry 64:18–26

3. Ren J, Li H, Palaniyappan L, Liu H, Wang J, Li C et al (2014) Repetitive transcranial magnetic stimulation versus electroconvulsive therapy for major depression: a systematic review and meta-analysis. Prog Neuropsychopharmacol Biol Psychiatry 51:181–189

4. Polesel DN, Fukushiro DF, Andersen ML, Nozoe KT, Mari-Kawamoto E, Saito LP et al (2014) Anxiety-like effects of meta-chlorophenylpiperazine in paradoxically sleep-deprived mice. Prog Neuropsychopharmacol Biol Psychiatry 49:70–77

5. Na KS, Lee KJ, Lee JS, Cho YS, Jung HY (2014) Efficacy of adjunctive celecoxib treatment for patients with major depressive disorder: a meta-analysis. Prog Neuropsychopharmacol Biol Psychiatry 48:79–85

6. Wang K, Song LL, Cheung EF, Lui SS, Shum DH, Chan RC (2013) Bipolar disorder and schizophrenia share a similar deficit in semantic inhibition: a meta-analysis based on Hayling Sentence Completion Test performance. Prog Neuropsychopharmacol Biol Psychiatry 46:153–160

7. Wu YL, Ding XX, Sun YH, Yang HY, Chen J, Zhao X et al (2013) Association between MTHFR C677T polymorphism and depression: an updated meta-analysis of 26 studies. Prog Neuropsychopharmacol Biol Psychiatry 46:78–85

8. Schild AH, Pietschnig J, Tran US, Voracek M (2013) Genetic association studies between SNPs and suicidal behavior: a meta-analytical field synopsis. Prog Neuropsychopharmacol Biol Psychiatry 46:36–42

9. Niitsu T, Fabbri C, Bentini F, Serretti A (2013) Pharmacogenetics in major depression: a comprehensive meta-analysis. Prog Neuropsychopharmacol Biol Psychiatry 45:183–194

10. Yao L, Lui S, Liao Y, Du MY, Hu N, Thomas JA et al. (2013) White matter deficits in first episode schizophrenia: an activation likelihood estimation meta-analysis. Prog Neuropsychopharmacol Biol Psychiatry 45:100–106

11. Bartley CA, Hay M, Bloch MH (2013) Meta-analysis: aerobic exercise for the treatment of anxiety disorders. Prog Neuropsychopharmacol Biol Psychiatry 45:34–39

12. Du MY, Wu QZ, Yue Q, Li J, Liao Y, Kuang WH et al. (2012) Voxelwise meta-analysis of gray matter reduction in major depressive disorder. Prog Neuropsychopharmacol Biol Psychiatry 36(1):11–16

13. Vederine FE, Wessa M, Leboyer M, Houenou J (2011) A meta-analysis of whole-brain diffusion tensor imaging studies in bipolar disorder. Prog Neuropsychopharmacol Biol Psychiatry 35(8):1820–1826

14. Mikkelsen B, Pedersen KK, Christiansen LV (1986) Prophylactic treatment of migraine with tolfenamic acid, propranolol and placebo. Acta Neurol Scand 73(4):423–427

15. Pradalier A, Serratrice G, Collard M, Hirsch E, Feve J, Masson M et al. (1989) Long-acting propranolol in migraine prophylaxis: results of a double-blind, placebo-controlled study. Cephalalgia 9(4):247–253

16. Hering R, Kuritzky A (1992) Sodium valproate in the prophylactic treatment of migraine: a double-blind study versus placebo. Cephalalgia 12(2):81–84

17. Mathew NT, Saper JR, Silberstein SD, Rankin L, Markley HG, Solomon S et al. (1995) Migraine prophylaxis with divalproex. Arch Neurol 52(3):281–286

18. Bendtsen L, Jensen R, Olesen J (1996) A non-selective (amitriptyline), but not a selective (citalopram), serotonin reuptake inhibitor is effective in the prophylactic treatment of chronic tension-type headache. J Neurol Neurosurg Psychiatry 61(3):285–290

19. Diener HC, Foh M, Iaccarino C, Wessely P, Isler H, Strenge H et al. (1996) Cyclandelate in the prophylaxis of migraine: a randomized, parallel, double-blind study in comparison with placebo and propranolol. The Study group. Cephalalgia 16(6):441–447

20. Kaniecki RG (1997) A comparison of divalproex with propranolol and placebo for the prophylaxis of migraine without aura. Arch Neurol 54(9):1141–1145

21. Klapper J (1997) Divalproex sodium in migraine prophylaxis: a dose-controlled study. Cephalalgia 17(2):103–108

22. Mathew NT, Rapoport A, Saper J, Magnus L, Klapper J, Ramadan N et al (2001) Efficacy of gabapentin in migraine prophylaxis. Headache 41(2):119–128

23. Storey JR, Calder CS, Hart DE, Potter DL (2001) Topiramate in migraine prevention: a double-blind, placebo-controlled study. Headache 41(10):968–975

24. Freitag FG, Collins SD, Carlson HA, Goldstein J, Saper J, Silberstein S et al. (2002) A randomized trial of divalproex sodium extended-release tablets in migraine prophylaxis. Neurology 58(11):1652–1659

25. Brandes JL, Saper JR, Diamond M, Couch JR, Lewis DW, Schmitt J et al. (2004) Topiramate for migraine prevention: a randomized controlled trial. JAMA 291(8):965–973

26. Diener HC, Tfelt-Hansen P, Dahlöf C, Láinez MJA, Sandrini G, Wang SJ et al. (2004) Topiramate in migraine prophylaxis: Results from a placebo-controlled trial with propranolol as an active control. J Neurol 251(8):943–950

27. Mei D, Capuano A, Vollono C, Evangelista M, Ferraro D, Tonali P et al. (2004) Topiramate in migraine prophylaxis: a randomised double-blind versus placebo study. Neurol Sci 25(5):245–250

28. Silberstein SD, Neto W, Schmitt J, Jacobs D (2004) Topiramate in migraine prevention: results of a large controlled trial. Arch Neurol 61(4):490–495

29. Brandes JL, Kudrow DB, Rothrock JF, Rupnow MF, Fairclough DL, Greenberg SJ (2006) Assessing the ability of topiramate to improve the daily activities of patients with migraine. Mayo Clin Proc 81(10):1311–1319

30. Shaygannejad V, Janghorbani M, Ghorbani A, Ashtary F, Zakizade N, Nasr V (2006) Comparison of the effect of topiramate and sodium valporate in migraine prevention: a randomized blinded crossover study. Headache 46(4):642–648

31. Silberstein SD, Hulihan J, Karim MR, Wu SC, Jordan D, Karvois D et al (2006) Efficacy and tolerability of topiramate 200 mg/d in the prevention of migraine with/without aura in adults: a randomized, placebo-controlled, double-blind, 12-week pilot study. Clin Ther 28(7):1002–1011

32. de Tommaso M, Marinazzo D, Nitti L, Pellicoro M, Guido M, Serpino C et al. (2007) Effects of levetiracetam vs topiramate and placebo on visually evoked phase synchronization changes of alpha rhythm in migraine. Clin Neurophysiol 118(10):2297–2304

33. Diener HC, Bussone G, Van Oene JC, Lahaye M, Schwalen S, Goadsby PJ (2007) Topiramate reduces headache days in chronic migraine: a randomized, double-blind, placebo-controlled study. Cephalalgia 27(7):814–823

34. Diener HC, Kurth T, Dodick D (2007) Patent foramen ovale and migraine. Curr Pain Headache Rep 11(3):236–240

35. Gupta P, Singh S, Goyal V, Shukla G, Behari M (2007) Low-dose topiramate versus lamotrigine in migraine prophylaxis (the Lotolamp study). Headache 47(3):402–412

36. Silberstein SD, Lipton RB, Dodick DW, Freitag FG, Ramadan N, Mathew N et al. (2007) Efficacy and safety of topiramate for the treatment of chronic migraine: a randomized, double-blind, placebo-controlled trial. Headache 47(2):170–180

37. Ashtari F, Shaygannejad V, Akbari M (2008) A double-blind, randomized trial of low-dose topiramate vs propranolol in migraine prophylaxis. Acta Neurol Scand 118(5):301–305

38. Dodick DW, Freitag F, Banks J, Saper J, Xiang J, Rupnow M et al. (2009) Topiramate versus amitriptyline in migraine prevention: a 26-week, multicenter, randomized, double-blind, double-dummy, parallel-group noninferiority trial in adult migraineurs. Clin Ther 31(3):542–559

39. Holroyd KA, Cottrell CK, O'Donnell FJ, Cordingley GE, Drew JB, Carlson BW et al. (2010) Effect of preventive (β blocker) treatment, behavioural migraine management, or their combination on outcomes of optimised acute treatment in frequent migraine: Randomised controlled trial. BMJ 341(7776):769

40. Lipton RB, Silberstein S, Dodick D, Cady R, Freitag F, Mathew N et al. (2011) Topiramate intervention to prevent transformation of episodic migraine: the topiramate INTREPID study. Cephalalgia 31(1):18–30

41. Afshari D, Rafizadeh S, Rezaei M (2012) A comparative study of the effects of low-dose topiramate versus sodium valproate in migraine prophylaxis. Int J Neurosci 122(2):60–68

42. Silberstein S, Goode-Sellers S, Twomey C, Saiers J, Ascher J (2013) Randomized, double-blind, placebo-controlled, phase II trial of gabapentin enacarbil for migraine prophylaxis. Cephalalgia 33(2):101–111

43. Nofal WH, Mahmoud MS, Al Alim AA (2014) Does preoperative gabapentin affects the characteristics of post-dural puncture headache in parturients undergoing cesarean section with spinal anesthesia? Saudi J Anaesth 8(3):359–363

44. Sarchielli P, Messina P, Cupini LM, Tedeschi G, Di Piero V, Livrea P et al. (2014) Sodium valproate in migraine without aura and medication overuse headache: a randomized controlled trial. Eur Neuropsychopharmacol 24(8):1289–1297

45. Sadeghian H, Motiei-Langroudi R (2015) Comparison of Levetiracetam and sodium Valproate in migraine prophylaxis: A randomized placebo-controlled study. Ann Indian Acad Neurol 18(1):45–48

46. Trzesniak C, Kempton MJ, Busatto GF, de Oliveira IR, Galvao-de Almeida A, Kambeitz J et al. (2011) Adhesio interthalamica alterations in schizophrenia spectrum disorders: A systematic review and meta-analysis. Prog Neuropsychopharmacol Biol Psychiatry 35(4):877–886

47. Farrer TJ, Hedges DW (2011) Prevalence of traumatic brain injury in incarcerated groups compared to the general population: a meta-analysis. Prog Neuropsychopharmacol Biol Psychiatry 35(2):390–394

48. Woon FL, Sood S, Hedges DW (2010) Hippocampal volume deficits associated with exposure to psychological trauma and posttraumatic stress disorder in adults: a meta-analysis. Prog Neuropsychopharmacol Biol Psychiatry 34(7):1181–1188

49. Zai CC, Tiwari AK, Basile V, de Luca V, Muller DJ, Voineskos AN et al. (2010) Oxidative stress in tardive dyskinesia: genetic association study and meta-analysis of NADPH quinine oxidoreductase 1 (NQO1) and Superoxide dismutase 2 (SOD2, MnSOD) genes. Prog Neuropsychopharmacol Biol Psychiatry 34(1):50–56

50. Rahimi R, Nikfar S, Abdollahi M (2009) Efficacy and tolerability of Hypericum perforatum in major depressive disorder in comparison with selective serotonin reuptake inhibitors: a meta-analysis. Prog Neuropsychopharmacol Biol Psychiatry 33(1):118–127

51. Lin PY (2007) Meta-analysis of the association of serotonin transporter gene polymorphism with obsessive-compulsive disorder. Prog Neuropsychopharmacol Biol Psychiatry 31(3):683–689

12

OnabotulinumtoxinA effectiveness on chronic migraine, negative emotional states and sleep quality

Elif Ilgaz Aydinlar[*], Pinar Yalinay Dikmen, Seda Kosak and Ayse Sagduyu Kocaman

Abstract

Background: OnabotulinumtoxinA (OnabotA) is considered effective in in patients with chronic migraine (CM) who failed on traditional therapies. This study was designed to evaluate the effect of OnabotA injection series on migraine outcome, negative emotional states and sleep quality in patients with CM.

Methods: A total of 190 patients with CM (mean (SD) age: 39.3 (10.2) years; 87.9% were female) were included. Data on Pittsburgh sleep quality index (PSQI), headache frequency and severity, number of analgesics used, Migraine Disability Assessment Scale.

(MIDAS) scores and Depression, Anxiety and Stress Scale (DASS-21) were evaluated at baseline (visit 1) and 4 consecutive follow up visits, each conducted after OnabotA injection series; at week 12 (visit 2), week 24 (visit 3), week 36 (visit 4) and week 48 (visit 5) to evaluate change from baseline to follow up.

Results: From baseline to visit 5, significant decrease was noted in least square (LS) mean headache frequency (from 19.5 to 8.4, $p = 0.002$), headache severity (from 8.1 to 6.1, $p = 0.017$), number of analgesics (from 26.9 to 10.4, $p = 0.023$) and MIDAS scores (from 67.3 to 18.5, $p < 0.001$). No significant change from baseline was noted in global PSOI and DASS-21 scores throughout the study.

Conclusions: Our findings revealed that OnabotA therapy was associated with significant improvement in migraine outcome leading to decrease in headache frequency and severity, number of analgesics used and MIDAS scores. While no significant change was noted in overall sleep quality and prevalence of negative emotional states, patients without negative emotional states at baseline showed improved sleep quality throughout the study.

Keywords: Chronic migraine, Sleep quality, Headache, Analgesic, MIDAS, DASS-21

Background

Chronic Migraine (CM) is a complex and severely disabling neurological disorder, characterized by occurrence of headache on ≥15 days per month for >3 months with at least five attacks fulfilling criteria of migraine without aura on ≥8 days per month [1].

Having a prevalence of 1–3% documented in population-based studies [2], CM is considered to be a more disabling and burdensome disorder than episodic migraine (EM), as associated with greater

* Correspondence: elif.aydinlar@acibadem.edu.tr
Department of Neurology, Acibadem University School of Medicine, Içerenkoy, Kayisdagi Cd, 34752 Atasehir/Istanbul, Turkey

migraine-related disability [3], more frequent hospital admissions [4–6], poorer health-related quality of life (HRQoL) [4–7], higher amount of lost work and household productivity [4–6, 8], and increased risk for comorbidities [9] and medication overuse [10].

Increased comorbidity between migraine and several psychiatric conditions has consistently been reported with higher prevalence of mood and anxiety disorders, personality disorders and post-traumatic stress disorder (PTSD) among migraineurs than in the general population [11–13]. Also, increased headache frequency was shown to be correlated with higher rate of depression, anxiety and post-traumatic stress disorder [5, 14–16].

Recent studies also indicate a higher prevalence of poor sleep quality in patients with than without migraine and association of frequency of migraine headache with poor sleep quality [17–22].

This seems notable given the association of co-morbidities with increased burden of CM in terms of productivity loss, impaired HRQoL, healthcare utilization and emotional burden[5] as well as treatment complications and poor clinical outcomes [13].

Despite availability of preventive and abortive treatments as the mainstays of treatment for migraines, one-third of migraine sufferers remain symptomatic due to frequent partial response to treatment that leads to physical disability and high risk of medication overuse [22–24]. Therefore, development of new and effective therapeutic alternatives is of particular significance in the management of CM [24, 25].

Onabotulinumtoxin A (OnabotA) recently was discovered to be effective in preventing recurrent migraines in patients with CM who failed on traditional therapies [22, 26, 27]. Hence, based on data from PREEMPT (Phase 3 REsearch Evaluating Migraine Prophylaxis Therapy) trials confirming its efficacy in reduction of number of headache days and migraine days in CM patients with favorable safety and tolerability [28–31], OnabotA (155–195 U) is specifically indicated as a prophylactic treatment for CM in adults [26, 32].

The present study was designed to evaluate the effect of OnabotA injection series on migraine outcome, negative emotional states and sleep quality in patients with CM.

Methods
Study population
A total of 190 consecutive patients with CM (mean (SD) age: 39.3 (10.2) years; 87.9% were female) were included in this single-center prospective cohort study conducted between May 2012 and May 2016. After baseline visit at study enrollment (visit 1), patients were followed up for 48 weeks via 4 consecutive follow up visits each conducted after a new OnabotA injection series; at week 12 (visit 2), week 24 (visit 3), week 36 (visit 4) and week 48 (visit 5), respectively. Most of the patients had a history of prophylactic treatment for migraine which was either insufficient or was discontinued due to intolerance.

Written informed consent was obtained from each subject following a detailed explanation of the objectives and protocol of the study which was conducted in accordance with the ethical principles stated in the "Declaration of Helsinki" and approved by the Acibadem University Clinical Research Ethics Committee.

Study parameters
Data on patient demographics (age, gender), educational status, diagnosis (CM, CM + medication overuse),

migraine duration (year), family history for migraine, previous migraine treatments, migraine triggers are collected at baseline visit (visit 1). Data on migraine outcome [headache frequency and severity, number of analgesics used and Migraine Disability Assessment Scale (MIDAS) scores], sleep quality [Pittsburgh sleep quality index (PSQI)] and negative emotional states [Depression, Anxiety, and Stress Scale-21 (DASS-21)] were evaluated at baseline and follow up visits. Medication overuse was baseline of simple analgesics on ≥ 15 days. Follow up period was composed of 4 consecutive visits each conducted after a new OnabotA injection series; at week 12 (visit 2), week 24 (visit 3), week 36 (visit 4) and week 48 (visit 5), respectively. Change from baseline to follow up was evaluated based on data from visit 1 to visit 3 (24 weeks) for PSQI, from visit 1 to visit 4 (36 weeks) for DASS-21 scores, while based on data from visit 1 to visit 5 (48 weeks) for headache frequency and severity, number of analgesics used and MIDAS score. Data at visit 2, visit 3, visit 4 and visit 5 refer to changes in parameters observed after 1st, 2nd, 3rd and 4th OnabotA injection series, respectively.

Diagnosis of CM
CM was diagnosed based on International Classification of Headache Disorders (third revision) (ICHD-3 beta) diagnostic criteria that require headache occurring on ≥15 days per month for >3 months with at least five attacks fulfilling criteria of migraine without aura on ≥8 days per month [1].

OnabotA injection series
Administration of OnabotA was performed as 31 fixed-site, fixed-dose intramuscular injections applied at seven specified head and neck muscle points every 12 weeks for a minimum of 24 weeks (2 treatment cycles) according to injection scheme proposed in the PREEMPT studies [28, 29, 33]. We additionally administered OnabotA among occipitalis, temporalis or trapezius muscles using a follow-the-pain strategy.

MIDAS
The MIDAS is a 5-question tool to quantitatively evaluate the headache-related disability in terms of the number of days in the past 3 months and activity limitations due to migraine. MDAS was developed by Stewart et al.[34] and validated and checked for reliability for Turkish by Ertas et al. [35] The score obtained can be graded as follows: grade I (0 to 5 days) indicative of little or no disability; grade II (6 to 10 days), mild disability; grade III (11 to 20 days), moderate disability; and grade IV (greater than 21 days), severe disability.

DASS-21

The DASS-21 is a 21-item questionnaire which includes three self-report scales designed to measure the negative emotional states of depression, anxiety and stress. The Depression scale includes items that measure symptoms typically associated with dysphoric mood (e.g., sadness or worthlessness). The Anxiety scale includes items that are primarily related to symptoms of physical arousal, panic attacks, and fear (e.g., trembling or faintness). Finally, the Stress scale includes items that measure symptoms such as tension, irritability, and a tendency to overreact to stressful event. Each item is scored on a 4-point scale (0 = Did not apply to me at all, to 3 = Applied to me very much or most of the time) to rate the extent to which they have experienced each state over the past week. Sum of the score of each item reveals the total score with higher scores indicating greater levels of distress. Each state is categorized into normal/mild/moderate/severe/extremely severe based on cut-off scores recommended for depression (0-4/5-6/7-10/11-13/14+), anxiety (0-3/4-5/6-7/8-9/10+) and stress (0-7/8-9/10-12/13-16/17+) [36–38]. Psychometric properties of the Turkish version of the DASS was studied by Hekimoglu et al. and DASS was shown to be an excellent instrument for measuring features of depression, hyperarousal, and tension in clinical groups [39].

PSQI

The PSQI, used to assess sleep quality, was developed by Buysse et al. [40] and validated and checked for reliability for Turkish by Agargun et al. [41]. The scale consists of 24 items; eighteen items are scored and yield seven component scores. Each component is scored between 0 and 3 and the total of these scores gives the scale score. The total score ranges between 0 and 21 and the higher the score is, the worse the sleep quality. A total score under 5 indicates 'good sleep quality', while a score above 5 shows 'poor sleep quality'.

Statistical analysis

Statistical analysis was made using IBM SPSS Statistics (IBM Corp. Released 2012. IBM SPSS Statistics for Windows, Version 21.0, Armonk, NY: IBM Corp). Change over time analysis was based on number of patients with available data on both baseline (visit 1) and follow-up visits (visit 2 to 5), and performed via repeated measures variance analysis and McNemar test for continuous and categorical variables, respectively. Since time to follow up visits showed variability among patients, change over time analysis of continuous variables were adjusted for time (visit 2 = 12 weeks; visit 3 = 24 weeks; visit 4 = 36 weeks; visit 5 = 48 weeks). No specific procedure was defined for missing data. Data were expressed as n(%), mean (standard deviation; SD), median (inter-quartile range, IQR) and mean (lower and upper boundaries of 95% confidence interval; CI) where appropriate. $p < 0.05$ was considered statistically significant.

Results

Patient disposition and baseline characteristics

Of 190 patients; 101 (53.2%) attended at least one follow-up visit. Overall 98 (51.6%) patients attended visit 2, 58 (30.5%) patient visit 3, 34 (17.9%) patients visit 4, and 20 (10.5%) patients attend visit 5, which were performed at week 12, week 24, week 36 and week 48, respectively.

During the study period overall four injection series were applied per patient within a total treatment time of 48 weeks (median (IQR) 62.4 (53.8–85.2) weeks).

Most of the participants were university graduates (41.1%), diagnosed with CM per se (48.9%) without triggers (76.8%) and for median (IQR) 3.0 (1.0–10.0) years. Family history for migraine was evident in 28.9% of patients; while most common previous medication was non steroid anti-inflammatory drugs (88.4%). Medication overuse was evident in 76.2% of patients (Table 1).

Migraine outcome

Overall, mean (SD; median) headache frequency was 17.9 (7.8;15.0) at visit 1 and 6.8 (5.1;5.0) at visit 5. Median (IQR) headache severity scores were 8.0 (7.0–9.0) and 7.0 (5.0–7.0), number of analgesics used were 20.0 (15.0–30.0) and 5.5 (2.0–10.0) and MIDAS scores were 57.0 (35.5–75.0) and 10.0 (2.0–15.0) at visit 1 and visit 5, respectively (Table 2).

Mean headache frequency was significantly decreased from LS mean 19.5 at visit 1 to 6.8 at visit 2 ($p < 0.001$), to 7.5 at visit 3 ($p < 0.001$), to 5.4 at visit 4 ($p < 0.001$) and to 8.4 at visit 5 ($p = 0.002$) (Table 3).

Mean headache severity was significantly decreased from 8.1 at baseline to 6.2 at visit 2 ($p < 0.001$), to 5.8 at visit 3 and visit 4 ($p < 0.001$ for each) and to 6.1 at visit 5 ($p = 0.017$) (Table 3).

Mean number of analgesics used was significantly decreased from 26.9 at baseline to 7.8 at visit 2 ($p < 0.001$), to 8.7 at visit 3 ($p < 0.001$), to 5.1 at visit 4 ($p < 0.001$) and to 10.4 at visit 5 ($p = 0.023$) (Table 3).

Mean MIDAS score was decreased significantly from 67.3 at baseline to 17.4 at visit 2 ($p < 0.001$), to 15.3 at visit 3 ($p < 0.001$), to 9.3 at visit 4 ($p < 0.001$) and to 18.5 at visit 5 ($p < 0.001$) (Table 3).

Negative emotional states

DASS-21 revealed normal scores for depression (60.0, 52.0, 60.0 and 57.1%), anxiety (56.5, 51.5, 41.2 and 57.1%) and stress (51.8, 54.5, 29.4 and 42.9%) in similar percentage of patients at visit 1, visit 2, visit 3 and visit 4, respectively (Table 4).

Table 1 Patient characteristics

Age (year), mean (SD)	39.3 (10.2)
Gender, n(%)	
Male	23 (12.1)
Female	167 (87.9)
Total	190 (100.0)
Educational status, n(%)	
Primary school	9 (4.7)
High school	22 (11.6)
University	78 (41.1)
MSc & PhD	9 (4.7)
Missing	72
Diagnosis n(%)	
Chronic migraine	93 (48.9)
Chronic migraine + medication overuse	97 (51.1)
Migraine duration (year), median (IQR)	3.0 (1.0–10.0)
Family history for migraine, n(%)	
Present	55 (28.9)
Absent	61 (32.1)
Missing	74
Previous migraine treatments, n(%)	
Non-steroid anti-inflammatory drugs	168 (88.4)
Antiepileptic	61 (32.1)
Antidepressants	57 (30.0)
Beta blockers	24 (12.6)
Calcium channel blockers	1 (0.5)
Migraine triggers, n(%)	
None	146 (76.8)
At least one trigger	44 (23.2)
Air/weather change	13 (6.8)
Anxiety/depression	15 (7.9)
Fasting	21 (11.1)
Food/beverage	12 (6.3)
Insomnia	33 (17.4)
Menstruation	22 (11.6)
Stress	35 (18.4)

IQR interquartile range

Mild-to-moderate depression (29.4% at visit 1, 28.6% at visit 4), anxiety (25.9% at visit 1, 28.6% at visit 4) and stress (35.3% at visit 1, 42.9% at visit 4) was evident in remarkable percentage of patients throughout the study period, while severe-to-extremely severe depression (10.6% at visit 1, 14.3% at visit 4), anxiety (17.7% at visit 1, 14.3% at visit 4) and stress (12.9% at visit 1, 14.3% at visit 4) were also noted in less than 15% of patients.

Based on patients with valid data for both baseline and follow up visits, no significant change was noted in percentage of patients categorized to have normal anxiety, depression and stress scores at each follow up visit (Table 5).

Sleep quality

Overall, median (IQR) global score at visit 1 and visit 5 were 9.0 (5.0–12.0) and 4.0 (1.0–7.0), respectively (Table 6).

Based on patients with valid data for both baseline and follow up visits, no significant difference was noted in global scores and thus overall sleep quality from baseline to visit 2 or visit 3. Considering component scores, mean (95% CI lower bound-upper bound) scores for subjective sleep quality (from baseline 1.7 (1.4–2.0) to 1.1 (0.8–1.5) at visit 2, $p = 0.002$), sleep latency (from baseline 1.7 (1.4–2.0) to 1.1 (0.8–1.5 at visit 2, $p = 0.002$) and sleep disturbance (from baseline 1.7 (1.4–2.0) to 1.2 (0.9–1.6) at visit 2, $p = 0.013$) components improved significantly from baseline to visit 2 (Table 7).

Sleep quality with respect to DASS-21 scores

Good sleep quality was noted at visit 1, visit 2 and visit 3 34.3, 40.0 and 57.1% of patients with normal depression scores at visit 1, in 38.7, 45.5 and 50.0% of patients with normal anxiety scores at visit 1, and in 33.3, 46.2 and 60.0% of patients with normal stress scores at visit 1, respectively (Table 8).

Adverse events and treatment alterations under OnabotA therapy

OnabotA therapy was associated with minor and temporary side effects (e.g., asymmetry of the position of the eyebrows and neck ache) in some patients. In one patient who has a very thin cervical region, dysphagia and difficulty in swallowing appeared while regressed after the third week of therapy. Treatment was continued in this patient with omission of further injections to the cervical area.

Treatment alterations included discontinuation of OnabotA therapy ($n = 2$), addition of antiepileptic ($n = 3$) or SSRI ($n = 9$) medications and discontinuation of ongoing antiepileptic ($n = 3$) or SSRI ($n = 1$) medications.

Discussion

Our findings revealed that administration of four OnabotA injection series over 48 weeks in chronic migraineurs was associated with a significant improvement in all migraine parameters including headache frequency and severity, number of analgesics used and MIDAS scores, while no significant change from baseline was noted in overall sleep quality and prevalence of negative emotional states. Patients without negative emotional states at baseline showed improved sleep quality throughout the study.

Table 2 Overall headache frequency and severity, analgesic use and MIDAS scores

	Headache frequency	Headache severity	Number of analgesics	MIDAS score
	Median (IQR)	Median (IQR)	Median (IQR)	Median (IQR)
Visit 1 ($n = 185$)	15.0(12.0–25.0)	8.0(7.0–9.0)	20.0(15.0–30.0)	57.0(35.5–75.0)
Visit 2 ($n = 89$)	5.0(3.0–10.0)	7.0(5.0–8.0)	5.0(2.0–10.0)	10.5(1.5–23.0)
Visit 3 ($n = 55$)	5.0(2.0–10.0)	6.0(5.0–7.0)	4.0(1.0–10.0)	9.0(3.0–24.0)
Visit 4 ($n = 31$)	4.0(1.0–9.0)	6.0(5.0–8.0)	4.0(1.0–10.0)	6.0(2.0–10.0)
Visit 5 ($n = 19$)	5.0(2.0–10.0)	7.0(5.0–7.0)	5.5(2.0–10.0)	10.0(2.0–15.0)

IQR inter-quartile range, *n* patient count without missing data

Significant reduction in monthly headache frequency, headache severity, number of analgesics used and MIDAS scores in our cohort support the efficacy of OnabotA in reduction of the frequency, intensity, and duration of chronic migraines as well as decreasing medication overuse among CM patients who failed on traditional preventive therapies [22, 25–27, 42–44].

Reduction in MIDAS scores, indicating lesser amount of lost work and personal time due to migraine [6], after OnabotA therapy in our cohort seems notable given that a day lived with severe migraine is considered to be as disabling as a day lived with dementia, quadriplegia or acute psychosis and more disabling than blindness, paraplegia, angina or rheumatoid arthritis [4, 45, 46].

CM has been associated with a high intake of abortive medications with estimated analgesic overuse in 50–80% of patients with CM that may lead to the development of medication overuse headache (MOH) [47]. Given the similar rates of medication overuse (76.2%) in our cohort at baseline, reduction in in number of analgesics used starting from the first injection and consistently throughout the study period emphasizes the potential role of OnabotA therapy in prevention of MOH via headache episode reduction [25, 42, 48–50].

In terms of monthly headache frequency, headache severity, number of analgesics used and MIDAS scores our findings support the association of OnabotA therapy with rapid improvement in migraine parameters usually after the first session as reported in past studies [26, 27, 30, 51–53].

The rapid improvement of migraine parameters after OnabotA therapy has been linked to the combined pharmacological and the placebo effect at the beginning of the treatment [51, 52], while increased benefit offered via repeated OnabotA injections over time is associated with a prophylactic cumulative effect [31, 54]. Also, patients who respond well to therapy early have been suggested to maintain and continue these reductions over at least 2 years [27, 55–57], while limited data are available on long-term efficacy of OnabotA therapy with evaluation of efficacy only up to1 year in most of clinical trials [42, 44, 50].

Alike to our findings, use of four OnabotA injections over 48 weeks in CM patients was reported to be associated with significant improvement in monthly headache days, migraine days and medication days that continued throughout the entire study period [42]. Nonetheless, in a longer-term study with seven OnabotA injections in CM patients, based on a decrease in initial efficacy of OnabotA therapy after the third injection, authors concluded that actual improvement and amelioration of daily headache under OnabotA therapy needs several months to be consolidated [52].

Long-term efficacy of OnabotA in CM patients has recently been evaluated in some studies based on administration of OnabotA therapy for 2 years [25], 4 years [43] and 7–9 injections series [52, 58]. However, while finding are consistent regarding long-term efficacy of therapy with no serious adverse events in responders, they varied in terms of durability of benefit, non-responder rates and the length and necessity of withdrawal of treatment at scheduled times [25, 43, 52, 58].

Both depression and anxiety have been proposed to be a risk factor for migraine chronification [13, 59, 60], while migraine headache frequency and headache severity were reported to be associated with higher rate of depression and anxiety disorders [4, 5, 14, 61]. Accordingly, identification of abnormal scores for depression, anxiety and stress in almost half of patients in our cohort is in line with higher rates of self-reported mood and anxiety disorders in patients with CM as compared with general population and EM patients [4, 5, 13, 14] with more than 40.0% of CM patients to meet criteria for moderate to severe anxiety and depression [4, 13].

Reduction in headache frequency via 24-week OnabotA therapy was reported to be associated with reduction in depression (via Beck Depression Inventory-II) and anxiety scores (Generalized Anxiety Disorder-7 scale) in a past among CM patients [62]. In fact, even a direct effect of OnabotA injection in amelioration of depressive symptoms has been suggested that probably occur via the facial feedback mechanism with consideration of OnabotA as a

Table 3 Change in severity, analgesic use, MIDAS scores and headache frequency at follow-up visits

		Headache severity	Number of analgesics	MIDAS score	Headache frequency
Baseline	n	89	80	66	89
	LS mean	8.1	26.9	67.3	19.5
Week 12	n	89	80	66	89
	LS mean (p)	6.2 (<0.001)	7.8 (<0.001)	17.4 (0.001)	6.8 ($p < 0.001$)
Week 24	n	52	50	47	55
	LS mean (p)	5.8 (<0.001)	8.7 (<0.001)	15.3 (<0.001)	7.5 (<0.001)
Week 36	n	31	28	24	30
	LS mean (p)	5.8 (<0.001)	5.1 (<0.001)	9.3 (<0.001)	5.4 (<0.001)
Week 48	n	19	18	17	19
	LS mean (p)	6.1 (0.017)	10.4 (0.023)	18.5 (<0.001)	8.4 (0.002)

LS mean least square mean, n patient count with valid data at each visit, P p value of repeated measures variance analysis with reference to baseline

safe adjunctive treatment to pharmacotherapy for major depressive disorder [63].

In this regard, it seems notable that despite significant reductions obtained via OnabotA therapy in both monthly headache frequency and headache severity in our cohort, no significant change from baseline occurred in depression, anxiety and stress rates throughout the study.

High rates of negative emotional states regardless of the ongoing OnabotA therapy in our patients seems notable given the impact of psychiatric comorbidities on disease prognosis, treatment, and clinical outcomes and higher prevalence of severe headache-related disability, headache impact and poor quality of life in migraineurs with than without psychiatric comorbidities [11, 13, 64]. Hence our findings emphasize consideration of co-morbid psychiatric disorders in diagnostic evaluation and formulation of treatment plan in CM patients, being aware of the likely negative impact of co-morbid psychiatric disorder on treatment outcomes, adherence and quality of life [5, 14, 65].

Identification of poor sleep quality at baseline in 72.9% of our patients seems consistent with high prevalence (30–79%) of co-morbid poor sleep quality among migraineurs [20, 66–68], particularly in those with 8 or more migraine days per month [17]. Higher prevalence of poor sleep quality was also noted in patients with migraine compared to those without migraine [17–21], while high migraine frequency was shown to correlate with poor sleep quality and a higher prevalence of poor sleepers in chronic migraineurs [21].

In a past study on the effects of OnabotA on jaw motor events during sleep in sleep bruxism patients, no significant change from baseline was noted in usual sleep variables such as sleep efficiency, arousal index, sleep stages, or awakenings per hour during follow-up recordings [69].

Similarly, our findings revealed no direct effect of OnabotA injection on overall sleep quality at week 12 and week 24, while significant improvement in subjective sleep quality, sleep latency and sleep disturbance at week 12. This seems notable given the reported association of higher migraine frequency with higher scores for certain domains of PSQI such as "cannot get to sleep within 30 minutes," "wake up in the middle of the night or early morning," and "bad dreams" among migraineurs [21].

Sleep-related migraine is considered to be associated with a more severe and disabling clinical course given the increased mean attack severity and monthly use of

Table 4 DASS-21 anxiety, depression and stress scores at study visits

	DASS-21-Depression score, n (%)				DASS-21-Anxiety score, n (%)				DASS-21-Stress score, n (%)			
Severity	Visit 1	Visit 2	Visit 3	Visit 4	Visit 1	Visit 2	Visit 3	Visit 4	Visit 1	Visit 2	Visit 3	Visit 4
Normal	51 (60.0)	13 (52.0)	9 (60.0)	4 (57.1)	48 (56.5)	17 (51.5)	7 (41.2)	4 (57.1)	44 (51.8)	18 (54.5)	5 (29.4)	3 (42.9)
Mild	10 (11.8)	6 (24.0)	2 (13.3)	0 (0)	9 (10.6)	5 (15.2)	3 (17.6)	1 (14.3)	14 (16.5)	6 (18.2)	5 (29.4)	1 (14.3)
Moderate	15 (17.6)	2 (8.0)	3 (20.0)	2 (28.6)	13 (15.3)	5 (15.2)	6 (35.3)	1 (14.3)	16 (18.8)	5 (15.2)	6 (35.3)	2 (28.6)
Severe	6 (7.1)	3 (12.0)	1 (6.7)	0 (0)	10 (11.8)	4 (12.1)	0 (0)	0 (0)	7 (8.2)	4 (12.1)	1 (5.9)	1 (14.3)
Extremely severe	3 (3.5)	1 (4.0)	0 (0)	1 (14.3)	5 (5.9)	2 (6.1)	1 (5.9)	1 (14.3)	4 (4.7)	0 (0)	0 (0)	0 (0)
Total	85 (100)	25 (100)	15 (100)	7 (100)	85 (100)	33 (100)	17 (100)	7 (100)	85 (100)	33 (100)	17 (100)	7 (100)

Table 5 Change in DASS-21 anxiety, depression and stress scores from baseline at study visits

Severity, n (%)	Change at visit 2		Change at visit 3		Change at visit 4	
DASS-21-Depression score	Visit 1	Visit 2	Visit 1	Visit 3	Visit 1	Visit 4
Normal	14 (56.0)	13 (52.0)	8 (53.3)	9 (60.0)	4 (57.1)	4 (57.1)
Abnormal	11 (44.0)	12 (48.0)	7 (46.7)	6 (40.0)	3 (42.9)	3 (42.9)
Total	25 (100)	25 (100)	15 (100)	15 (100)	7 (100)	7 (100)
P value[a]	1.000		1.000		1.000	
DASS-21-Anxiety score	Visit 1	Visit 2	Visit 1	Visit 3	Visit 1	Visit 4
Normal	18 (54.5)	17 (51.5)	7 (41.2)	7 (41.2)	3 (42.9)	4 (57.1)
Abnormal	15 (45.5)	16 (48.5)	10 (58.8)	10 (58.8)	4 (57.1)	3 (42.9)
Total	33 (100)	33 (100)	17 (100)	17 (100)	7 (100)	7 (100)
P value[a]	1.000		1.000		1.000	
DASS-21-Stress score	Visit 1	Visit 2	Visit 1	Visit 3	Visit 1	Visit 4
Normal	18 (54.5)	18 (54.5)	4 (23.5)	5 (29.4)	3 (42.9)	3 (42.9)
Abnormal	15 (45.5)	15 (45.5)	13 (76.5)	12 (70.6)	4 (57.1)	4 (57.1)
Total	33 (100)	33 (100)	17 (100)	17 (100)	7 (100)	7 (100)
P value[a]	1.000		1.000		1.000	

[a]McNemar test Comparisons for visit 5 is not performed due to small number patients with valid data

symptomatic drugs in patients with than without sleep related migraine despite similar monthly headache frequency [70].

Although data on sleep quality are available for only two OnabotA injections in our cohort, given that patients without negative emotional states at baseline showed improved sleep quality throughout the study, maintenance of co-morbid negative emotional states throughout the study seems to be associated with lack of improvement in overall sleep quality, despite significantly decreased migraine frequency.

Nonetheless, it should also be noted that while the presence of negative emotional states such as depression was reported to be reciprocally associated with poor sleep quality [66, 71] and migraine history and comorbid

anxiety and depression were shown as predictors of sleep quality [20] in some studies, poor sleep quality was shown to be associated uniquely with migraine itself, regardless of comorbid depression, anxiety or sleep disorders in other studies, particularly among EM patients [17, 44, 72, 73].

Certain limitations to this study should be considered. First, due to observational nature, non-randomized allocation and thereby the likelihood of main selection bias and confounding is possible. Second, although provide data on real-life clinical practice, potential lack of generalizability seems another important limitation due to single-center design of the study. Third, lack of intervention considering timing and number of follow up visits in accordance with the observational nature caused

Table 6 Overall PSQI scores at study visits

	Global score	Sleep quality, n(%)		Component scores						
				Subjective sleep quality	Sleep latency	Sleep duration	Habitual sleep efficiency	Sleep disturbances	Use of sleep medications	Daytime dysfunction
	Median (IQR)	Good	Poor	Median (IQR)	Median (IQR)	Median (IQR)	Median (IQR)	Median (IQR)	Median (IQR)	Median (IQR)
Visit 1 (n = 59)	9.0 (5.0–12.0)	16 (27.1)	43 (72.9)	2.0 (1.0–2.0)	1.0 (1.0–2.0)	1.0 (0.0–2.0)	1.0 (0.0–2.0)	2.0 (1.0–2.0)	0.0 (0.0–1.0)	1.0 (0.0–2.0)
Visit 2 (n = 28)	7.0 (3.0–9.5.0)	11 (39.3)	17 (60.7)	1.0 (1.0–2.0)	1.0 (1.0–2.0)	1.0 (0.0–2.0)	0.5 (0.0–2.0)	1.0 (1.0–2.0)	0.0 (0.0–1.0)	1.0 (0.0–2.0)
Visit 3 (n = 14)	10.0 (5.0–15.0)	4 (28.6)	10 (71.4)	2.0 (1.0–2.0)	2.0 (0.0–2.0)	2.0 (1.0–3.0)	1.5 (1.0–2.0)	2.0 (1.0–2.0)	0.0 (0.0–0.0)	2.0 (0.0–2.0)
Visit 4 (n = 7)	8.0 (7.0–15.0)	1 (14.3)	6 (85.7)	1.0 (1.0–2.0)	1.0 (0.0–2.0)	2.0 (1.0–3.0)	2.0 (1.0–3.0)	1.0 (1.0–2.0)	0.0 (0.0–2.0)	2.0 (1.0–2.0)
Visit 5 (n = 3)	4.0 (1.0–7.0)	2 (66.7)	1 (33.3)	1.0 (0.0–1.0)	0.0 (0.0–1.0)	0.0 (0.0–1.0)	0.0 (0.0–1.0)	1.0 (1.0–2.0)	0.0 (0.0–0.0)	1.0 (0.0–2.0)

IQR inter-quartile range (percentile 25 – percentile 75), *SD* standard deviation, *n* patient count without missing data

Table 7 Change in PSQI scores at follow up visits

		Global score	Sleep quality		Component scores						
					Subjective sleep quality	Sleep latency	Sleep duration	Habitual sleep efficiency	Sleep disturbance	Use of sleep medication	Daytime dysfunction
		Mean (95% CI)	n(%)		Mean (95% CI)						
Visit 2 (week 12)	n[a]	25	28		24	24	24	24	24	24	24
	baseline	9.5(7.8;11.3)	good	9 (32.1)	1.7(1.4;2.0)	1.7(1.4;2.0)	1.3(0.8;1.8)	1.4(0.9;2.0)	1.7(1.4;2.0)	0.6(0.1;1.0)	1.4(0.8;1.9)
			poor	19 (67.9)							
	current	8.0(5.8;10.1)	good	11 (39.3)	1.1(0.8;1.5)	1.1(0.8;1.5)	1.3(0.9;1.8)	1.3(0.7;1.9)	1.2(0.9;1.6)	0.7(0.2;1.2)	1.0(0.6;1.4)
			poor	17 (60.7)							
	p value	0.185[1]		0.727[2]	**0.002[1]**	**0.002[1]**	0.824[1]	0.724[1]	**0.013[1]**	0.531[1]	0.192[1]
Visit 3 (week 24)	n[a]	13	13		13	13	13	13	13	13	13
	baseline	9.4(6.8;12.1)	good	3 (21.4)	1.8(1.3;2.3)	1.8(1.3;2.3)	1.3(0.5;2.1)	1.6(0.8;2.4)	1.8(1.4;2.2)	0.4(−0.;1.2)	1.3(0.3;2.4)
			poor	11 (78.6)							
	current	10.5(6.0;15.0)	good	4 (28.6)	1.7(1.2;2.2)	1.7(1.2;2.2)	1.6(0.6;2.6)	1.6(0.7;2.4)	1.8(1.1;2.4)	0.9(−0.1;1.8)	1.7(0.8;2.5)
			poor	10 (71.4)							
	p value	0.531[1]		1.000[2]	0.590[1]	0.590[1]	0.570[1]	0.940[1]	0.882[1]	0.278[1]	0.205[1]

CI confidence interval
[a]number of patients without missing data (data available for both baseline and the specific follow up visit)
[1]Repeated measures variance analysis, [2]McNemar test. Comparisons for visit 4 and, visit 5 could not be performed due to small number patients with valid data
Values in bold indicate statistical significance (p <0.05)

relatively limited follow-up data and the frequency of patient visits to be not uniform with considerable loss to follow up rate challenging analysis of sleep and mood variables. Fourth, analysis of data on negative emotional states and sleep quality were based on self-report rather than objective measures. However, our analysis was based on use of validated questionnaires along with evidence on high concordance between self-report instruments and clinical diagnosis of psychiatric disorders [13]. Lack of follow up data on sleep quality after second OnabotA injection, lack of data on inter-individual variations in headache characteristics with likely impact on therapeutic response as well as lack of data on adverse events are other limitations which otherwise would extend the knowledge achieved in the current study.

Conclusions

In conclusion, our findings in a cohort of chronic migraineurs revealed that OnabotA injection was associated with significant improvement in migraine outcome

Table 8 Sleep quality with respect to DASS-21 anxiety, depression and stress scores

	Visit 1			Visit 2			Visit 3		
	good SQ	poor SQ	Total	good SQ	poor SQ	Total	good SQ	poor SQ	Total
	n(%)								
DASS 21-depression score									
Normal	12 (34.3)	23 (65.7)	35 (100)	4 (40.0)	6 (60.0)	10 (100)	4 (57.1)	3 (42.9)	7 (100)
Abnormal	4 (16.7)	20 (83.3)	24 (100)	2 (22.2)	7 (77.8)	9 (100)	0 (0)	6 (100)	6 (100)
Total	16 (27.1)	43 (72.9)	59 (100)	6 (31.6)	13 (68.4)	19 (100)	4 (30.8)	9 (69.2)	13 (100)
DASS 21-anxiety score									
Normal	12 (38.7)	19 (61.3)	31 (100)	5 (45.5)	6 (54.5)	11 (100)	3 (50.0)	3 (50.0)	6 (100)
Abnormal	4 (14.3)	24 (85.7)	28 (100)	3 (25.0)	9 (75)	12 (100)	1 (14.3)	6 (85.7)	7 (100)
Total	16 (27.1)	43 (72.9)	59 (100)	8 (34.8)	15 (65.2)	23 (100)	4 (30.8)	9 (69.2)	13 (100)
DASS 21-stress score									
Normal	10 (33.3)	20 (66.7)	30 (100)	6 (46.2)	7 (53.8)	13 (100)	3 (60.0)	2 (40.0)	5 (100)
Abnormal	6 (20.7)	23 (79.3)	29 (100)	2 (20)	8 (80)	10 (100)	1 (12.5)	7 (87.5)	8 (100)
Total	16 (27.1)	43 (72.9)	59 (100)	8 (34.8)	15 (65.2)	23 (100)	4 (30.8)	9 (69.2)	13 (100)

SQ sleep quality
Visit 4 to 5 was not evaluated because of small number of data

leading to decrease in headache frequency and severity, number of analgesics used and MIDAS scores. While no significant change was noted in overall sleep quality and prevalence of negative emotional states with OnabotA injections, patients without negative emotional states at baseline showed improved sleep quality throughout the study. There is a need for future larger-scale long-term longitudinal studies addressing the durability as well as predictors of efficacy of OnabotA in CM patients.

Abbreviations
CM: Chronic migraine; DASS-21: Depression, anxiety, and stress scale-21; HRQoL: Health-related quality of life; ICHD: International classification of headache disorders; MIDAS: Migraine disability assessment scale; MOH: Medication overuse headache; OnabotA: OnabotulinumtoxinA; PREEMPT: Phase 3 research evaluating migraine prophylaxis therapy; PSQI: Pittsburgh sleep quality index; PTSD: Post-traumatic stress disorder

Funding
None.

Authors' contributions
EIA contributed to conception/design of the research; EIA, PYD, ASK and SK contributed to acquisition, analysis, or interpretation of the data; EIA, PYD, ASK and SK drafted the manuscript; EIA, PYD and ASK critically revised the manuscript; and EIA agrees to be fully accountable for ensuring the integrity and accuracy of the work. All authors read and approved the final manuscript.

Competing interests
The authors declare that they have no competing interests.

References
1. International Headache Society. Revised International Headache Society criteria for chronic migraine. Available at: https://www.ichd-3.org/appendix/a1-migraine/a1-3-chronic-migraine-alternative-criteria Accessed 25 Apr 2016
2. Natoli JL, Manack A, Dean B, Butler Q, Turkel CC, Stovner L, Lipton RB (2010) Global prevalence of chronic migraine: a systematic review. Cephalalgia 30: 599–609
3. Bigal ME, Rapoport AM, Lipton RB, Tepper SJ, Sheftell FD (2003) Assessment of migraine disability using the Migraine Disability Assessment (MIDAS) questionnaire. A comparison of chronic migraine with episodic migraine. Headache 43:336–342
4. Blumenfeld AM, Varon SF, Wilcox TK, Buse DC, Kawata AK, Manack A, Goadsby PJ, Lipton RB (2011) Disability, HRQoL and resource use among chronic and episodic migraineurs: results from the international burden of migraine study (IBMS). Cephalalgia 31:301–315
5. Buse DC, Manack A, Serrano D, Turkel C, Lipton RB (2010) Sociodemographic and comorbidity profiles of chronic migraine and episodic migraine sufferers. J Neurol Neurosurg Psychiatry 81:428–432
6. Stewart WF, Wood GC, Manack A, Varon SF, Buse DC, Lipton RB (2010) Employment and work impact of chronic migraine and episodic migraine. J Occup Environ Med 52:8–14
7. Meletiche DM, Lofland JH, Young WB (2001) Quality of life differences between patients with episodic and transformed migraine. Headache 41: 573–578
8. Bigal ME, Serrano D, Reed M, Lipton RB (2008) Chronic migraine in the population: burden, diagnosis, and satisfaction with treatment. Neurology 71:559–566
9. Katsarava Z, Buse DC, Manack AN, Lipton RB (2012) Defining the differences between episodic migraine and chronic migraine. Curr Pain Headache Rep 16:86–92

10. Bigal ME, Rapoport AM, Sheftell FD, Tepper SJ, Lipton RB (2004) Transformed migraine and medication overuse in a tertiary headache centre-clinical characteristics and treatment outcomes. Cephalalgia 24:483–490
11. Jette N, Patten S, Williams J, Becker W, Wiebe S (2008) Comorbidity of migraine and psychiatric disorders: a national population-based study. Headache 48:501–516
12. Lanteri-Minet M, Radat F, Chautard M-H, Lucas C (2005) Anxiety and depression associated with migraine: influence on migraine subjects' disability and quality of life, and acute migraine management. Pain 118:319–326
13. Buse DC, Silberstein SD, Manack AN, Papapetropoulos S, Lipton RB (2013) Psychiatric comorbidities of episodic and chronic migraine. J Neurol 260: 1960–1969
14. Zwart JA, Dyb G, Hagen K, Ødegård KJ, Dahl AA, Bovim G, Stovner LJ (2003) Depression and anxiety disorders associated with headache frequency. The Nord-Trøndelag Health Study. Eur J Neurol 10:147–152
15. Juang KD, Wang SJ, Fuh JL, Lu SR, Su TP (2000) Comorbidity of depressive and anxiety disorders in chronic daily headache and its subtypes. Headache 40:818–823
16. Peterlin BL, Tietjen G, Meng S, Lidicker J, Bigal M (2008) Post-traumatic stress disorder in episodic and chronic migraine. Headache 48:517–522
17. Seidel S, Hartl T, Weber M, Matterey S, Paul A, Riederer F, Gharabaghi M, Wöber-Bingöl C, Wöber C, PAMINA Study Group (2009) Quality of sleep, fatigue and daytime sleepiness in migraine—a controlled study. Cephalalgia 29:662–669
18. Sadeghniiat K, Rajabzadeh A, Ghajarzadeh M, Ghafarpour M (2013) Sleep quality and depression among patients with migraine. Acta Med Iran 51: 784–788
19. Morgan I, Eguia F, Gelaye B, Peterlin BL, Tadesse MG, Lemma S, Berhane Y, Williams MA (2015) Sleep disturbances and quality of life in Sub-Saharan African migraineurs. J Headache Pain 16:18
20. Zhu Z, Fan X, Li X, Tan G, Chen L, Zhou J (2013) Prevalence and predictive factors for poor sleep quality among migraineurs in a tertiary hospital headache clinic. Acta Neurol Belg 113:229–235
21. Lin YK, Lin GY, Lee JT, Lee MS, Tsai CK, Hsu YW, Lin YZ, Tsai YC, Yang FC (2016) Associations between sleep quality and migraine frequency: a cross-sectional case-control study. Medicine (Baltimore) 95:e3554
22. National Institute of Neurological Disorders and Stroke. Migraine information. Available at: www.ninds.nih.gov/disorders/migraine/migraine. htm. Accessed Apr 25 2016
23. Dodick DW (2005) Triptan nonresponder studies: implications for clinical practice. Headache 45:156–162
24. Lionetto L, Negro A, Palmisani S, Gentile G, Del Fiore MR, Mercieri M, Simmaco M, Smith T, Al-Kaisy A, Arcioni R, Martelletti P (2012) Emerging treatment for chronic migraine and refractory chronic migraine. Expert Opin Emerg Drugs 17:393–406
25. Negro A, Curto M, Lionetto L, Martelletti P (2015) A two years open-label prospective study of OnabotulinumtoxinA 195 U in medication overuse headache: a real-world experience. J Headache Pain 17:1
26. Rothrock JF (2012) Botox-A for suppression of chronic migraine: commonly asked questions. Headache 52:716–717
27. Sanassi LA (2016) Botulinum toxin: a lift for chronic migraines. JAAPA 29:1–4, Review
28. Aurora SK, Dodick DW, Turkel CC, DeGryse RE, Silberstein SD, Lipton RB, Diener HC, Brin MF, PREEMPT 1 Chronic Migraine Study Group (2010) OnabotulinumtoxinA for treatment of chronic migraine: results from the double-blind, randomized placebo-controlled phase of the PREEMPT 1 trial. Cephalalgia 30:793–803
29. Diener HC, Dodick DW, Aurora SK, Turkel CC, DeGryse RE, Lipton RB, Silberstein SD, Brin MF, PREEMPT 2 Chronic Migraine Study Group (2010) OnabotulinumtoxinA for treatment of chronic migraine: results from the double-blind, randomized, placebo-controlled phase of the PREEMPT 2 trial. Cephalalgia 30:804–814
30. Dodick DW, Turkel CC, DeGryse RE, Aurora SK, Silberstein SD, Lipton RB, Diener HC, Brin MF (2010) OnabotulinumtoxinA for treatment of chronic migraine: pooled results from the double-blind, randomized placebo-controlled phases of the PREEMPT clinical program. Headache 50:921–936
31. Aurora SK, Dodick DW, Diener HC, DeGryse RE, Turkel CC, Lipton RB, Silberstein SD (2014) OnabotulinumtoxinA for chronic migraine: efficacy, safety, and tolerability in patients who received all five treatment cycles in the PREEMPT clinical program. Acta Neurol Scand 129:61–70

32. Allergan Inc (2013) BOTOX (onabotulinumtoxinA) full prescribing information. Allergan Inc, Irvine

33. Blumenfeld A, Silberstein SD, Dodick DW, Aurora SK, Turkel CC, Binder WJ (2010) Method of injection of onabotulinumtoxinA for chronic migraine: a safe, well-tolerated, and effective treatment paradigm based on the PREEMPT clinical program. Headache 50:1406–1418

34. Sawyer J (2001) Development and testing of the migraine disability assessment (MIDAS) questionnaire to assess headache-related disability. Neurology 15:20–28

35. Ertas M, Siva A, Dalkara T, Uzuner N, Dora B, Inan L, Idiman F, Sarica Y, Selcuki D, Sirin H, Oguzhanoglu A, Irkec C, Ozmenoglu M, Ozbenli T, Ozturk M, Saip S, Neyal M, Zarifoglu M, Turkish MIDAS group (2004) Validity and reliability of the Turkish migraine disability assessment (MIDAS) questionnaire. Headache 15:786–793

36. Lovibond SH, Lovibond PF (1995) Manual for the depression anxiety stress scales, 2nd edn. Psychology Foundation, Sydney

37. Brown TA, Chorpita BF, Korotitsch W, Barlow DH (1997) Psychometric properties of the depression anxiety stress scales (DASS) in clinical samples. Behav Res Ther 35:79–89

38. Antony MM, Bieling PJ, Brian J, Cox BJ, Enns MW, Swinson RP (1998) Psychometric properties of the 42-item and 21-item versions of the depression anxiety stress scales in clinical groups and a community sample. Psychol Assess 10:176–181

39. Hekimoglu L, Altun ZO, Kaya EZ, Bayram N, Bilgel N (2012) Psychometric properties of the Turkish version of the 42 item depression anxiety stress scale (DASS-42) in a clinical sample. Int J Psychiatry Med 44:183–198

40. Buysse DJ, Reynolds CF 3rd, Monk TH, Berman SR, Kupfer DJ (1998) The Pittsburgh sleep quality index: a new instrument for psychiatric practice and research. Psychiatry Res 28:193–213

41. Agargun MY, Kara H, Anlar O (1996) Pittsburgh Uyku kalitesi indeksi'nin gecerliliği ve güvenilirligi. Turk Psikiyatri Derg 7:107–115 [Turkish]

42. Kollewe K, Escher CM, Wulff DU, Fathi D, Paracka L, Mohammadi B, Karst M, Dressler D (2016) Long-term treatment of chronic migraine with OnabotulinumtoxinA: efficacy, quality of life and tolerability in a real-life setting. J Neural Transm (Vienna) 123:533–540

43. Cernuda-Morollón E, Ramón C, Larrosa D, Alvarez R, Riesco N, Pascual J (2015) Long-term experience with onabotulinumtoxinA in the treatment of chronic migraine: what happens after one year? Cephalalgia 35:864–868

44. Jackson JL, Kuriyama A, Hayashino Y (2012) Botulinum toxin A for prophylactic treatment of migraine and tension headaches in adults: a meta-analysis. JAMA 307:1736–1745

45. Harwood RH, Sayer AA, Hirschfeld M (2004) Current and future worldwide prevalence of dependency, its relationship to total population, and dependency ratios. Bull World Health Organ 82:251–258

46. Menken M, Munsat TL, Toole JF (2000) The global burden of disease study: implications for neurology. Arch Neurol 57:418–420

47. Deiner HC, Limmroth V (2004) Medication overuse headache: a worldwide problem. Lancet Neurol 3:475–483

48. Silberstein SD, Blumenfield AM, Cady RK, Turner IM, Lipton RB, Deiner HC, Aurora SK, Sirimanne M, DeGryse RE, Turkel CC, Dodick DW (2013) OnabotulinumtoxinA for treatment of chronic migraine: PREEMPT 24-week pooled subgroup analysis of patients who had acute headache medication overuse at baseline. J Neurol Sci 331:48–56

49. Saper JR, Dodick D, Gladstone JP (2005) Management of chronic daily headache: challenges in clinical practice. Headache 45(Suppl 1):S74–S85, Review

50. Finkel AG (2015) Botulinum toxin and the treatment of headache: a clinical review. Toxicon 107:114–119

51. Negro A, Curto M, Lionetto L, Crialesi D, Martelletti P (2015) OnabotulinumtoxinA 155 U in medication overuse headache: a two years prospective study. Springerplus 4:826

52. Guerzoni S, Pellesi L, Baraldi C, Pini LA (2015) Increased efficacy of regularly repeated cycles with onabotulinumtoxinA in MOH patients beyond the first year of treatment. J Headache Pain 17:48

53. Demiryurek BE, Ertem DH, Tekin A, Ceylan M, Aras YG, Gungen BD (2016) Effects of onabotulinumtoxinA treatment on efficacy, depression, anxiety, and disability in Turkish patients with chronic migraine. Neurol Sci 37:1779–1784

54. Silberstein SD, Dodick WD, Aurora SK, Dienere H-C, DeGryse RE, Lipton RB, Turkel CC (2015) Per cent of patients with chronic migraine who responded per onabotulinumtoxinA treatment cycle: PREEMPT. J Neurol Neurosurg Psychiatry 86:996–1001

55. Khalil M, Zafar HW, Quarshie V, Ahmed F (2014) Prospective analysis of the use of onabotulinumtoxinA (BOTOX) in the treatment of chronic migraine; real-life data in 254 patients from Hull, UK. J Headache Pain 15:54

56. Lipton RB, Varon SF, Grosberg B, McAllister PJ, Freitag F, Aurora SK, Dodick DW, Silberstein SD, Diener HC, DeGryse RE, Nolan ME, Turkel CC (2011) OnabotulinumtoxinA improves quality of life and reduces impact of chronic migraine. Neurology 77:1465–1472

57. Baney J (2011) How effective is long-term use of botox for chronic migraine? Neurol Rev 19:18A

58. Blumenfeld AM, Inocelda A, Purdy C, Dalfonso L, Magar R (2015) The durability of onabotulinumtoxinA for the treatment of chronic migraine: CLARITY Pilot Study. Toxicon 93(Suppl):S11

59. Bigal M (2009) Migraine chronification-concept and risk factors. Discov Med 8:145–150

60. Ashina S, Buse DC, Maizels M, Manack A, Serrrano D, Turkel CC, Lipton RB (2010) Self-reported anxiety as a risk factor for migraine chronification: results from the American Migraine Prevalence and Prevention (AMPP) study. Headache 50(Suppl 1):4

61. Fishbain DA, Cutler R, Rosomoff HL, Rosomoff RS (1997) Chronic pain-associated depression: antecedent or consequence of chronic pain? A review. Clin J Pain 13:116–137

62. Boudreau GP, Grosberg BM, McAllister PJ, Lipton RB, Buse DC (2015) Prophylactic onabotulinumtoxinA in patients with chronic migraine and comorbid depression: an open-label, multicenter, pilot study of efficacy, safety and effect on headache-related disability, depression, and anxiety. Int J Gen Med 8:79–86

63. Parsaik AK, Mascarenhas SS, Hashmi A, Prokop LJ, John V, Okusaga O, Singh B (2016) Role of botulinum toxin in depression. J Psychiatr Pract 22:99–110

64. Silberstein SD, Dodick D, Freitag F, Pearlman SH, Hahn SR, Scher AI, Lipton RB (2007) Pharmacological approaches to managing migraine and associated comorbidities—clinical considerations for monotherapy versus polytherapy. Headache 47:585–599

65. Blier P, Abbott FV (2001) Putative mechanisms of action of antidepressant drugs in affective and anxiety disorders and pain. J Psychiatry Neurosci 26:37–43

66. Ghajarzadeh M, Jalilian R, Togha M, Azimi A, Hosseini P, Babaei N (2014) Depression, poor sleep, and sexual dysfunction in migraineurs women. Int J Prev Med 5:1113–1118

67. Kelman L, Rains JC (2005) Headache and sleep: examination of sleep patterns and complaints in a large clinical sample of migraineurs. Headache 45:904–910

68. Alberti A (2006) Headache and sleep. Sleep Med Rev 10:431–437

69. Shim YJ, Lee MK, Kato T, Park HU, Heo K, Kim ST (2014) Effects of botulinum toxin on jaw motor events during sleep in sleep bruxism patients: a polysomnographic evaluation. J Clin Sleep Med 10:291–298

70. Gori S, Lucchesi C, Baldacci F, Bonuccelli U (2015) Preferential occurrence of attacks during night sleep and/or upon awakening negatively affects migraine clinical presentation. Funct Neurol 30:119–123

71. Gori S, Morelli N, Maestri M, Fabbrini M, Bonanni E, Murri L (2005) Sleep quality, chronotypes and preferential timing of attacks in migraine without aura. J Headache Pain 6:258–260

72. Gori S, Lucchesi C, Maluccio MR, Morelli N, Maestri M, Bonanni E, Murri L (2012) Inter-critical and critical excessive daily sleepiness in episodic migraine patients. Neurol Sci 33:1133–1136

73. Walters AB, Hamer JD, Smitherman TA (2014) Sleep disturbance and affective comorbidity among episodic migraineurs. Headache 54:116–124

13

Mindfulness and pharmacological prophylaxis after withdrawal from medication overuse in patients with Chronic Migraine

Licia Grazzi[1*], Emanuela Sansone[2], Alberto Raggi[2], Domenico D'Amico[1], Andrea De Giorgio[3], Matilde Leonardi[2], Laura De Torres[2], Francisco Salgado-García[4] and Frank Andrasik[4]

Abstract

Background: Chronic Migraine (CM) is a disabling condition, worsened when associated with Medication Overuse (MO). Mindfulness is an emerging technique, effective in different pain conditions, but it has yet to be explored for CM-MO. We report the results of a study assessing a one-year course of patients' status, with the hypothesis that the effectiveness of a mindfulness-based approach would be similar to that of conventional prophylactic treatments.

Methods: Patients with CM-MO (code 1.3 and 8.2 of the International Classification of Headache Disorders-3Beta) completed a withdrawal program in a day hospital setting. After withdrawal, patients were either treated with Prophylactic Medications (Med-Group), or participated in a Mindfulness-based Training (MT-Group). MT consisted of 6 weekly sessions of guided mindfulness, with patients invited to practice 7–10 min per day. Headache diaries, the headache impact test (HIT-6), the migraine disability assessment (MIDAS), state and trait anxiety (STAI Y1-Y2), and the Beck Depression Inventory (BDI) were administered before withdrawal and at each follow-up (3, 6, 12 after withdrawal) to patients from both groups. Outcome variables were analyzed in separate two-way mixed ANOVAs (Group: Mindfulness vs. Pharmacology x Time: Baseline, 3-, 6-, vs. 12-month follow-up).

Results: A total of 44 patients participated in the study, with the average age being 44.5, average headache frequency/month was 20.5, and average monthly medication intake was 18.4 pills. Data revealed a similar improvement over time in both groups for Headache Frequency (approximately 6–8 days reduction), use of Medication (approximately 7 intakes reduction), MIDAS, HIT-6 (but only for the MED-Group), and BDI; no changes on state and trait anxiety were found. Both groups revealed significant and equivalent improvement with respect to what has become a classical endpoint in this area of research, i.e. 50% or more reduction of headaches compared to baseline, and the majority of patients in each condition no longer satisfied current criteria for CM.

Conclusions: Taken as a whole, our results suggest that the longitudinal course of patients in the MT-Group, that were not prescribed medical prophylaxis, was substantially similar to that of patients who were administered medical prophylaxis.

Keywords: Chronic migraine, Medication overuse, Pharmacological prophylaxis, Mindfulness

* Correspondence: licia.grazzi@istituto-besta.it
[1]Neurological Institute "C. Besta" IRCCS Foundation, Headache and Neuroalgology Unit, Via Celoria 11, 20133 Milan, Italy
Full list of author information is available at the end of the article

Mindfulness and pharmacological prophylaxis after withdrawal from medication overuse in patients...

115

Background

Headache disorders are common disabling conditions that, in the last Global Burden of Disease study, were rated as the sixth cause of disability [1]. Further, medication overuse headache was rated as the 18th and, among those aged under 50, migraine was rated as the third cause of disability [2]. Chronic Migraine (CM), is construed as a negative evolution of episodic migraine, based on the findings that approximately 2.5% of episodic migraineurs progress to CM each year [3], with a prevalence of approximately 2% [3, 4]. CM is diagnosed when headache episodes occur more than 15 days/month (with at least 8 displaying migraine headache features) for more than three months [5], and is frequently associated with overuse of acute medications. This has been hypothesized to be one of the chief factors contributing to migraine chronification [6, 7] and, when overuse of medicine reaches a level to warrant a diagnosis of Medication Overuse (MO), it further complicates CM making it particularly difficult to manage. Chronic Migraine associated with Medication Overuse (CM-MO) is diagnosed when the intake of headache medications for headache episodes is greater than 15 days/month for simple analgesics, or exceeds 10 days/month for triptans, opioids, ergotamine or combinations of certain drugs [5]. A recent review of the literature evidenced that analgesics and opioids are associated with a higher risk of developing MO and the authors concluded that the so-called "migraine-specific" treatments, namely triptans and ergots, should be preferred as they are less frequently associated with development of overuse and disease chronification [8].

Patients with CM-MO present therapeutic challenges and require multidisciplinary care, including pharmacological and non-pharmacological therapeutic approaches [9]. Various pharmacological therapies have more recently been developed to help these patients better manage their condition [10–13], but symptom resolution is not always optimal and up to one third of patients relapse by 12 months [14–16]. Medication withdrawal is strongly recommended and its use can be viewed as a "reset" that then affords patients a greater likelihood of positively responding to appropriate prophylactics [13, 17, 18]. It is most helpful when patients are provided education and support about proper use of medications and taught strategies for avoiding relapse [19]. Studies have shown that such approaches can produce significant improvements that endure for extended periods, up to 5 years [20, 21].

CM-MO results in pervasive negative consequences, where personal suffering is accompanied by reduced quality of life and disability, and decreased abilities to participate in daily work and/or family activities, which often results in increasing symptoms of depression [12, 22–24]. Clinicians and researchers working in the field of headache disorders are becoming increasingly aware of the consequences of this condition, the resultant need for a multifactorial approach and treatment [25]. The joint use of pharmacological and non-pharmacological techniques has been shown to improve the health status of migraine patients and to enhance clinical outcomes by teaching and reinforcing patients to implement alternative procedures for addressing and coping with headache attacks [9, 26–30].

Among the wide array of available non-pharmacological treatments, mindfulness has been recently included in rehabilitation programs for chronic pain conditions [31–36]. Its efficacy has been addressed in a recent review of the psychological therapies in the neurorehabilitation of pain syndromes [37], where it has been judged as effective (Grade Level A) for chronic pain syndromes with heterogeneous physiopathology, exclusive of headache disorders. However when this review was prepared researchers had only begun to explore the utility of mindfulness for headache, so no firm recommendations could be made. The success with other pain conditions, however, has spurred researchers in the field of headache to increasingly turn their attention to mindfulness training as another viable alternative approach for supplementing patient care. The main goal of this approach is to increase patient awareness of their pain and improve their abilities to manage headache before resorting to their former medications [38–45]. As concluded in two recent reviews on the use of mindfulness-based approaches in headache disorders [46, 47], this kind of approach seems promising. In brief, literature findings [40–45] suggest that various mindfulness-based approaches may be helpful for headache sufferers, and that it may be of value also for those with CM-MO. However, the available studies are limited by an inadequate consideration of some of the most important endpoints in chronic headache research, namely the frequency of headache and the consumption of medications for acute headaches management. Further, other meaningful indicators of effectiveness, such as pain intensity, headache duration, disability, quality of life and some mental health-related variables, such as stress, anxiety, pain acceptance or self-efficacy, have yet to be fully explored. A second relevant shortcoming is the limited duration of follow-up reported in these studies, which has ranged between 3 weeks and 3 months. Finally, what is not clear is the ability of a mindfulness-based approach by *itself* to impact key primary as well as secondary migraine headache parameters, as well as promote reductions in consumption of acute medications. Two research areas, thus, warrant further attention: first, identifying optimal components and delivery schedules, by adequately specifying the intervention protocols; second, conducting rigorous controlled trials that assess the durability of effects over extended time periods, with appropriate control conditions and a clear specification of primary and secondary outcomes.

As a way to begin to address these uncertainties we conducted an exploratory clinical trial, one that compared conventional prophylactic pharmacological treatment *alone* to a mindfulness-based treatment *alone* for patients diagnosed with CM-MO and incorporated a more extended follow-up period. We carefully monitored the clinical course of these patients after all had undergone a structured withdrawal, with the hypothesis that the mindfulness-based approach would be similar in effectiveness when compared to conventional prophylactic treatment, for reducing headache frequency, consumption of acute medications, headache impact, symptoms of depression, and of anxiety.

Methods

Participants

Eligible patients were those diagnosed with CM-MO – i.e. code 1.3 and associated medication overuse, following the international criteria included in point 8.2 of the International Classification of Headache Disorder III edition, beta version (ICHD-3-beta) [5] – who presented consecutively for treatment at the Headache Centre of the Neurological Institute C. Besta of Milan, Italy, between February 2014 and June 2015. These patients were aged between 18 and 65 years and had a history of CM lasting for at least ten years that was associated with overuse of Triptans and non-steroidal anti-inflammatory drugs (NSAIDs) for a minimum of the past five years. Patients with comorbid major psychiatric disorders, namely psychotic disorders and personality disorders, determined on the basis of clinical history and psychiatric evaluation, or pregnancy were excluded.

Procedures

All patients were first admitted to our out-patient day hospital service, where they participated in a 5-day structured medication withdrawal program that utilized intravenous therapy, including steroids and ademetionine [28, 48]. During withdrawal, patients were instructed to avoid the use of medications to manage any acute pain attacks. Upon completion of the structured medication withdrawal, all patients were encouraged to increase their physical activity and perform aerobic exercises, for 45 min twice per week, maintain a suitable level of hydration, and strive to consume 3 meals each day on a regular basis (emphasizing breakfast). Prior to discharge from the day treatment program, patients were informed of the

possibility to participate in a new clinical trial, in which they could receive "medication alone" or "mindfulness training alone" (Med-Group or MT-Group).

Patients participating in the Med-Group received only prophylactic medications. The preventive compound was chosen on the basis of clinical history and medical comorbidities [49–52], such as done in routine care. Patients included in the MT-group, participated in a series of mindfulness training sessions and were not prescribed any form of prophylaxis. The mindfulness protocol we used was implemented on the basis of the Mindfulness-Based-Stress-Reduction MBSR program (MBSR) by Jon Zabat-Zinn [53]. Together with a close variant – the mindfulness-based cognitive therapy (MBCT) [54] – this is the most largely applied for various forms of recurrent pain [46], which we partially modified with regard to the frequency and the duration of sessions to increase the likelihood of adherence to treatment by patients. Training was provided in small groups (5–6 patients), that met in a relaxed and quiet room every consecutive Monday for 6 weekly sessions, each of about 45 min duration. All sessions were guided by an experienced neurologist trained in mindfulness practice. The order in which the different techniques and phases were administered– with the due caution and flexibility – was as follows. First, patients were provided a detailed explanation about the treatment protocol; i.e. what it is and what it is not, and in which clinical conditions it may be of most value. Second, patients were trained to assume a relaxed position that promoted good and regular breathing, while their eyes remained closed, with them maintaining a relaxed sitting position. Third, during the first meditations (approximately up to the second/third session), patients were invited to focus on attention on their breathing, on the present and on silence to enhance awareness of current mind and body sensations. Fourth, once patients learned to focus on the present, they erre requested to enhance awareness of their thoughts (third and fourth session), accepting them in a non-judgmental way. Fifth, in the last sessions (generally the last two), when patients had gathered higher awareness of their thoughts and the capacity to accept them, they were invited to preserve themselves from interfering thoughts, and to focus on the present and on the sensations they received from their bodies. When distractions occurred, patients were informed to resume attention to breathing and body awareness and observe the interfering content in a non-judgmental way [55]. Finally patients were encouraged to supplement their training with regular home self-practice, of 7–10 min per day (an amount typically recommended in studies of this type). The importance of practicing this form of meditation in an effortless manner was pointed out. Unlike prior investigations [41], we purposely limited the number of techniques to promote mastery of a few (versus exposure to numerous modalities where patients may be unable to master any to a meaningful degree) and keep time demands low and similar to that for pharmacological treatment.

This was an exploratory study, conducted in a working clinic that draws patients from a large coverage area, and the neurologist who guided the mindfulness sessions was one of the authors (LG), who had undergone extensive training in mindfulness at the Association for Meditation and Awareness under the supervision of Prof. Corrado Pensa. In this clinical setting it was not possible to implement random assignment, due to limited resources in terms of personnel and space. Another barrier lies in patients' provenance and past history: in fact, our center is a high-level specialty one, and patients seeking treatment come from all over the country, with some of them being followed-up for many years, thus making it difficult to enroll patients in a way that is strictly consistent with the requirements of a RCT. Therefore, certain aspects were not blinded: in particular, the investigators knew which patients attended mindfulness sessions and which not, as those that did not attend the sessions needed to be supervised with regard to eventual side effects of prophylactic medications. Participation was, thus, on a voluntary basis, with patients self-selecting their preferred treatment condition. Patients opting for mindfulness training alone were informed of the importance of being available to attend weekly sessions on a consistent basis upon discharge. Patients unable to commit to the stated schedule were invited to participate in the medical prophylaxis alone condition. Follow-up evaluations were carried out by another neurologist (DD) to limit possible source of bias with clinical outcomes, and questionnaire completion was supervised by a psychologist (ES). Given these considerations we view this investigation as more along the lines of an *effectiveness trial* (versus an efficacy trial) [56]. The consequence of this is that our results have to be taken as preliminary and the efficacy has to be tested in future randomized trials.

The study was approved by the Institute's Ethical Committee and written informed consent was obtained from each patient prior to enrollment in the study protocol. Follow-up assessments were conducted at 3, 6 and 12 months for all available patients. During this period, patients were instructed to continue their prior treatments. Patients in both groups were encouraged to restrict use of acute medications to headaches judged to be very disabling, operationally defined as a pain intensity rated as 8 or greater on a 0–10 (no pain – pain as bad as it could be). Patients were instructed to take Eletriptan (40 mg) and/or Almotriptan (12.5 mg) as the

first-line treatment, and indomethacin (50 mg) as the second line; with regard to other NSAIDs, they were urged to take those medications that had already proved to be effective. Finally, in any case, they were strongly recommended to avoid opioids to the extent possible.

Measures

Headache diaries [25], completed on a daily basis, provided the primary measure of outcome, i.e., headache frequency, and the consumption of acute medications (NSAIDs and triptans). The amount of single intakes was recorded, irrespective of the kind of medication.

The Headache Impact Test (HIT-6) [57] is a 6-item scale that measures lost time in 3 domains and other areas of impact (e.g., pain severity, fatigue, and mood), based on patient recall for the immediate past 4 weeks. Each item is rated on a scale ranging from "never" to "always." Total scores range from 36 to 78 with higher scores indicating greater impact: scores ≥ 60 are indicative of a severe impact.

The Migraine Disability Assessment (MIDAS) [58] is the most widely used measure of disability in headache research and we included it to facilitate comparisons with prior research. It is composed of 7 questions, all referenced to the preceding 3 months. The first 5 inquire about the number of days during which headache presence disrupted (partially or totally) paid and school work, household work, and leisure/family/social duties. Summing these individual values yields a total disability score, which correspond to four severity level: 0–5, little or no disability; 6–10, mild disability; 11–20, moderate disability; 21 or above, severe disability. The remaining two items address the overall headache frequency and average pain intensity, measured on a 0–10 scale. As headache frequency and intensity were prospectively obtained from daily diaries, and the validity of headache data recalled over three months is questionable [59], we elected to not report these data here.

Beck Depression Inventory (BDI) [60]. We used the 13-item version, which asks participants to rate the extent to which they are experiencing each of the 13 common symptoms of depression included. Items are rated on a scale from 0 to 3 (where 3 represents the highest severity), with the maximum score being 39. When used as a screening device, a cut-off score of 9/10 seems best suited for indicating the presence/absence of depression [61].

The State-Trait Anxiety Inventory (STAI) Y1 and Y2 [62] is composed of two sections, each containing 20 items, that address state and trait anxiety, i.e., the transitory feelings that respondents experience in the moment in which they complete the questionnaire vs. the relatively stable and enduring personal features reflective of a predisposition to anxiety. Raw scores range between

20 and 80 for each scale, with higher scores indicating higher anxiety levels. The raw scores can be transformed into norm-based T-Scores (mean 50, SD 10) to enable comparability across gender and age groups [63].

Data analyses

Mean baseline values for all demographic and dependent variables for the 2 treatment conditions were compared by t-tests. The primary and secondary outcome variables were analyzed in separate two-way mixed ANOVAs (Group: Mindfulness vs. Pharmacology x Time: Baseline, 3-, 6-, vs. 12-month follow-up), followed by post-hoc tests, with appropriate adjustments made when significant effects were obtained in order to guard against inflation of the familywise error rate. Partial eta squared (η^2_p) values were calculated for all significant findings, conservatively interpreting them as small (.01–.08), medium (.09–.24), and large ($\geq$.25).

We additionally evaluated clinical significance by determining the percentage of patients that, compared to baseline evaluation, achieved a 50% or greater reduction in migraine frequency and the percentage of patients who no longer met the diagnostic criteria for CM at each of the three follow-up evaluations. We then compared the ratios between the two groups of patient (MT-Group and Med-Group), for each of these 2 additional measures, at each time-point using Chi-Squared analyses. The p-value for significance for all tests was set at .05.

Results

Fifty patients met inclusion criteria during the study period, but six declined to participate due to lack of time or interest. Forty-four patients were therefore enrolled in this trial, 22 in each condition. In the Med-Group, five patients received valproate, eight botulinum toxin, five pizotifen, one amitriptyline, two received a combination of beta blockers and amitriptyline and one was given beta blockers and valproate. Table 1 reports the mean baseline values for all enrolled patients, collectively and by group assignment, along with current age and age at onset of headache. No differences were found between the 2 groups for any measures (the same was true when comparing baseline values for those who completed the trial; n = 39 versus those who did not, n = 3). At baseline, a similar percentage of patients were overusing triptans: 8 of 22 patients (36.4%) in the Med-Group and 6 of 22 patients (27.3%) in the MT-Group ($\chi^2(1)$ = 0.42, p = .52). The 2 groups did differ with respect to overuse of NSAIDS: 22 of 22 (100%) for Med-Group vs. 18 of 22 for MT-Group ($\chi^2(1)$ = 4.40, p = .04).

Figure 1 shows the flow of patients in each of the two groups: complete follow-up data at 12 months was available for 19 patients in the Med-Group and for 20 in the MT-Group.

Primary and secondary outcomes

Mean values for all measures at all time points are reported for patients who completed the entire trial (see Table 2). Four of the seven separate mixed within-between subjects ANOVAs revealed significance only for the main effect of time— Headache Frequency, Medication intake, MIDAS, and BDI-13 (see Table 3). Analysis of the HIT-6 data revealed not only a main effect for time, but also for the interaction of time and group. Neither analysis for STAI-S or STAI-T revealed any significant effects (so these variables are not discussed further here). Pair wise post-hoc comparisons with Bonferroni corrections revealed all 3 follow-up points as significantly improved with respect to baseline values, but no differences among the 3 follow-up periods, for Headache Frequency, Medication intake, and BDI-13. MIDAS scores were significantly different from baseline

Table 1 Mean (and SD) baseline values for all measures for patients who began the trial, all 44 combined and separately for condition assignment, and statistical comparisons among the groups

Variable	Total (N = 44)		MT-Group (N = 22)		Med-Group (N = 22)		t (42)	P
	M	SD	M	SD	M	SD		
Age	44.5	9.2	45.6	9.3	43.5	9.2	0.75	.457
Age at Onset	20.4	9.0	21.5	10.5	19.3	7.3	0.80	.428
Headache frequency/month	20.5	7.9	19.2	7.8	21.9	7.8	-1.14	.263
Monthly medication intake	18.4	6.5	18.0	6.4	18.8	6.7	-0.41	.681
HIT	66.3	5.2	65.5	5.5	67.1	4.9	-1.05	.301
MIDAS	73.1	39.9	65.3	41.4	81.0	37.6	-1.32	.194
BDI-13	13.3	6.1	13.1	5.8	13.6	6.6	-0.32	.754
STAI-S	48.2	7.3	47.1	6.6	49.4	7.9	-1.06	.297
STAI-T	52.3	9.6	52.1	9.3	52.5	10.0	-0.13	.901

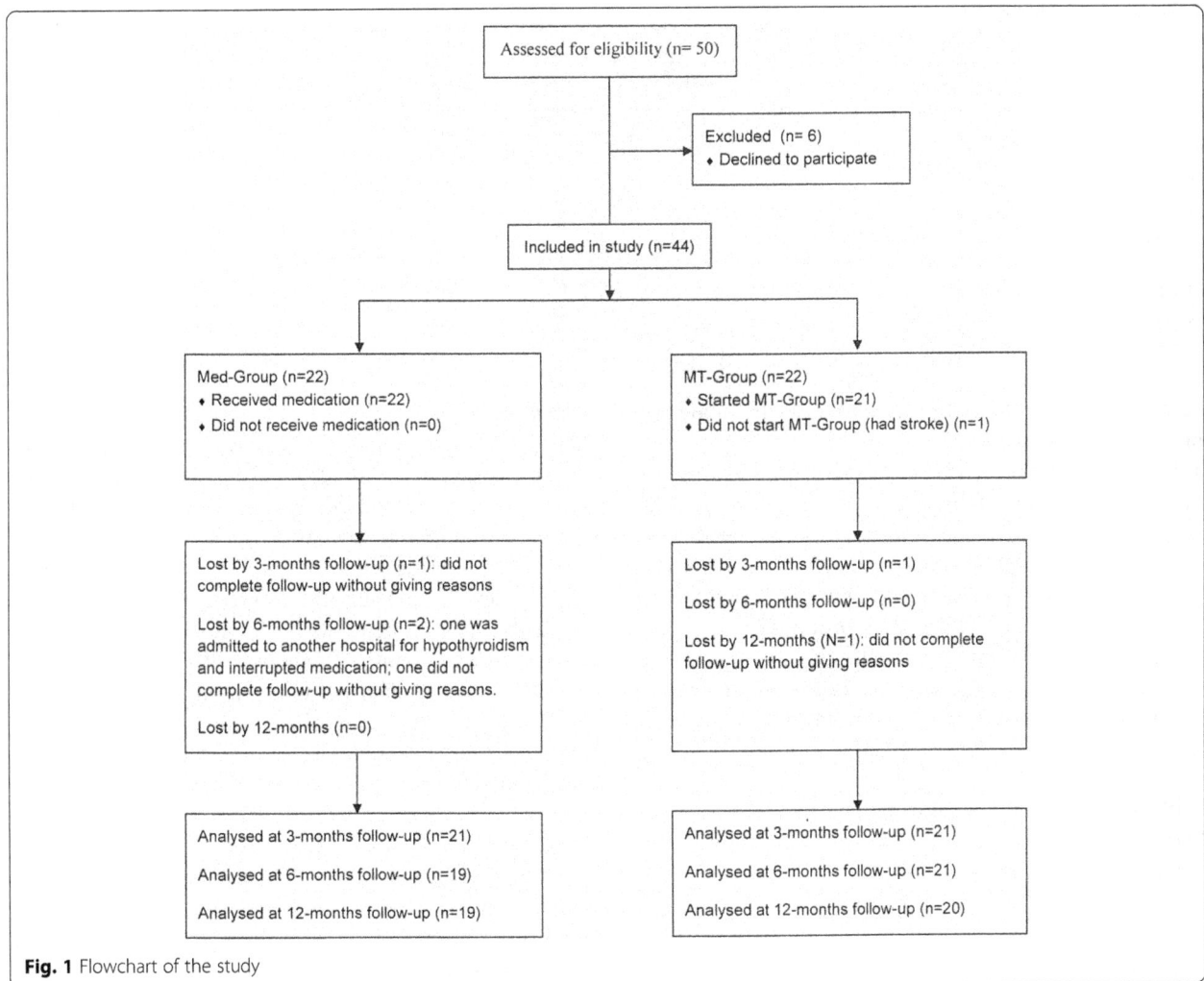

Fig. 1 Flowchart of the study

for the 3- and 6-month follow-up, but not for the 12-month follow-up (see Table 4). Figure 2 graphically presents the outcomes for headache frequency and consumption of medication for management of acute headaches over the 12-month follow-up period.

To investigate the source of the significant interaction effect for the HIT-6, we conducted all pairwise comparisons for all time points for each group separately (see Table 5 and Fig. 3). Pairwise comparisons, with Sidak correction, revealed no differences between any time points for the MF-Group. For the MED-Group the 3-month and 12-month values were significantly reduced when compared to baseline. No other differences emerged.

Table 2 Mean values and SD's for mindfulness (MT-Group) and pharmacology (MED-Group) at each measurement period

	MT-Group				Med-Group			
	Baseline	3-MO	6-MO	12-MO	Baseline	3-MO	6-MO	12-MO
Headaches Frequency	18.5 ± 7.2	8.3 ± 3.5	10.4 ± 6.9	12.4 ± 8.5	18.5 ± 7.2	8.9 ± 8.0	11.4 ± 8.0	10.4 ± 7.2
Medications intake	17.7 ± 5.9	8.1 ± 4.6	8.9 ± 4.2	10.3 ± 5.4	15.4 ± 4.4	8.8 ± 8.4	11.0 ± 7.6	8.6 ± 4.8
HIT-6	65.3 ± 5.7	62.0 ± 5.7	60.7 ± 10.8	64.5 ± 7.0	66.9 ± 5.2	60.7 ± 7.7	62.6 ± 6.3	61.5 ± 4.8
MIDAS	65.4 ± 43.5	39.0 ± 36.7	41.5 ± 51.7	53.7 ± 52.6	82.9 ± 40.0	26.7 ± 23.5	38.8 ± 25.4	51.5 ± 50.2
BDI-13	13.4 ± 5.9	9.0 ± 6.3	9.0 ± 5.3	10.3 ± 6.8	13.3 ± 6.8	6.2 ± 6.3	8.0 ± 5.9	7.6 ± 6.4
STAI-T	52.3 ± 9.8	48.6 ± 8.4	48.6 ± 7.7	50.9 ± 9.5	52.8 ± 10.2	48.5 ± 9.4	51.3 ± 9.9	48.4 ± 9.6
STAI-S	47.0 ± 6.8	45.4 ± 6.4	45.5 ± 6.9	49.9 ± 9.3	49.6 ± 7.8	47.2 ± 6.1	48.3 ± 10.7	48.6 ± 8.7

N = 19 for MT-Group and N = 20 for MED-Group
Note. Values are expressed as means ± SD

Table 3 Mixed within-between ANOVA results

Variable	Main effects for time			Main effect for group		Interaction (Time X Group)		
	Wilks' lambda	P	partial η^2	F	p	Wilks' lambda	p	partial η^2
Headaches frequency	.43	< .001	.57	0.00	.959	.93	.453	.07
Medications intake	.31	< .001	.69	0.04	.842	.83	.094	.17
HIT	.67	.002	.34	0.02	.902	.76	.020	.24
MIDAS	.43	< .001	.57	0.02	.902	.86	.141	.14
BDI-13	.49	< .001	.51	1.12	.297	.93	.475	.07
STAI-S	.82	.064	.19	0.70	.408	.93	.481	.07
STAI-T	.82	.068	.18	0.00	.952	.89	.246	.11

Percent improvement and percent of patients no longer meeting criteria for CM

Table 6 reports the percentage of patients showing 50% or more reduction of headaches compared to baseline and of patients no longer meeting criteria for CM for each of the time-points. For both of the clinical endpoints, there were no differences between patients in the MT-Group and those in the Med-Group. With regard to the percent improvement variable, the trend had a U-shaped curve in both groups, while the trend had a J-shaped curve with regard to the number of patients no longer meeting the criteria for CM.

Table 4 Post-hoc comparisons across time for significant time main effects

Variable	M	SD	M diff	P
Freq				
Baseline (ref)	18.5	7.1		
3-month	8.6	6.1	9.9	< .001
6-month	10.9	7.4	7.6	< .001
12-month	11.4	7.9	7.1	< .001
Medications intake				
Baseline (ref)	16.6	5.3		
3-month	8.4	6.6	8.2	< .001
6-month	9.9	6.1	6.7	< .001
12-month	9.5	5.1	7.1	< .001
MIDAS				
Baseline (ref)	73.9	42.2		
3-month	33.0	31.2	40.9	< .001
6-month	40.2	40.6	33.7	< .001
12-month	52.6	50.8	21.3	ns
BDI-13				
Baseline (ref)	13.3	6.2		
3-month	7.6	6.4	5.7	< .001
6-month	8.5	5.5	4.9	< .001
12-month	9.0	6.7	4.4	.001

Note: Only comparisons to baseline scores are presented in this table, as all other pairwise comparisons were not statistically significant

Discussion

Our preliminary data show that both groups of patients, treated with only a single, non-combination intervention—conventional pharmacological approach only versus a mindfulness-based approach only—revealed significant decreases in number of monthly headache days, monthly consumption of medication for acute headache management, MIDAS, and depressive symptoms up to 12-months follow-up. The change in mean BDI-13 scores (collapsing across groups), appears to be of clinical significance, as the baseline values, which fell into the stringent range (13/14) for tentatively identifying moderate to severe clinical depression, had by 12 months fallen overall within the lowest end of the range suggesting the possible presence of moderate/severe depression (9/10). Although MIDAS scores decreased from baseline by 28.8% at 12 months, the mean score at this time point (averaged across both conditions) continued to fall within the highest severity grade Level (IV). Headache impact was reduced to a statistically significant degree at 3- and 12-month follow-up, but only for the MED-Group. It is important to point out that at all time points, neither group revealed clinically meaningful reductions on this measure because means continued to fall within the highest severity category for this scale (all means ≥ 60). Given the long-standing duration of chronic headache activity by our patients, it is not surprising that headache impact and depression did not reveal more marked changes, even at 1 year follow-up. Changes of a psychological nature often take additional time to fully manifest [26]. Anxiety scores remained unchanged over time. Although anxiety disorders and CM are known to be comorbid [64] – STAI scores revealed the absence of significant anxiety problems in either group, thus leaving little room for change ("basement" or floor effect).

The proportion of patients achieving a 50% reduction in headaches frequency (a measure commonly used to evaluate "clinically significant improvements") was similar at all time-points (at 12 months: 50% in the MT-Group, 52.6% in the Med-Group), and the same was true

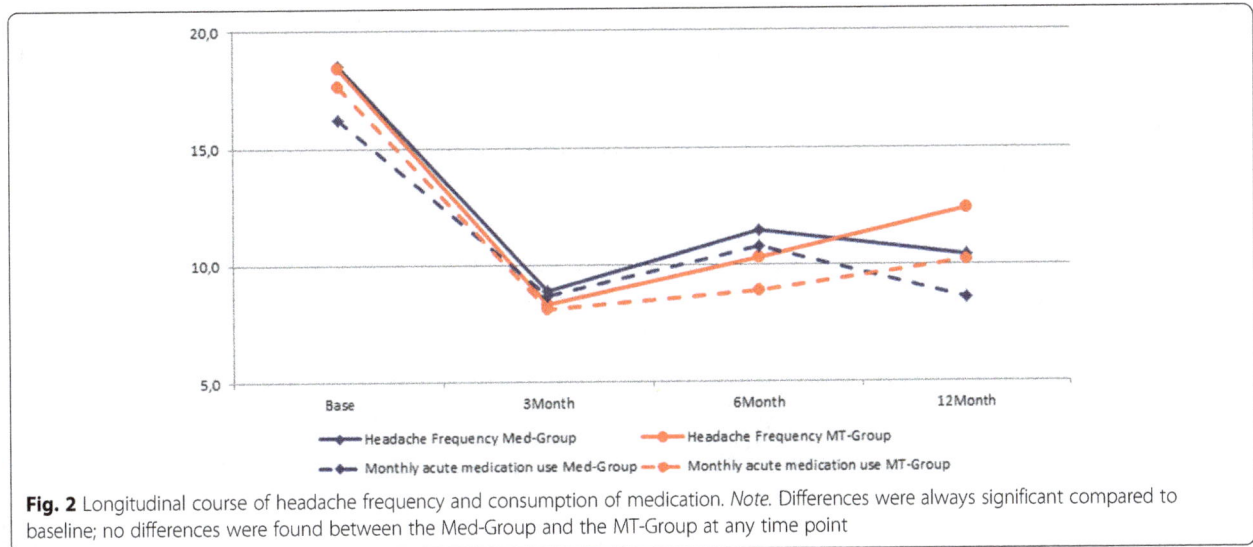

Fig. 2 Longitudinal course of headache frequency and consumption of medication. *Note.* Differences were always significant compared to baseline; no differences were found between the Med-Group and the MT-Group at any time point

for the proportion of patients no longer meeting the CM criteria (at 12 months: 65% in the MT-Group, 73.7% in the Med-Group). Taken as a whole, our results suggest that the longitudinal course of patients receiving Mindfulness-based treatment, and who were instructed to refrain from medical prophylaxis (which was verified by the dairy records participants maintained throughout the study), was overall very similar to that for patients who were administered conventional medical prophylaxis, with few exceptions noted.

Our preliminary data extend the findings of Wells and colleagues [40], whose mindfulness intervention was focused on episodic migraine and reported more limited findings. To our knowledge, only one previous study has examined the utility of mindfulness-based treatments for chronic forms of headache (CM or Tension-Type Headache, with the distribution not being reported) wherein

mindfulness was also examined as an "add-on" therapy and consisted of a host of other therapeutic components, some derived from a mindfulness framework but many derived from other theoretical models [41]. These investigators found significant differences between MBSR + pharmacotherapy and pharmacotherapy alone with respect to perceived pain intensity and quality of life. However, it is not clear if their treatment impacted headache frequency, which is our primary measure and the primary outcome recommended by the most recent IHS clinical trial guidelines [65], or other outcome measures such as those that we included, i.e., use of acute medications, disability burden and mood. The fact that positive effects (although not always reaching significant changes) were observed in our study for these varied measures in patients who received our brief mindfulness training alone (in the absence of prophylactic medications)

Table 5 Pairwise comparisons between time points of HIT for each treatment group

Group	Comparisons		Mean difference (A-B)	SE	p	95% CI of difference	
	Time A	Time B				LL	UL
Mindfulness	Baseline	3 M	3.25	1.56	.240	-1.10	7.60
		6 M	4.55	2.21	.247	-1.58	10.68
		12 M	0.80	1.73	.998	-4.00	5.60
	3 M	6 M	1.30	1.87	.983	-3.91	6.51
		12 M	-2.45	1.81	.705	-7.48	2.58
	6 M	12 M	-3.75	1.43	.073	-7.73	0.23
Pharmacological	Baseline	3 M	6.21	1.60	.003	1.75	10.67
		6 M	4.32	2.26	.328	-1.97	10.60
		12 M	5.42	1.77	.024	0.50	10.34
	3 M	6 M	-1.90	1.92	.910	-7.24	3.45
		12 M	-0.79	1.86	.999	-5.95	4.37
	6 M	12 M	1.11	1.47	.974	-2.97	5.18

Note. Multiple comparisons were adjusted with Sidak correction

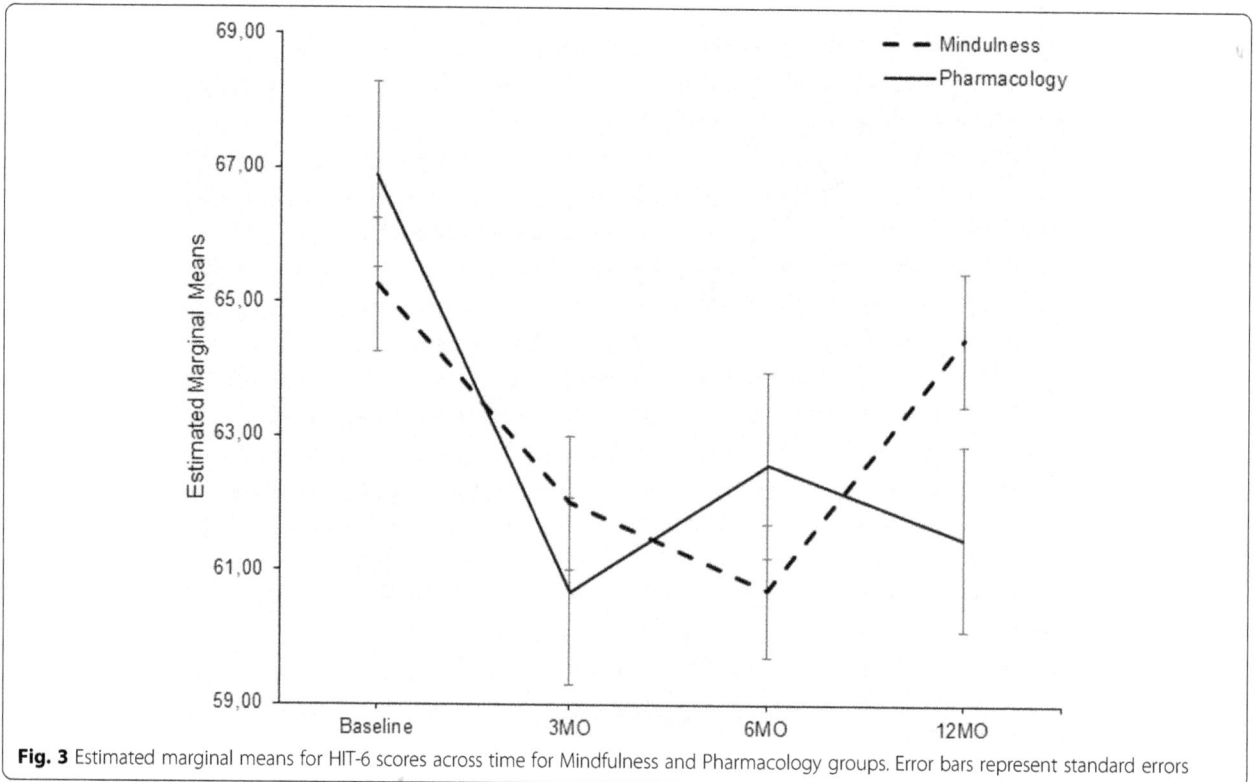

Fig. 3 Estimated marginal means for HIT-6 scores across time for Mindfulness and Pharmacology groups. Error bars represent standard errors

suggests that mindfulness-based treatment may be comparable to standard pharmacological prophylaxis as far as its global positive clinical improvement. However, the absence of random assignment and the fact that our study was not cast as a non-inferiority trial leaves this possibility more as a hypothesis, one in need of further testing.

Mood is one of the most important non-headache factors associated with migraine chronification [7, 64] and reducing headache frequency can lead to reductions in depression [29, 66]. Nonetheless, the relevance of depressive symptoms remains somewhat controversial. In fact, in previous studies on CM-MO samples [24, 67] depression scores – measured with the updated BDI-II [68] and not with the original BDI – were not correlated with frequency of headaches and, when implemented in a predictive model together with headache frequency

and pain intensity, BDI-II scores had higher value in predicting disability and quality of life scores. Our finding that Mindfulness practice (as well as medication) had a modest positive effect on levels of reported depression over time is compatible with a conclusion previously drawn in studies addressing depression and mindfulness-based treatments [69–73]. These findings show that the effect of mindfulness-based approaches on symptoms of depression were superior to psycho-educational intervention and non-inferior to individual cognitive behavioral therapy, that they yielded similar results compared to antidepressant therapies and, finally, that the effect is maximized when the treatment is combined. Considering that only 40% of patients in the MED-group received a therapy having some kind of mood-modulating effect, the finding that the impact on mood component was similar is in line with the previous report, and suggests that mindfulness-based treatments, combined with appropriate antidepressant therapy, might yield an increased impact on symptoms of depression.

Although mean BDI values for both groups were in the range of a significant levels of depression prior to treatment, we hesitate to speculate further about the meaningfulness of the changes reported here given that our measure of depression is intended primarily as a screening instrument and does not take the place of a careful clinical diagnosis.

Table 6 Percent improvement and percent of patients no longer meeting criteria for CM at each time-point

		MT-Group	Med-Group	Chi-Squared (P-value)
50% reduction	3 Months	57.1%	76.2%	1.71 (P = .190)
	6 Months	47.6%	26.3%	1.93 (P = .165)
	12 Months	50.0%	52.6%	0.03 (P = .869)
No longer CM	3 Months	95.2%	90.0%	0.41 (P = .520)
	6 Months	76.2%	78.9%	0.04 (P = .835)
	12 Months	65.0%	73.7%	0.35 (P = .557)

More recent conceptions, wherein migraine is being recognized as a condition in which biological, social and psychological aspects are very interconnected [25] has helped to increase awareness of the need to modify therapeutic approaches to include newer and sometimes "non-conventional" options (behaviorally and cognitively based), along with "traditional" treatments (i.e., medical) to better help patients to manage their condition, reduce their medication intake, and minimize the incidences of relapse in overuse after withdrawal [25, 74].

Mindfulness is designed to promote the ability to focus on and accept the present situations and the difficulties of every day. As demonstrated by Kabat-Zinn [75], patients who have been educated to use mindfulness may better manage stressful situations, increase their self-efficacy, and learn to manage pain more adequately avoiding the compulsion between pain and medication intake which easily sets in motion the vicious cycle of pain and medication and to the condition of overuse. Mindfulness research, especially as regards headache, remains in the infancy stage, with many aspects in need of further investigation. Among these are determining which of the myriad of bio-psycho-social factors may underlie treatment effectiveness, including, for example, changes in perception of and reactions to pain sensations and emotion, self-efficacy and coping abilities, physiology, cerebral structures and circuits [19, 38, 46, 47].

Although our findings are encouraging and suggestive of the independent value of mindfulness for headache care, certain design limitations preclude us making unequivocal claims. Our inability to randomize patients to conditions serves as a limiting factor, with results perhaps applying only to those particularly motivated to commit to an extended training period for mindfulness. Our headache center is designed primarily as a fee for service clinic, where patient preferences must be considered. However, as pointed out by Nash et al [56] trials of this type, more aptly termed "effectiveness trials" (versus the more standard "efficacy trials") clearly have a place in the early stage of treatment development. In this case, we hope our findings serve to expand recently published data on patients with primary headaches supporting the clinical value of mindfulness in the most severely affected patients in the migraine spectrum; i.e., those with chronic migraine coupled with medication overuse. Another consideration is our inability to document the extent to which patients adhered to each treatment (no dose monitoring for the MED group and no checks for amount of mindfulness practice or the depth of learning patients acquired). Nonetheless, we believe our findings support the value of conducting further more well-controlled studies (incorporating random assignment, larger samples sizes, and checks on integrity of treatment) are warranted to more fully explore the benefits, boundaries, and mechanisms of action for mindfulness in treating chronic migraine by itself and when it is complicated by medication overuse and medical or psychological comorbidities. Finally, our sample was composed of patients with CM and with no psychiatric comorbidities. Two literature reviews showed that migraineurs, compared to the general population, are much more likely to suffer from psychiatric comorbidities (up to 60-70% for mood and anxiety disorders) and that women with migraine with aura are at an increased risk of suicide attempt [76, 77]. Conversely, the evidence on the relationships between mood disorders expression and suicidal ideation seems contrasting, with some studies finding and others not finding any connections [78, 79]. Patients included in our sample seem to be clearly different from those described in these previous studies, as they did not have psychiatric comorbidity – although some degree of low mood was found – and actually we had no reasonable ground to suspect any suicidal ideation among the participants herein included. Caution is therefore recommended before generalizing our results to the entire population of CM patients: for all of the above reasons, our results should be taken as preliminary.

Conclusions

Our results provide initial support for the beneficial effect of Mindfulness-based treatment in the management of chronic migraine that is accompanied with medication overuse, a headache form which represents a clinical challenge. Our results further suggest that a Mindfulness-based treatment may be comparable to standard pharmacological prophylaxis with regard to relevant primary outcomes such as headaches frequency reduction and reduction in the consumption of acute medications.

Abbreviations
BDI: Beck depression inventory; CM: Chronic migraine; CM-MO: Chronic migraine associated with medication overuse; HIT-6: Headache impact test; ICHD-3Beta: International Classification of Headache Disorder III edition, beta version; MBCT: Mindfulness-based cognitive therapy; MBSR: Mindfulness based stress reduction; Med-Group: Medication alone group; MIDAS: Migraine disability assessment; MO: Medication overuse; MT-Group: Mindfulness training alone group; NSAIDs: Non-steroidal anti-inflammatory drugs; STAI: State-trait anxiety inventory; TAU: Therapy as usual; TTH: Tension-type headache

Funding
The study was supported by the Neurological Institute C. Besta IRCCS Foundation and by the European Commission, Seventh Framework Programme, Grant No. 316795 (MARATONE).

Authors' contributions
LG – Enrolment of patients, MT administration, prescription of prophylaxis. ES – Enrolment of patients, outcome measures collection, revision of the manuscript. AR – Preparation of the first draft of the manuscript and data analysis. DD – Selection and follow-up of patients, revision of the entire manuscript. ADG – Preparation of the protocol. ML – Supervision of the manuscript. LDT – Supervision of the manuscript. FSG – Data analysis. FA – Revision of the entire manuscript and data analysis. All authors read and approved the final manuscript.

Competing interests
The authors declare that they have no competing interests.

Author details
[1]Neurological Institute "C. Besta" IRCCS Foundation, Headache and Neuroalgology Unit, Via Celoria 11, 20133 Milan, Italy. [2]Neurological Institute "C. Besta" IRCCS Foundation, Neurology, Public Health and Disability Unit, Milan, Italy. [3]eCampus University, Faculty of Psychology, Novedrate, Italy. [4]Department of Psychology, Univeristy of Memphis, Memphis, TN, USA.

References
1. Global Burden of Disease Study 2013 Collaborators (2015) Global, regional, and national incidence, prevalence, and years lived with disability for 301 acute and chronic diseases and injuries in 188 countries, 1990-2013: a systematic analysis for the Global Burden of Disease Study 2013. Lancet 386: 743–800
2. Steiner TJ, Stovner LJ, Vos T (2016) GBD 2015: migraine is the third cause of disability in under 50s. J Headache Pain 17:104
3. Manack AN, Buse DC, Lipton RB (2011) Chronic migraine: Epidemiology and disease burden. Curr Pain Headache Rep 15:70–78
4. Giannini G, Favoni V, Bauleo S, Ferrante T, Pierangeli G, Albani F, Bacchi Reggiani ML, Baruzzi A, Cortelli P, Cevoli S (2012) SPARTACUS: underdiagnosis of chronic daily headache in primary care. Neurol Sci 33:181–183
5. Headache Classification Committee of the International Headache Society (2013) The International Classification of Headache Disorders, 3rd edition (beta version). Cephalalgia 33:629–808
6. Cevoli S, Sancisi E, Grimaldi D, Pierangeli G, Zanigni S, Nicodemo M, Cortelli P, Montagna P (2009) Family history for chronic headache and drug overuse as a risk factor for headache chronification. Headache 49:412–418
7. Bigal M (2009) Migraine chronification-concept and risk factors. Discov Med 8:145–150
8. Thorlund K, Sun-Edelstein C, Druyts E, Kanters S, Ebrahim S, Bhambri R, Ramos E, Mills EJ, Lanteri-Minet M, Tepper S (2016) Risk of medication overuse headache across classes of treatments for acute migraine. J Headache Pain 17:107
9. Andrasik F, Grazzi L, Usai S, Buse DC, Bussone G (2009) Non-pharmacological approaches to treating chronic migraine with medication overuse. Neurol Sci 30:89
10. Diener HC, Dodick DW, Goadsby PJ (2009) Utility of topiramate for the treatment of patients with chronic migraine in the presence or absence of acute medication overuse. Cephalalgia 29:1021–1027
11. Aurora SK, Dodick DW, Turkel CC, DeGryse RE, Silberstein SD, Lipton RB (2010) OnabotulinumtoxinA for treatment of chronic migraine: Results from the double-blind, randomized placebo-controlled phase of the PREEMPT 1 trial. Cephalalgia 30:793–803
12. D'Amico D, Grazzi L, Usai S, Raggi A, Leonardi M, Bussone G (2011) Disability in chronic daily headache: state of the art and future directions. Neurol Sci 32:S71–S76
13. Evers S, Jensen R (2011) Treatment of medication overuse headache-Guideline of the EFNS headache panel. Eur J Neurol 18:1115–1121
14. Raggi A, Giovannetti AM, Leonardi M, Sansone E, Schiavolin S, Curone M, Grazzi L, Usai S, D'Amico D (2017) Predictors of 12-Months Relapse After Withdrawal Treatment in Hospitalized Patients With Chronic Migraine Associated With Medication Overuse: A Longitudinal Observational Study. Headache 57:60–70
15. Biagianti B, Grazzi L, Usai S, Gambini O (2014) Dependency-like behaviors and pain coping styles in subjects with chronic migraine and medication overuse: Results from a 1-year follow-up study. BMC Neurol 14:181
16. Rossi P, Faroni JV, Nappi G (2008) Medication overuse headache: Predictors and rates of relapse in migraine patients with low medical needs. A 1-year prospective study. Cephalalgia 28:1196–1200
17. Grazzi L, Andrasik F, Usai S, Bussone G (2009) Treatment of chronic migraine with medication overuse. Is drug withdrawal crucial? Neurol Sci 30:S85–S88
18. Rossi P, Faroni JV, Nappi G (2011) Short-term effectiveness of simple advice as a withdrawal strategy in simple and complicated medication overuse headache. Eur J Neurol 18:396–401
19. Candy R, Farmer K, Beach ME, Tarrasch J (2008) Nurse-based education: an office-based comparative model for education of migraine patients. Headache 48:564–569
20. Grazzi L (2008) Behavioural approach to the difficult patient. Neurol Sci 29: S96–S98
21. Andrasik F, Grazzi L, Usai S, Kass S, Bussone G (2009) Disability in chronic migraine with medication overuse: Treatment effects through 5 years. Cephalalgia 30:610–614
22. Holroyd KA, Drew JB, Cottrell CK, Romanek KM, Heh V (2007) Impaired functioning and quality of life in severe migraine: The role of catastrophizing and associated symptoms. Cephalalgia 27:1156–1165
23. Wang SJ, Wang PJ, Fuh JL, Penh KP, Ng K (2013) Comparisons of disability, quality of life, and resource use between chronic and episodic migraineurs: A clinic based study in Taiwan. Cephalalgia 33:171–181
24. Raggi A, Curone M, Schiavolin S, Di Fiore P, Leonardi M, Grazzi L (2015) Chronic migraine with medication overuse: Association between disability and quality of life measures, and impact of disease on patients' lives. J Neurol Sci 348:60–66
25. Andrasik F, Flor H, Turk DC (2005) An expanded view of psychological aspects in head pain: the biopsychosocial model. Neurol Sci 26:S87–S89
26. Grazzi L, Andrasik F, D'Amico D, Leone M, Usai S, Kass SJ (2002) Behavioral and pharmacologic treatment of transformed migraine with analgesic overuse: Outcome at 3 years. Headache 42:483–490
27. Rains JC, Penzien DB, Lipchik GL (2006) Behavioral facilitation of medical treatment for headache-part II. Theor Models Behav Strategies Improv Adherence Headache 46:1395–1403
28. Andrasik F (2007) What does the evidence show? Efficacy of behavioral treatments for recurrent headache in adults. Neurol Sci 28:S70–S77
29. Nestoriuc Y, Martin A, Rief W, Andrasik F (2008) Biofeedback Treatment for Headache Disorders: A Comprehensive Efficacy Review. Appl Psychophysiol Biofeedback 33:125–140
30. Rausa M, Palomba D, Cevoli S, Lazzerini L, Sancisi E, Cortelli P, Pierangeli G (2016) Biofeedback in the prophylactic treatment of medication overuse headache: a pilot randomized controlled trial. J Headache Pain 17:87
31. Rosenzweig S, Greeson JM, Reibel DK, Jasser SA, Beasley D (2010) Mindfulness based stress reduction for chronic pain condition: Variation in treatment outcomes and role of home meditation practice. J Psychosom Res 68:29–36
32. Chiesa A, Serretti A (2010) Systematic review of neurobiological and clinical features of mindfulness meditations. Psychol Med 40:1239–1252
33. Abdollah O, Fatemeh Z (2014) Effect of mindfulness-based stress reduction on pain severity and mindful awareness in patients with tension headache: a randomized controlled clinical trial. Nurs Midwifery Stud 3:e21136
34. Makenzie E, Wachholtz A (2014) Meditation Based Treatment Yielding Immediate Relief for Meditation-Naïve Migraineurs. Pain Manag Nurs 15:36–40
35. McCracken LM, Gauntlett-Gilbert J, Vowles KE (2007) The role of mindfulness in a contextual cognitive-behavioral analysis of chronic pain-related suffering and disability. Pain 131:63–69
36. Morone NE, Greco CM, Weiner DK (2008) Mindfulness meditation for the treatment of chronic low back pain in older adults: a randomized controlled pilot study. Pain 134:310–319
37. Castelnuovo G, Giusti EM, Manzoni GM, Saviola D, Gatti A, Gabrielli S, Lacerenza M, Pietrabissa G, Cattivelli R, Spatola CA, Corti S, Novelli M, Villa V, Cottini A, Lai C, Pagnini F, Castelli L, Tavola M, Torta R, Arreghini M, Zanini L, Brunani A, Capodaglio P, D'Aniello GE, Scarpina F, Brioschi A, Priano L, Mauro A, Riva G, Repetto C, Regalia C, Molinari E, Notaro P, Paolucci S, Sandrini G, Simpson SG, Wiederhold B, Tamburin S (2016) Psychological Treatments and Psychotherapies in the Neurorehabilitation of Pain: Evidences and Recommendations from the Italian Consensus Conference on Pain in Neurorehabilitation. Front Psychol 7:115
38. Reiner K, Tibi L, Lipsitz JD (2013) Do mindfulness- based intervention reduce pain intensity? A critical review of the literature. Pain Med 14:230–242
39. Tonelli AN, Buse DC, Lipton RB (2011) Chronic migraine: epidemiology and disease burden. Curr Pain Headache Rep 15:70–78
40. Wells RE, Burch R, Paulsen RH, Wayne PM, Houle TT, Loder E (2014) Meditation for Migraines: A Pilot Randomized Controlled Trial. Headache 54:1484–1495
41. Bakhshani NM, Amirani A, Amirifard H, Shahrakipoor M (2015) The

Effectiveness of Mindfulness-Based Stress Reduction on Perceived Pain Intensity and Quality of Life in Patients With Chronic Headache. Glob J Health Sci 8:142–151

42. Day MA, Thorn BE, Ward LC, Rubin N, Hickman SD, Scogin F, Kilgo GR (2014) Mindfulness-based cognitive therapy for treatment of headache pain: A pilot study. Clin J Pain 30:152–161

43. Day MA, Thorn BE, Rubin NJ (2014) Mindfulness-based cognitive therapy for the treatment of headache pain: A mixed-methods analysis comparing treatment responders and treatment non-responders. Complement Ther Med 22:278–285

44. Omidi A, Zargar F (2015) Effects of mindfulness-based stress reduction on perceived stress and psychological health in patients with tension headache. J Res Med Sci 20:1058–1063

45. Cathcart S, Galatis N, Immink M, Proeve M, Petkov J (2014) Brief mindfulness-based therapy for chronic tension-type headache: A randomized controlled pilot study. Behav Cogn Psychother 42:1–15

46. Andrasik F, Grazzi L, D'Amico D, Sansone E, Leonardi M, Raggi A, Salgado-Garcia F (2016) Mindfulness and headache: a "new" old treatment, with new findings. Cephalalgia 36:1192–1205

47. Wells RE, Smitherman TA, Seng EK, Houle TT, Loder EW (2014) Behavioral and mind/body interventions in headache: Unanswered questions and future research directions. Headache 54:1107–1113

48. Grazzi L, Andrasik F, D'Amico D, Usai S, Kass S, Bussone G (2004) Disability in Chronic Migraine Patients With Medication Overuse: Treatment Effects at 1-Year Follow-up. Headache 44:678–683

49. D'Amico D, Tepper SJ (2008) Prophylaxis of migraine: general principles and patient acceptance. Neuropsychiatr Dis Treat 4:1155–1167

50. Ferrari A, Baraldi C, Sternieri E (2015) Medication overuse and chronic migraine: a critical review according to clinical pharmacology. Expert Opin Drug Metab Toxicol 11:1127–1144

51. Zheng H, Chen M, Huang D, Li J, Chen Q, Fang J (2015) Interventions for migraine prophylaxis: protocol of an umbrella systematic review and network meta-analysis. BMJ Open 5:e007594

52. Forde G, Duarte RA, Rosen N (2016) Managing Chronic Headache Disorders. Med Clin North Am 100:117–141

53. Kabat-Zinn J (2013) Full catastrophe living, third edition: using the wisdom of your body and mind to face stress, pain, and illness. Random House, New York

54. Segal Z, Williams JM, Teasdale J (2002) Mindfulness-based cognitive therapy for depression: a new approach to preventing relapse. Guilford Press, New York

55. Kabat Zinn J, Lipworth L, Burney R (1985) The clinical use of mindfulness meditation for the self-regulation of chronic pain. J Behav Med 8:163–190

56. Nash JM, McCrory DC, Nicholson RA, Andrasik F (2005) Efficacy and effectiveness approaches in behavioral treatment trials. Headache 45:507–512

57. Kosinski M, Bayliss MS, Bjorner JB, Ware JE Jr, Garber WH, Batenhorst A, Cady R, Dahlöf CG, Dowson A, Tepper S (2003) A six-item short-form survey for measuring headache impact: the HIT-6. Qual Life Res 12:963–974

58. Stewart WF, Lipton RB, Whyte J, Dowson A, Kolodner K, Liberman JN (1999) An international study to assess reliability of the Migraine Disability Assessment (MIDAS) score. Neurology 53:988–994

59. Andrasik F, Holroyd KA (1980) Reliability and concurrent validity of headache questionnaire data. Headache 20:44–46

60. Beck AT (1967) The diagnosis and management of depression. Universisty of Pennsylvania Press, Philadelphia

61. Furlanetto LM, Mendlowicz MV, Romildo Bueno J (2005) The validity of the Beck Depression Inventory-Short Form as a screening and diagnostic instrument for moderate and severe depression in medical inpatients. J Affect Disord 86:87–91

62. Spielberger CD (1989) State-Trait Anxiety Inventory: Bibliography, 2nd edn. Consulting Psychologists Press, Palo Alto

63. Predabissi L (1989) Santinello M. Inventario per l'ansia di stato e di tratto Nuova versione italiana dello S.T.A.I. – Forma Y, Organizzazioni Speciali, Firenze

64. Buse DC, Silberstein SD, Manack AN, Papapetropoulos S, Lipton RB (2013) Psychiatric comorbidities of episodic and chronic migraine. J Neurol 260:1960–1969

65. Tfelt-Hansen P, Pascual J, Ramadan N, Dahlöf C, D'Amico D, Diener HC (2012) Guidelines for controlled trials of drugs in migraine: Third edition. A guide for investigators. Cephalalgia 32:6–38

66. Boudreau GP, Grosberg BM, McAllister PJ, Lipton RB, Buse DC (2015) Prophylactic onabotulinumtoxinA in patients with chronic migraine and comorbid depression: An open-label, multicenter, pilot study of efficacy, safety and effect on headache-related disability, depression, and anxiety. Int J Gen Med 9:79–86

67. D'Amico D, Grazzi L, Bussone G, Curone M, Di Fiore P, Usai S, Leonardi M, Giovannetti AM, Schiavolin S, Raggi A (2015) Are depressive symptomatology, self-efficacy, and perceived social support related to disability and quality of life in patients with chronic migraine associated to medication overuse? Data from a cross-sectional study. Headache 55:636–645

68. Beck AT, Steer RA, Brown G (1996) BDI-II. Beck Depression Inventory: Second Edition. The Psychological Corporation, San Antonio

69. Meadows GN, Shawyer F, Enticott JC, Graham AL, Judd F, Martin PR, Piterman L, Segal Z (2014) Mindfulness-based cognitive therapy for recurrent depression: A translational research study with 2-year follow-up. Aust N Z J Psychiatry 48:743–755

70. Sundquist J, Lilja Å, Palmér K, Memon AA, Wang X, Johansson LM, Sundquist K (2015) Mindfulness group therapy in primary care patients with depression, anxiety and stress and adjustment disorders: randomised controlled trial. Br J Psychiatry 206:128–135

71. Mayor S (2015) Mindfulness based therapy is as effective as antidepressants in preventing depression relapse, study shows. BMJ 350:h2107

72. Chiesa A, Castagner V, Andrisano C, Serretti A, Mandelli L, Porcelli S, Giommi F (2015) Mindfulness-based cognitive therapy vs. psycho-education for patients with major depression who did not achieve remission following antidepressant treatment. Psychiatry Res 226(2-3):474–483

73. Kuyken W, Hayes R, Barrett B, Byng R, Dalgleish T, Kessler D, Lewis G, Watkins E, Brejcha C, Cardy J, Causley A, Cowderoy S, Evans A, Gradinger F, Kaur S, Lanham P, Morant N, Richards J, Shah P, Sutton H, Vicary R, Weaver A, Wilks J, Williams M, Taylor RS, Byford S (2015) Effectiveness and cost-effectiveness of mindfulness-based cognitive therapy compared with maintenance antidepressant treatment in the prevention of depressive relapse or recurrence (PREVENT): a randomised controlled trial. Lancet 386:63–73

74. Gaul C, Visscher CM, Bhola R, Sorbi MJ, Galli F, Rasmussen AV (2011) Team players against headache: multidisciplinary treatment of primary headaches and medication overuse headache. J Headache Pain 12:511–519

75. Kabat Zinn J (2003) Mindfulness-based interventions in context: past, present, and future. Clin Psychol Sci Pract 10:144–156

76. Pompili M, Di Cosimo D, Innamorati M, Lester D, Tatarelli R, Martelletti P (2009) Psychiatric comorbidity in patients with chronic daily headache and migraine: a selective overview including personality traits and suicide risk. J Headache Pain 10:283–290

77. Pompili M, Serafini G, Di Cosimo D, Dominici G, Innamorati M, Lester D, Forte A, Girardi N, De Filippis S, Tatarelli R, Martelletti P (2010) Psychiatric comorbidity and suicide risk in patients with chronic migraine. Neuropsychiatr Dis Treat 6:81–91

78. Serafini G, Pompili M, Innamorati M, Gentile G, Borro M, Lamis DA, Lala N, Negro A, Simmaco M, Girardi P, Martelletti P (2012) Gene variants with suicidal risk in a sample of subjects with chronic migraine and affective temperamental dysregulation. Eur Rev Med Pharmacol Sci 16:1389–1398

79. Breslau N (1992) Migraine, suicidal ideation, and suicide attempts. Neurology 42:392–395

14

OnabotulinumtoxinA injections in chronic migraine, targeted to sites of pericranial myofascial pain: an observational, open label, real-life cohort study

Danièle Ranoux[1]*Ⓘ, Gaelle Martiné[2], Gaëlle Espagne-Dubreuilh[2], Marlène Amilhaud-Bordier[3], François Caire[1] and Laurent Magy[4]

Abstract

Background: OnabotulinumtoxinA has proven its efficacy in reducing the number of headache days in chronic migraine (CM) patients. The usual paradigm includes 31 pericranial injection sites with low dose (5 U) per site. The aim of this study is to present the results obtained using a simpler injection protocol of onabotulinumtoxinA, with injection sites targeted to pericranial myofascial sites of pain.

Methods: Observational, open label, real-life, cohort study. We enrolled 63 consecutive patients fulfilling the diagnostic criteria of CM, and refractory to conventional treatments. The patients were injected using a "follow-the-pain" pattern into the corrugator and/or temporalis and/or trapezius muscles. The doses per muscle were fixed. According to the number of muscles injected, the total dose could vary from 70 to 150 U per session. Patients were considered responders if they had a ≥ 50% decrease in number of headache days in at least two consecutive injection cycles.

Results: Forty one patients (65.1% in intention to treat analysis) responded to treatment. In 70.7% of responders, the effect size was even higher, with a reduction ≥70% in the number of headache days. The associated cervical pain and muscle tenderness, present in 33 patients, was reduced by ≥50% in 31 patients (94%). Triptan consumption dramatically decreased (81%) in responders. The trapezius was the most frequently injected muscle. We observed no serious adverse event. The mean patient satisfaction rate was 8.5/10.

Conclusions: This study provides additional robust evidence supporting the efficacy of onabotulinumtoxinA injections in CM. Furthermore, the paradigm we used, with reduced number of injection sites targeted to pericranial myofascial sites of pain, may provide evidence in favor of the implication of myofascial trigger points in migraine chronicization.

Background

Chronic migraine (CM) is defined as headache occurring on 15 or more days per month for more than 3 months, which has the features of migraine headache on at least 8 days per month [1]. This disabling condition affects approximately 1–2% of the general population [2] and has a much stronger impact on quality of life and employment than episodic migraine [3]. The reason why episodic migraine becomes chronic remains poorly understood. The most recent data highlight the role of decreased activity of the descending pain-modulating network, and of sensitization of central structures including the thalamus, periaqueductal grey matter, and spinal trigeminal ganglion [4]. Some risk factors for chronicization of migraine have been identified, including frequency of migraine attacks, obesity, excessive use of opioids and barbiturates, caffeine overuse, stressful life events, sleeps disorders and cutaneous allodynia

* Correspondence: daniele.ranoux@gmail.com
[1]Department of Neurosurgery, Centre Hospitalier Universitaire de Limoges, Limoges, France

[5]. Most patients with CM overuse medication, but it is unclear whether this fact is a cause or a consequence of chronicization of migraine, and in ICHD-3 (International Classification of Headache Disorders 3) beta version the diagnosis of CM can be made regardless of whether the patient overuses medication or not [1].

Treatment of CM is challenging, since triptans or ergot derivatives are inconsistently effective. It requires a multifaceted approach, including lifestyle modifications, management of triggering factors, education, support, and behavioral therapy [4]. Drug withdrawal is considered mandatory by most physicians who believe that acute medication overuse is the major cause of migraine chronicization. Some studies, however, have demonstrated that CM patients' condition could be improved without drug withdrawal [6]. Furthermore, the modalities of medication discontinuation are still a matter of debate [7]. Pharmacological treatment options are limited, relying on classical oral prophylactic drugs. With the exception of topiramate, however, these agents have not been specifically evaluated in patients with CM. Non-pharmacological options include invasive procedures such as occipital nerve stimulation, even if the first randomized studies did not confirm the promising preliminary data [8]. In 2010, two large, placebo-controlled trials, PREEMPT (Phase III Research Evaluating Migraine Prophylaxis Therapy) 1 and 2, demonstrated that OnabotulinumtoxinA (OnaA) (Botox®, Allergan Inc) significantly decreased the severity and frequency of CM headache [9, 10]. The design of these studies has been criticized [11, 12], stressing several methodological weaknesses such as the change of primary outcome measure between the two studies, and possibly inadequate blinding. Furthermore, the placebo effect was particularly strong in these trials. These results, however, led the Food and Drug Administration to approve Botox® use in CM, and the recent update of the American Academy of Neurology guidelines recommends (level A) the use of OnaA in CM to reduce the number of headache days [13].

The PREEMPT trials injection scheme relies on the observation that OnaA injections applied for hyperfunctional facial lines are able to alleviate migraine symptoms [14], and consists in 31 injection sites throughout pericranial muscles. We postulated that, instead of injecting small doses in multiple sites, it could be more appropriate to inject higher dosage in a limited number of muscles known to be a source of myofascial pain in CM patients, such as the corrugator, temporalis and trapezius muscles [15–20].

We present here the clinical outcome of a cohort of 63 patients treated with this paradigm of injection.

Methods
Patients

In France, OnaA has not yet been approved for the treatment of CM. Since 2008, in a compassionate use, we offered these patients to receive OnaA injections on an off-label basis. Patients were eligible to OnaA treatment if they fulfilled International Headache Society (IHS) criteria for CM, regardless of whether they had an excessive abortive drug intake or not. This is in line with the current ICHD3 definition of CM in which medication overuse no longer excludes the diagnosis of CM [1]. The patients were considered refractory if they did not have any response to at least two prophylactic antimigrainous agents. They had to sign informed consent to receive OnaA treatment, and the off-label status of this drug in France was stressed. Patients were initially evaluated and followed-up by one of the authors or were alternatively referred by neurologists or pain specialists from elsewhere.

Study design (Figure 1)

This study was an observational, open-label, cohort-study conducted in accordance with the principles of the Helsinki Declaration. We prospectively and systematically recorded data from the patients and analyzed them retrospectively. During a first phase, called *adaptation period*, the injector (DR) used a follow-the-pain approach in order to determine the optimal injection scheme for each individual. The possible injection sites were the corrugator, temporalis, and trapezius muscles. Patients were systematically asked about the usual topography and time course of migraine attacks, and the existence of pain or stiffness of the cervical muscles. Examination searched for muscle tenderness and the existence of myofascial trigger points (TrPs). The decision to inject a single muscle relied on data from questioning and examination. The existence of referred pain patterns characteristic of TrPs on questioning as well as the identification of TrPs on examination were arguments to inject a given muscle. As an atlas of muscle referred pain, we used the manual by Travell and Simons [21]. For example, the existence of pain in any or all of the upper teeth during most migraine attacks in an individual was considered suggestive of myofascial involvement of the temporalis muscle. If the pain was predominantly located in, or started from the frontotemporal area, or if TrPs were demonstrated in corrugator and temporalis muscles, or if the topography of pain was suggestive of myofascial involvement, both muscles were injected bilaterally. When the patients had predominant pain in the back of the head, or when their headache pain frequently started and/or ended in the trapezius muscles, both trapezius muscles were injected. All muscle groups were injected if pain was both frontotemporal and cervico-occipital. When this first set of injections was efficacious, patients were re-injected in the same manner at the time when the frequency of headache days definitely increased. In the absence of efficacy, the paradigm was modified using the same follow-the-

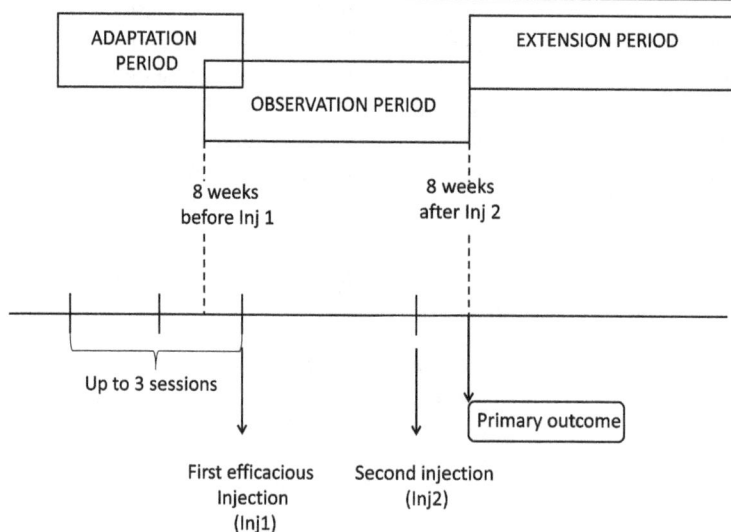

Fig. 1 Flow-chart. During a first phase, called *adaptation period*, we used a follow-the-pain approach in order to determine the optimal injection scheme for each individual. Once the best procedure was determined for each patient, it was reproduced at each subsequent injection session. This adaptation phase could necessitate up to three sessions. The *observation period* started 8 weeks before the first efficacious injection and ended 2 months after the second consecutive efficacious injection, or in case of inefficacy. Throughout the adaptation and the observation phases, patients kept a headache diary where they were asked to note the days with headache and the use of rescue medication. The *extension period* included all treatment cycles after the observation phase. During this period, the injector was allowed to modify the dosage and sites of injections

pain approach. Once the best procedure was determined for each patient, it was reproduced at each subsequent injection session. This adaptation phase could necessitate up to three sessions. The *observation period* started 8 weeks before the first efficacious injection and ended 2 months after the second consecutive efficacious injection, or in case of inefficacy. Throughout the adaptation and the observation phases, patients kept a headache diary where they were asked to note the days with headache and the use of rescue medication. The use of prophylactic drugs was allowed, but the dosage was maintained during the two phases. The *extension period* included all treatment cycles after the observation phase. During this period, the injector was allowed to modify the dosage and sites of injections using an even more tailored, follow-the pain approach.

OnaA injections: Dosage, dilution

The doses per muscle, as well as the injection technique, were predetermined according to our previous experience in CM (DR, unpublished data), and were off-label as well. The corrugator muscle is located in the supratrochlear region. The patient was asked to furrow his/her brow to activate the muscle, allowing an easy insertion of the needle. In order to inject the temporalis muscle, the patient was invited to chew gum, allowing to identify the most active part of the temporalis muscle. The patient was then asked to stop chewing, keeping the teeth clenched. The needle was inserted into the muscle,

the extremity of the needle being directed backwards. Then, the patient was invited to relax and the dose was administered into that point. For the trapezius muscle, the injections were also protocol-driven. The dose was distributed into 3 equally-distant sites along the lower part of this muscle. So, we targeted sites of myofascial pain, which are thought to contain TrPs [22] but did not make any effort to target TrPs themselves as sites of injection.

Variation of the dosage was not allowed during the observation phase. The doses of OnaA administered to the corrugator, temporalis and trapezius muscles were respectively 5 U, 30 U, and 40 U. Thus, the overall administered dose could vary from 70 U by session if only the facial muscles were injected to 150 U if all muscle groups were injected. The 100 U vial of Botox® was reconstituted with 2 ml of saline for cervical muscles and with 1 ml for facial muscles. The choice of employing an increased concentration for the corrugator and temporalis muscles aimed to limit unwanted diffusion of the toxin to the adjacent muscles and the subsequent side effects such as ptosis. It has been demonstrated that the injected volume is a major factor affecting the diffusion of botulinum toxin, independently from the dose. In other words, the more concentrated the toxin, the more limited the spreading of botulinum toxin [23]. Additionally, when the total dose is distributed in aliquots of smaller doses along the muscle, the diffusion of the product increases inside the muscle [23]. That is why we used a higher dilution for the trapezius muscles,

OnabotulinumtoxinA injections in chronic migraine, targeted to sites of pericranial myofascial...

129

as well as a multipoint injection procedure, in order to increase the diffusion of the toxin within such a large muscle.

Outcome measures

In accordance with current guidelines of clinical trials in CM [24], the primary outcome measure was mean change from baseline in frequency of headache days (as recorded in the patient diary) for the 2 months-period ending with week 8. Baseline was defined as the 2 months-period before the first efficient injection. The patients were considered responders if they had a ≥ 50% decrease in headache day frequency in at least two consecutive sets of injections.

The secondary outcome measures were the proportion of patients with a ≥ 70% decrease in headache day frequency, the decrease in triptan consumption, the time to efficacy onset, the duration of therapeutic effect (this was possible because retreatment was administered only when the patients needed to be reinjected ie at the time when the frequency of headache days definitely increased), and the assessment of patient satisfaction on a 0 to10 numerical scale (0 = no improvement, and 10 = maximum possible improvement). Data from the follow-up beyond the 2 first efficient injections were recorded.

Statistical analysis

Fisher exact test was used to compare frequencies between groups. Student t test was used to compare the means of two samples. A p value <0.05 was considered significant.

Results

Sixty three consecutive patients were referred to our center for refractory CM from 2008 to 2015. All screened patients consented to receive OnaA injections and signed informed consent. They were 43 females and 14 males, aged 17 to 85 years (mean: 44.3).

The results are summarized in Tables 1 and 2. Five patients dropped out early after the first injection session due to inefficacy (n = 2), living far from the hospital (n = 1), other health problems (n = 1), or personal reasons (n = 1). One other patient, aged 85 years, was excluded because of cognitive troubles making the assessment of response to OnaA difficult. Those 6 patients were included in the intention-to-treat (ITT) analysis. Sixteen patients did not respond. Forty one patients (65.1% in the ITT analysis, 72% in the per-

Table 1 Primary outcome measure

| Dropped out | Non responders | Responders | Proportion of responders | |
			ITT analysis	Per-protocol analysis
N 6	16	41	65.1%	72%

ITT Intention To Treat

Table 2 Secondary outcome measures

	Number	Percent of responders
Patients with ≥70% reduction in headache day frequency	29	70.7%
Patients with ≤1 headache day/ month	9	22%
Patients with ≥50% reduction in intercritic cervicalgia	31	94% [a]
	Mean	
Percentage of reduction in triptans consumption vs baseline	81% [b]	
Patient satisfaction mean on a numerical scale from 0 to 10 (min-max)	8,6 (6.5–10)	

[a]Percentage of the 33 patients with cervicalgia at baseline
[b]Percentage of the 28 patients who took triptans at baseline

protocol analysis) reached the primary efficacy endpoint (a ≥ 50% decrease in headache day frequency in at least two consecutive injection cycles). In 29 out of these 41 patients (70.7%), the reduction in headache days was ≥70%, with 9 patients (22% of responders) virtually headache-free (≤ 1 headache day per month.

Cervical pain and muscle tenderness were particularly frequent at baseline, present in 33 responders, and was reduced by ≥50% in 31 of them (94%) after treatment.

The optimal treatment regimen, determined during the adaptation period, included injections into the corrugator, temporalis and trapezius muscles bilaterally (total dose: 150 U) in the majority of patients (33/41, 80.5%). In five patients the treatment was administered into both trapezius muscles only (total dose: 80 U). The last three patients were injected into the corrugator and temporalis muscles only (total dose: 70 U). The trapezius muscle appeared to be a key target for OnaA injections in CM, since 38 patients out of 41 (92.7%) required injections into this muscle to improve.

At baseline, 15 patients did not take any triptans because of contraindication, loss of efficacy, or because triptans had never been effective. In responders, among the 28 triptan consumers, rescue drug consumption dramatically decreased (mean: 81%). Most patients reported a much better efficacy of the triptans on residual migraine attacks compared to the pre-treatment period.

There was no statistically significant difference between the responder and non-responder groups in terms of age, gender, mean baseline number of headache days, consumption of triptans at baseline, or the presence of prodromal, percritic or intercritic cervical muscle pain and tension (Table 3). By contrast, the presence of the three characteristics in the same patient (combination of a painful tension of the cervical muscles between, preceding and accompanying the attacks) was significantly more frequent in the responder group compared to the non responder group (p = 0.002).

Table 3 Description of the population and comparison of data in responders vs non responders

	All (N = 57)	Responders (N = 41)	Non responders (N = 16)	Comparison
Mean age (min-max)	44.3 (17–72)	43.2 (17–72)	48.4 (22–64)	NS
Female/Male	43/14	32/9	11/5	NS
Migraine with aura/without aura	7/50	6/35	1/15	NS
No triptans use	15	13	2	NS
Medication overusers	33	19	14	NS
Mean baseline number of headache days per month	23.12	22.63	24.36	NS
Baseline consumption of triptans/month	17.8	15.76	20.66	NS
Intercritic cervicalgia	42 (73.7%)	33	9	NS
Percritic cervicalgia	45	35	10	NS
Prodromal cervicalgia	35	30	5	NS
Combination of intercritic, percritic and prodromal cervicalgia	30	27	3	$P = 0.002$

NS non-significant

Surprisingly, the onset of efficacy was abrupt in most patients, the maximum of benefit being reached in a few days, after a latency ranging from 5 to 30 days (mean = 14.8 days). The duration of action ranged from 3 to 4 months.

The injections were well tolerated. The only significant adverse event we observed was local myalgia when the trapezius muscle was injected. This pain occurred 1 to 5 days after injection, and could last up to 15 days. It was qualified as severe in 4 patients (9.7%) and, interestingly, did not recur, or recurred very moderately, during the subsequent injection cycles. We observed no eyelid ptosis, perhaps due to the high concentration (1 ml/100 OnaA Units) used in our study to inject facial muscles. The patient satisfaction was particularly high, with a mean score of 8.6 (6.5–10) on a 0–10 numerical scale.

Extension phase

Two of the 16 patients considered to be non-responders claimed receiving retreatment because their migraine headaches were shorter-lasting, less severe, and easier to treat. Among the 41 responders, 34 are still under treatment, with a mean number of injection cycles of 5.95 (2–18). In those patients, the clinical benefit was maintained between each injection session and lasted three to 4 months. Seven patients discontinued treatment: 2 because they had achieved a sustained clinical benefit and the others due to personal reasons or lack of compliance. In this phase, patients were not required to keep a headache diary, but there was a trend towards a lengthening of intercycle intervals, and an increase in size effect with time. According to the patient pain pattern, additional muscles were injected in some patients, such as procerus, splenius capitis, suboccipitalis and masseter muscles.

Discussion

Myofascial pain syndromes have been described in CM patients in various pericranial sites including the neck muscles, the supratrochlear and corrugator region, and the temporalis muscles [15–20]. This preliminary study shows that OnaA injections targeted to those sites provide a high rate of response (65.1%, ITT) in CM. Furthermore, the magnitude of the response was large, with 70.7% of the responders exhibiting a ≥ 70% decrease in headache day frequency in at least two consecutive sessions of injections, and 22% being virtually headache-free. Finally, we observed a dramatic decrease (81%) in triptan consumption in responders.

Most patients had not experienced an improvement of this magnitude in years, as attested by the high degree of patient satisfaction (mean 8.6/10).

Our study, as well as the other recently published real-world experiments addressing the same issue [25–31], has some limitations, including the small sample size and the absence of a placebo arm. Placebo effect is particularly high in headache conditions, especially when the treatment is administered by injection. In order to lower the impact of placebo effect on our results, we considered patients as responders only if OnaA treatment was efficacious in two consecutive sets of injections. In addition, some features in the response can hardly be explained only by the placebo effect, such as (i) the reproducibility of results at each injection session (up to 18 per patient); (ii) the fact that the response to treatment in single patients differed according to the muscles injected (for example, some patients did not respond to frontotemporal injections in the adaptation phase, but responded to trapezius muscles injection). Finally, the long latency to efficacy onset we observed (up to 30 days) is unusual for a placebo effect.

Previous real-life studies provided conflicting results, with a ≥ 50% reduction in number of headache days achieved in a range as wide as 17.4 to 63% of patients [25–31]. With a figure of 65.1%, our results are in the higher part of this range, which may be due to the technical choice we have made. Indeed, our plan of injection differed from the PREEMPT protocol they used. We injected only the corrugator muscle on the forehead, not the frontalis or the procerus muscles. The temporalis muscle was injected in one site rather than in four, and the only cervical muscle injected was the trapezius muscle, with a higher dose (40 U versus 15 U). This resulted in a simplified paradigm with a maximum of 10 injections sites. Since the pivotal PREEMPT studies, a variety of injection techniques have been proposed, with modification of doses or sites of injections. Negro et al. [32] have demonstrated a dose-depending effect of OnaA in patients with CM and medication overuse headache, with a superior efficacy of OnaA 195 U compared to 155 U. Our results suggest that parameters others than the global injected dosage may be of relevance, such as the selection of a limited number of muscles using an individualized follow-the-pain approach, as well as an adequate dosage per muscle. Only a controlled, randomized study would be able to compare the efficacy of PREEMPT paradigm to such a tailored protocol, targeted to sites of myofascial pain. We suggest, however, that the paradigm we used may constitute a promising way to improve the outcome of CM patients treated with OnaA.

This injection paradigm was elaborated with reference to the theory which assumes that the muscle sites with myofascial pain act as triggers to initiate or perpetuate migraine. In support of this hypothesis, it has been demonstrated that inactivation of cervical trigger points by anesthetic infiltrations or manual therapy resulted in reduced migraine number and intensity [18, 19, 32–34]. The present study is to our knowledge the first to use OnaA injections targeted to pericranial muscle pain in CM patients. However, in a 2011 review paper, Gerwin mentioned his personal unpublished experience using a similar approach. He reports that he injects OnaA into the TrPs in the head, neck, and shoulder muscles identified by physical examination, and finds that 50% of patients treated in this way are headache-free, with an additional 30% significantly improved [35]. Both approaches are very close together. The only difference is that we did not target TrPs as the sites of injection. Identification of TrPs within a given muscle was just for us a mean to correctly select the muscles to inject. In a key paper about myofascial headache, Fernandez-de-las-penas [22] suggests the crucial role of TrPs in generating muscle pain. Indeed, evidence supports that active TrPs release algogenic substances that are susceptible to

promote the sensitization of muscle nociceptive nerve terminals, which may be responsible for muscle pain. In turn, the sensitized nerve ending liberate vasoactive neuropeptides such as calcitonine gene-related peptide (CGRP), Substance P and Glutamate, leading to a local neurogenic inflammation [22]. Since it is currently established that OnaA inhibits exocytosis of acetylcholine as well as multiple neurotransmitters including serotonin, dopamine, noradrenaline, gammaaminobutyric acid (GABA), enkephalin, glycine, substance P, ATP and calcitonin gene-related peptide (CGRP) [36], we can assume that OnaA may act in CM through a reduction of the peripheral sensitization within the injected muscles. It is however unlikely that the action of OnaA is limited to a peripheral effect. Indeed, the fact that OnaA induces a reduction of migraine attacks frequency implies that a central action also exists in one way or another. Some studies have suggested that myofascial inputs may activate the trigeminovascular system and therefore trigger migraine attacks in migraine sufferers [18]. It can therefore be suggested that an indirect central effect may result from the reduction of nociceptive myofascial input towards central neurons. In addition, we cannot rule out a direct central effect through the retrograde transport of OnaA, which has been demonstrated in numerous preclinical studies [37]. It is unclear, however, whether OnaA axonal transport has a clinical relevance in humans.

Cervicalgia present between migraine attacks was a major concern in our patients, present in 73.7% of cases. This is in keeping with studies that found a higher prevalence of neck pain disorders in patients with chronic rather than episodic migraine [38]. The significance of the cervical muscle tenderness observed in chronic headache is not fully understood, but is thought to result from myofascial pain [22]. We found that the combination of prodromal, percritic and intercritic cervicalgia was a predictive factor of response to OnaA treatment in CM patients, suggesting that the more severe the cervical myofascial disorder, the better the outcome. We also found that 94% of patients with neck muscle tenderness had a ≥ 50% reduction in cervicalgia intensity. Both findings are in line with our assumption that OnaA acts in CM at least partly by relieving the myofascial component of pain. We also showed that most patients reported a better efficacy of triptans after OnaA treatment. We think this supports the view that OnaA acts on myofascial pain, which is by definition unresponsive to triptan. Once relieved, the remaining pain is purely migrainous and is therefore triptan-responsive.

We found that the latency of therapeutic effect was long-lasting, with a mean of 14.8 days (up to 30 days). This finding was unexpected, since the delay of action of OnaA is estimated around a few days in the classical indications of OnaA such as dystonia and spasticity [39]. To our knowledge, only one other study addressed this issue [28]. The authors found that the first signs of therapeutic effect started after a mean of 5.5 days, which suggests a progressive onset of improvement. The pattern of response in our patients was quite different. Patients reported a delayed, but rapidly occurring improvement. This difference may be due to the injection paradigm we used, targeted to sites of myofascial pain. If so, the long delay to onset we observed could be an argument supporting a central participation in the mechanism of action of OnaA in CM.

Our results also raise the concern of the role of drug withdrawal in the management of CM. In the present study, we found that OnaA treatment itself led to a dramatic reduction of migraine rescue medication intake (81%). Thus, we propose that, in CM patients, (i) drug abuse may be a consequence of the ancillary myofascial pain rather than the cause of migraine chronicization, and (ii) OnaA treatment should be discussed before considering medication withdrawal.

Conclusions

We conclude that specifically targeting myofascial pain sites with selective OnaA injections may be a safe and effective option in CM treatment. Further larger, placebo-controlled studies are needed to compare the present protocol with the fixed "multipoint-low dose per point" PREEMPT protocol. If our results were confirmed by further studies, it could be suggested that myofascial pain and TrPs may contribute to headache pain in CM patients and constitute an important factor of migraine chronicization.

Authors' contributions
Conception and Design: DR, FC, LM. Injections: DR. Acquisition of Data: DR, GM, GED, MAB. Analysis and Interpretation of Data: DR, FC, LM, GM, GED, MAB. Drafting the Article: DR. Revising it for Intellectual Content: DR, FC, LM. All authors read and approved the final manuscript.

Competing interests
Danièle Ranoux received honoraria consultancy from Allergan, travel support and educational grants from Allergan, Merz and Ipsen. The other authors have no competing interests to declare. Publication fees for this manuscript are supported by the Teaching Hospital of Limoges, France.

Author details
[1]Department of Neurosurgery, Centre Hospitalier Universitaire de Limoges, Limoges, France. [2]Pain Center, Centre Hospitalier Universitaire de Limoges, Limoges, France. [3]Pain Center, Centre Hospitalier de Guéret, Guéret, France. [4]Department of Neurology, Centre Hospitalier Universitaire de Limoges, Limoges, France.

References
1. Headache Classification Committee of the International Headache Society (2013) The international classification of headache disorders, 3rd edition (beta version). Cephalalgia 33:629–808
2. Natoli JL, Manack A, Dean B, Butler Q, Turkel CC, Stovner L, Lipton RB (2010) Global prevalence of chronic migraine: a systematic review. Cephalalgia 30:599–609
3. Diener HC, Dodick DW, Goadsby PJ, Lipton RB, Lessen J, Silberstein SD (2012) Chronic migraine- classification, characteristics and treatment. Nat Rev Neurol 8:162–171
4. Bernstein C, Burstein R (2012) Sensitization of the trigeminovascular pathway: perspective and implications to migraine pathophysiology. J Clin Neurol 8:89–99
5. Bigal ME, Lipton RB (2009) What predicts the change from episodic to chronic migraine? Curr Opin Neurol 22:269–276
6. Hagen K, Albretsen C, Vilming ST, Salvesen R, Grønning M, Helde G, Gravdahl G, Zwart JA, Stovner LJ (2009) Management of medication overuse headache: 1-year randomized multicenter open-label trial. Cephalalgia 29:221–232
7. Créac'h C, Frappe P, Cancade M, Laurent B, Peyron R, Demarquay G, Navez M (2011) In-patient versus out-patient withdrawal programmes for medication overuse headache: a 2-year randomized trial. Cephalalgia 31:1189–1198
8. Palmisani S, Al-Kaisy A, Arcioni R, Smith T, Negro A, Lambru G, Bandikatla V, Carson E, Martelletti P (2013) A six year retrospective review of occipital nerve stimulation practice-controversies and challenges of an emerging technique for treating refractory headache syndromes. J Headache Pain 6(14):67
9. Aurora SK, Dodick DW, Turkel CC, DeGryse RE, Silberstein SD, Lipton RB, Diener HC, Brin MF, on behalf of PREEMPT 1 Chronic Migraine Study Group (2010) OnabotulinumtoxinA for treatment of chronic migraine: results from the double-blind, randomized, placebo-controlled phase of the PREEMPT 1 trial. Cephalalgia 30:793–803 Curr Pain Headache Rep 15:336-8
10. Diener HC, Dodick DW, Aurora SK, Turkel CC, DeGryse RE, Lipton RB, Silberstein SD, Brin MF, on behalf of PREEMPT 2 Chronic Migraine Study Group (2010) OnabotulinumtoxinA for treatment of chronic migraine: results from the double-blind, randomized, placebo-controlled phase of the PREEMPT 2 trial. Cephalalgia 30:804–814
11. Russell MB (2011) Clinical trials on onabotulinumtoxinA for the treatment of chronic migraine. J Headache Pain 12:135–136
12. Solomon S (2013) Onabotulinumtoxin a for treatment of chronic migraine: the unblinding problem. Headache 53:824–826
13. Simpson DM, Hallett M, Ashman EJ, Comella CL, Green MW, Gronseth GS, Armstrong MJ, Gloss D, Potrebic S, Jankovic J, Karp BP, Naumann M, So YT, Yablon SA (2016) Practice guideline update summary: Botulinum neurotoxin for the treatment of blepharospasm, cervical dystonia, adult spasticity, and headache: report of the guideline development Subcommittee of the American Academy of neurology. Neurology 86:1818–1826
14. Binder WJ, Brin MF, Blitzer A, Pogoda JM (2002) Botulinum toxin type a (BOTOX) for treatment of migraine. Dis Mon 48:323–335
15. Calandre EP, Hidalgo J, Garcia-Leiva JM, Rico-Villademoros F (2006) Trigger points evaluation in migraine patients: an indication of peripheral sensitization linked to migraine predisposition? Eur J Neurol 13:244–249
16. Fernandez-de-Las-Penas C, Cuadrado ML, Gerwin RD, Pareja JA (2006) Myofascial disorders in the trochlear region in unilateral migraine: a possible initiating or perpetuating factor. Clin J Pain 22:548–553
17. Fernandez-de-Las-Penas C, Cuadrado ML, Pareja JA (2006) Myofascial trigger points, neck mobility and forward head posture in unilateral migraine. Cephalalgia 26:1061–1070
18. Garcia-Leiva HJ, Rico-Villademoros F, Moreno V, Calandre EP (2007) Effectiveness of ropivacaine trigger points inactivation in the prophylactic management of patients with severe migraine. Pain Med 8:65–70
19. Giamberardino MA, Tafuri E, Savini A, Fabrizio A, Affaitati G, Lerza R, Di Ianni L, Lapenna D, Mezzetti A (2007) Contribution of myofascial trigger points to migraine symptoms. J Pain 8:869–878
20. Fallucco M, Janis JE, Hagan RR (2012) The anatomical morphology of the supraorbital notch: clinical relevance to the surgical treatment of migraine headaches. Plast Reconstr Surg 130:1227–1233
21. Simons DG, Travell JG, Simons LS (1999) Myofascial pain and dysfunction: the trigger point manual, vol 1. Lippincott Williams & Wilkins, Philadelphia
22. Fernández-de-las-Peñas (2015) Myofascial head pain. Curr Pain Headache Rep 19:28
23. Ramirez-Castaneda J, Jankovic J, Comella C, Dashtipour K, Fernandez HH, Mari Z (2013) Diffusion, spread, and migration of botulinum toxin. Mov Disord 28:1775–1783
24. Silberstein S, Tfelt-Hansen P, Dodick DW, Limmroth V, Lipton RB, Pascual J, Wang SJ (2008) Guidelines for controlled trials of prophylactic treatment of chronic migraine in adults. Cephalalgia 28:484–495
25. Khalil M, Zafar HW, Quarshie V, Ahmed F (2014) Prospective analysis of the use of OnabotulinumtoxinA (BOTOX) in the treatment of chronic migraine; real-life data in 254 patients from hull, U.K. J Headache Pain 15:54

26. Grazzi L, Usai S (2015) Onabotulinum toxin a (Botox) for chronic migraine treatment: an Italian experience. Neurol Sci 36(Suppl 1):33–35

27. Silberstein SD, Dodick DW, Aurora SK, Diener HC, DeGryse RE, Lipton RB, Turkel CC (2015) Per cent of patients with chronic migraine who responded per onabotulinumtoxinA treatment cycle: PREEMPT. J Neurol Neurosurg Psychiatry 86:996–1001

28. Kollewe K, Escher CM, Wulff DU, Fathi D, Paracka L, Mohammadi B, Karst M, Dressler D (2016) Long-term treatment of chronic migraine with OnabotulinumtoxinA: efficacy, quality of life and tolerability in a real-life setting. J Neural Transm (Vienna) 123:533–540

29. Russo M, Manzoni GC, Taga A, Genovese A, Veronesi L, Pasquarella C, Sansebastiano GE, Torelli P (2016) The use of onabotulinum toxin a (Botox®) in the treatment of chronic migraine at the Parma headache Centre: a prospective observational study. Neurol Sci 37:1127–1131

30. Vikelis M, Argyriou AA, Dermitzakis EV, Spingos KC, Mitsikostas DD (2016) Onabotulinumtoxin-A treatment in Greek patients with chronic migraine. J Head Pain. 17:84

31. Butera C, Colombo B, Bianchi F, Cursi M, Messina R, Amadio S, Guerriero R, Comi G, Del Carro U (2016) Refractory chronic migraine: is drug withdrawal necessary before starting a therapy with onabotulinum toxin type a? Neurol Sci 37:1701–1706

32. Negro A, Curto M, Lionetto L, Martelletti P (2016) A two years open-label prospective study of OnabotulinumtoxinA 195 U in medication overuse headache: a real-world experience. J Head Pain 17:1

33. Tflet-Hanson P, Lous I, Olesen J (1981) Prevalence and significance of muscle tenderness during common migraine headache. Headache 21:49–54

34. Mellick GA, Mellick LB (2003) Regional head and face pain relief following lower cervical intramuscular anesthetic injection. Headache 43:1109–1111

35. Gerwin R (2011) Treatment of chronic migraine headache with onabotulinumtoxinA. Curr Pain Headache Rep 15:336–338

36. Aoki KR, Francis J (2011) Updates on the antiociceptive mechanism hypothesis of botulinum toxin a. Parkinsonism Relat Disord 17(Suppl 1):S28–S33

37. Matak I, Lacković Z (2014) Botulinum toxin a, brain and pain. Prog Neurobiol 119-120:39–59

38. Florencio LL, Chaves TC, Carvalho GF, Gonçalves MC, Casimiro EC, Dach F, Bigal ME, Bevilaqua-Grossi D (2014) Neck pain disability is related to the frequency of migraine attacks: a cross-sectional study. Headache 54:1203–1210

39. Thenganatt MA, Fahn S (2012) Botulinum toxin for the treatment of movement disorders. Current Neurol Neurosci Rep 91:399–409

15

The enigma of site of action of migraine preventives: no effect of metoprolol on trigeminal pain processing in patients and healthy controls

Julia M. Hebestreit and Arne May[*]

Abstract

Background: Beta-blockers are a first choice migraine preventive medication. So far it is unknown how they exert their therapeutic effect in migraine. To this end we examined the neural effect of metoprolol on trigeminal pain processing in 19 migraine patients and 26 healthy controls. All participants underwent functional magnetic resonance imaging (fMRI) during trigeminal pain twice: Healthy subjects took part in a placebo-controlled, randomized and double-blind study, receiving a single dose of metoprolol and placebo. Patients were examined with a baseline scan before starting the preventive medication and 3 months later whilst treated with metoprolol.

Results: Mean pain intensity ratings were not significantly altered under metoprolol. Functional imaging revealed no significant differences in nociceptive processing in both groups. Contrary to earlier findings from animal studies, we did not find an effect of metoprolol on the thalamus in either group. However, using a more liberal and exploratory threshold, hypothalamic activity was slightly increased under metoprolol in patients and migraineurs.

Conclusions: No significant effect of metoprolol on trigeminal pain processing was observed, suggesting a peripheral effect of metoprolol. Exploratory analyses revealed slightly enhanced hypothalamic activity under metoprolol in both groups. Given the emerging role of the hypothalamus in migraine attack generation, these data need further examination.

Keywords: Metoprolol, Beta-blocker, Thalamus, Migraine, fMRI, Pain, Pharmacological modulation, Preventive treatment, Nociceptive trigeminal system, Pain

Background

Beta-blockers such as metoprolol and propranolol are first choice migraine preventive medication. While the clinical efficacy of beta-blockers in reducing migraine attack frequency is certainly established [1–4], it is still poorly understood how they exert their therapeutic effect. So far, no imaging studies investigated the central effects of beta-blockers and our knowledge about the mechanisms derives from preclinical studies. Metoprolol belongs to the group of β-adrenergic blockers and select-

ively blocks β1 receptors. Beta-blockers attenuate the effects of adrenaline and noradrenaline [5, 6] and thereby downregulate the stimulating effect of the sympathetic nervous system. This downregulation was examined in several measures of cortical information processing that have been shown to be abnormal in migraineurs, such as visual evoked potentials, auditory evoked potentials and contingent negative variations [7]. Beta-blockers seem to have a regulatory effect upon all of these. In the visual system of migraineurs, metoprolol decreased the amplitude of visual evoked potentials [8]. Another study found a decrease of intensity dependence of auditory evoked cortical potentials in migraineurs [9] and this decrease was related to clinical improvement. It has therefore been proposed that modulating the excitability of the cortex is how beta-blockers reduce the

* Correspondence: a.may@uke.de
Department of Systems Neuroscience, Center for Experimental Medicine, University Medical Center Eppendorf, Martinistr. 52, 20246 Hamburg, Germany

migraine attack frequency. Another neurophysiological approach to observe cortical information processing is the analysis of contingent negative variation (CNV), an event-related, slow cerebral potential following activation in the striato-thalamo-cortical loop. In untreated migraineurs the CNV is significantly increased and lacks habituation. Several studies found that beta-blockers normalize the CNV [10] and further that normalization of high CNV was positively correlated with treatment response [10–12]. These studies suggest that the effects refer to a general effect of beta-blockers on cortical excitability and abnormal cortical information processing in migraine. Accordingly it has been hypothesized that beta-blockers exert their preventive action in migraine by modulating cortical excitability and processing [11]. However, the aforementioned studies applied methods with a focus on specific network activity rather than a focus on the location where metoprolol potentially exerts its action in the brain. A plausible explanation for the described abnormalities in sensory processing in migraineurs is a dysfunction of processing in thalamo-cortical neurons [13–15]. Evidence that preventive action of beta-blockers is effective through β_1-adrenoceptor inhibition in nociceptive neurons in the thalamus comes from electrophysiological animal studies. Shields and Goadsby (2005) reported that thalamo-cortical activity evoked by superior sagittal sinus stimulation was inhibited after locally applied propranolol [16].

To address this issue and to achieve a more integrated picture of central effects of metoprolol, we employed pharmacological functional magnetic resonance imaging in combination with a human model of headache attacks. The aim of this study is to assess the effects of metoprolol on brain activation patterns during trigeminal pain in migraine patients, as well as healthy human subjects, determined by fMRI. Based on earlier studies we hypothesize that metoprolol has an inhibiting effect on trigeminal pain processing, especially in the thalamus and/or thalamocortical networks.

Methods

Subjects

Patients

Twenty five migraineurs were recruited from the Headache Outpatient Department of the University Medical Center Eppendorf, Hamburg. Four patients dropped out after the first session, 2 were excluded because of corrupted data. The final sample therefore encompassed 19 patients (18 females; mean age: 35 ± 2.2 years). Patients fulfilled International Classification of Headache Disorders, 3rd Edition (beta version) criteria of episodic respectively chronic migraine with or without aura [17]. Another inclusion criteria was indication for a preventive medication (more than 3 attacks/months) and the decision to start a treatment with metoprolol. Exclusion criteria were any other neurologic or internal disease, the use of other medications and any contraindication for the MRI examination such as claustrophobia or pregnancy. Clinical characteristics of the patients' population are included in Table 1.

Healthy subjects

Thrity one healthy subjects were recruited via online advertisements. Exclusion criteria were the presence of any pain disorder (including migraine), neurological and psychiatric disorders as well as any contraindications for metoprolol or the MRI examination. Data of 4 subjects had to be excluded from the analysis for corrupted data and 1 subject dropped out after the first session. Twenty six subjects (14 females; mean age: 25 ± 0.7 years) were included in the final analyses.

Standard protocol approvals, registrations, and patient consents

The study was approved by the local ethics committee (PV4084, PV4102) and all subjects gave written informed consent. Subjects were remunerated for participation.

Table 1 Clinical characteristics of the patients population ($n = 19$)

	Episodic migraineurs	Chronic migraineurs	Healthy subjects
Male / female, n	1 / 12	0 / 6	12 / 14
Mean age, y	35	34	25
Patients with aura, n	4	1	N/A
Headaches on scan day I, n	4	2	N/A
Headaches on scan day II, n	3	0	N/A
Headache frequency scan 1, mean d/m	12	19	N/A
Headache frequency scan 2, mean d/m	6	8	N/A
Successful treatment (50% reduction), n	5	4	N/A
Disease duration, mean y	19	16	N/A

Study design

Healthy subjects

Every subject participated in two identical sessions that were separated by at least 2 weeks to account for the wash-out effect. In a placebo-controlled, crossover, randomized and double-blind fashion, participants took an oral dose of either 75 mg metoprolol or placebo. After a 50 min waiting period to reach the peak plasma concentration of metoprolol [18, 19] during the MR measurement, blood samples were drawn. Procedure of the healthy subjects group is depicted in Fig. 1.

Patients

Patients also participated in two identical sessions. One session took place before they started the preventive treatment with metoprolol, the second session when they had taken metoprolol on a regular basis for at least 2 months.

Experimental paradigm

The paradigm was identical for healthy subjects and patients in both sessions. In their first session subjects completed a training session to get acquainted with the task before starting the MR session. The standardized trigeminal nociceptive stimulation in the MR scanner (Fig. 2) has been described in detail in previous publications [20, 21]. In summary the paradigm consisted of 4 stimuli: 3 gaseous stimuli and one visual stimulus. Three gaseous stimuli were either ammonia as a nociceptive trigeminal stimulus, rose odor as an olfactory stimulus and air as a control stimulus, applied through a Teflon tube to the left nostril. A rotating checkerboard as a visual stimulus and the gaseous stimuli were applied 15 times each, in a pseudorandomized order. Each stimulation was followed by two visual rating scales, where the subject rated the stimulus painfulness (following the ammonia stimuli) and unpleasantness or intensity (rose and air stimuli) and unpleasantness. Painfulness/intensity was rated on a visual numeric analogue scale from 0 to 100, whereas for unpleasantness rating a bipolar scale from −50 (no sensation) to 50 (very unpleasant) was used. The stimulation paradigm is illustrated in Fig. 2.

Medication (Metoprolol)

Participants received either metoprolol (75 mg; Metoprolol-ratiopharm®; ratiopharm GmbH, Ulm, Germany) or placebo (Mannitol 99.5 T, highly-dispersed silicon dioxide 0.5 T) in the first session and the alternate substance in the second session. In between measurements a 2-week washout period took place. 50 min after administration blood samples were drawn to determine metoprolol plasma concentration. Blood pressure and heart rate were monitored during the whole session.

Plasma concentration

At each session a blood sample was drawn from the forearm of the subject using a 4.9 ml vacuum tube containing ethylenediaminetetraacetic acid (EDTA). Afterwards the blood was centrifuged at 2.0 rmp for 20 min at 4 °C and stored at −20 °C until analysis. The Institute of Experimental Pharmacology and Toxicology (Center of Experimental Medicine, University Medical Center Hamburg-Eppendorf, Germany) conducted the analysis of blood plasma concentration via liquid chromatography/mass spectrometry [22].

MRI data acquisition

All magnet-resonance imaging was acquired on a Siemens Trio 3 T scanner (Siemens AG, Erlangen, Germany) using a 32-channel head coil. High resolution T1 weighted structural images (voxel size 1 m^3) were obtained using a magnetization-prepared rapid gradient echo sequence. After the structural image, functional images were acquired by an echo planar imaging sequence (repetition time 2.62 s, echo time 30 milliseconds, flip angle 80°, field of view 220 × 220 mm). Each volume consisted of 40 axial slices (slice thickness

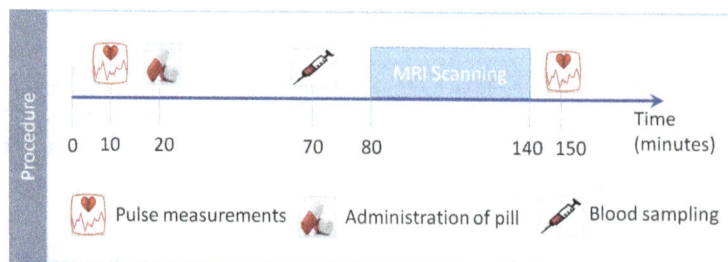

Fig. 1 Procedure in healthy subjects group. Timeline of procedures taking place at both scanning sessions (metoprolol and placebo session). Each session started out with pulse measurement and administration of a pill, either treatment or a placebo in a blinded fashion. A blood sample was drawn after a waiting period of 50 min that allowed the drug to reach its maximum plasma concentration while the participant completed the experiment in the scanner. Blood samples were drawn to determine plasma concentration of metoprolol. Then a paradigm of nociceptive trigeminal stimulation was conducted during fMRI, followed by a second pulse measurement after completion

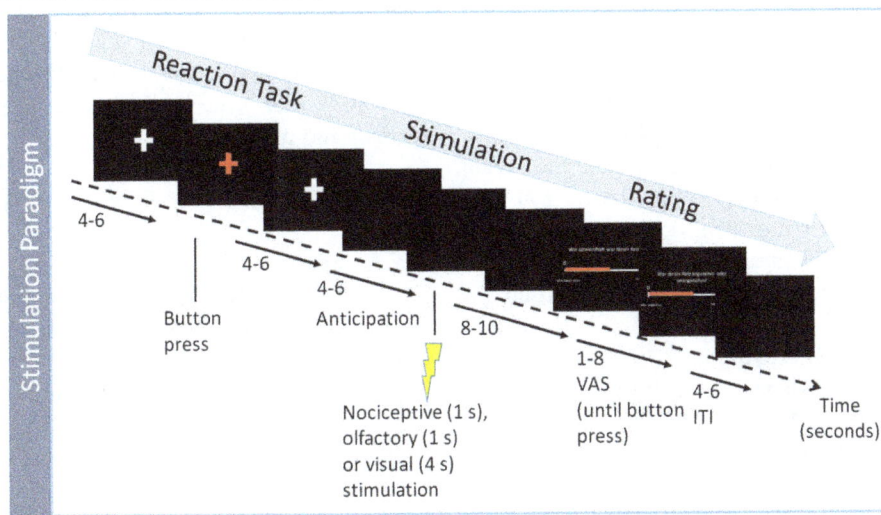

Fig. 2 Single trial of stimulation paradigm. Each trial started with a short reaction task, followed by an anticipation phase of jittered length and stimulation with one of the 4 stimuli: 3 gaseous (ammonia, rose odour and air) or a visual stimulus (rotating checkerboard). At the end of each trial subjects rated stimulus painfulness/intensity and pleasantness on two visual analogue scales (VAS). Abbreviations: ITI, Inter-trial interval

2 mm, gap 1 mm). For the whole experiment, scantime was about 55 min.

Behavioral data analysis

Behavioral data analyses were performed using SPSS Statistics version 22.00 (IBM Corp., Armonk, NY). Ratings were assessed with a visual analogue rating scale (VAS) and mean pain ratings (following trigemino-nociceptive stimulation) were calculated per subject, per session (treatment, no treatment). A paired t-tested was applied in order to compare average pain intensity ratings between sessions at a statistical threshold of $p < 0.05$.

MRI data processing

Data processing was performed similarly in the healthy subjects and the patients group.

Preprocessing

The Statistical Parametric Mapping software SPM12 (Wellcome Trust Centre of Neuroimaging, London, UK) was used for data processing. Standard algorithms and parameters were used, unless specified differently. The first 5 volumes of each session were discarded to account for T1 saturation effects. Anatomical images of each subject were co-registered with the corresponding functional images. The functional images were slice time corrected and realigned to the mean functional image, then normalized into MNI (Montreal Neurological Institute) space and finally smoothed using a 6 mm^3 Gaussian kernel.

Single subject analysis

The general linear model on single subject level included 22 regressors, 11 per session. For each session, experimental regressors included all 4 conditions (ammonia, rose odor, air puffs and visual rotating checker board) as well as button presses. At event onset, these were modeled by convolving stick functions with the canonical hemodynamic response function. Additionally, 6 movement regressors of no interest, resulting from the realignment step, were included per session. The contrast ammonia > air was defined as contrast of interest and also compared between medication and placebo on single subject level.

Group analysis

For group analyses the single subject contrast images were entered into the second level. In each group (patients and healthy subjects), potential changes in nociceptive processing caused my metoprolol were assessed by a one-sample t-test that compared BOLD signals (during painful stimulation) between both sessions. Results are reported at a voxel-wise FWE-corrected threshold of $p < 0.05$. Following the a-priori hypothesis that metoprolol acts on the thalamus [16] a small volume correction (SVC: $p_{(FWE)} < 0.05$) was performed. A thalamus mask obtained from the Harvard-Oxford cortical/subcortical structural atlas (http://www.cma.mgh.harvard.edu/fsl_atlas.html) was used for this analysis. Furthermore we were interested if there are any regions activated under metorpolol during pain in patients and healthy subjects alike. For this exploratory analyses a liberal threshold of 0.005 uncorrected was applied.

Results

Behavior

Ammonia stimuli, measured by the VAS scale (±SEM), were rated as painful in the healthy subjects group with a mean of 63.3 (± 2.9) in the metoprolol and 66.7 (±2.4) in the placebo session. In the patients group the mean intensity in the treatment session was 72.5 (± 2.7) and 72.2 (± 2.6) before treatment. Behavioral analysis of intensity ratings did not yield any significant results, neither in the patients, nor in the healthy subjects group.

Physiology in healthy subjects group

The mean metoprolol plasma concentration in healthy subjects, measured in the metoprolol session was 191 ng/mL (SD = 0.8). Additionally we compared the mean drop of heart rate (beats/min) in both sessions (Fig. 3). In each session, we subtracted the heart rate measured after the experiment, from the heart rate measured before the medication/placebo pill was administered (heart rate T2 – heart rate T1). In the metoprolol session the mean drop of the heart rate was 16.4 (±1.8), whereas in the placebo session it was 8.6 (±1.4). The fall of the heart rate in the metoprolol session was significantly larger than in the placebo session ($p < 0.001$).

Imaging

Main effects of painful trigeminal stimulation

In both groups, we detected significantly increased neural activation ($p < 0.05$, voxel-wise FWE-corrected) during nociceptive trigeminal stimulation in several pain related cortical and subcortical areas. The increase in BOLD signal responses included the bilateral thalamus, insular cortex, midcingulate and anterior cingulate cortex (MCC, ACC), cerebellum as well as somatosensory cortices and brainstem areas.

Differences in pain processing between metoprolol and placebo

We found no difference between the metoprolol and placebo session in BOLD signal intensity ($p < 0.05$, voxel-wise FWE-corrected) during trigeminal pain. Contrary to earlier studies, we did not find any inhibition in BOLD signal intensity of the thalamus after metoprolol treatment compared to placebo (SVC). The opposite contrast did not reveal any differences either.

Exploratory analyses

To further explore the effect of metoprolol on trigeminal pain processing with regard to similarities under metoprolol (during nociceptive input) in both groups, patients and healthy subjects, we lowered the threshold to 0.005 uncorrected. In both groups, i.e. patients and healthy subjects, we found the BOLD signal intensity of the hypothalamus increased under metoprolol during pain, compared to no medication, placebo respectively (Fig. 4). Following these results, we had a closer look at the relationship of hypothalamic activity (MNI coordinates (peak) and size of the significant cluster: x = –8, y = –8, z = 9, k = –10), in patients with the treatment effect of metoprolol. As depicted in Fig. 5, we found a negative

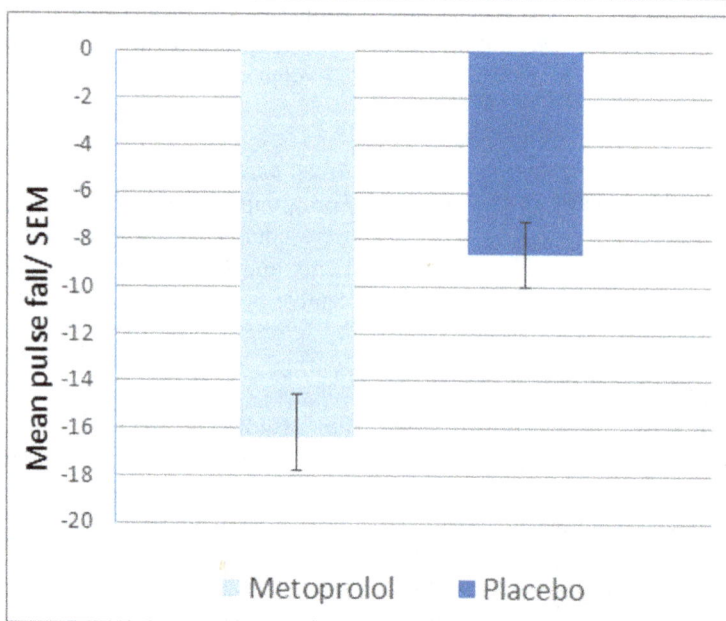

Fig. 3 Pulse under metoprolol and placebo in healthy subjects. Pulse of the subjects were measured at two time points in each session and subtracted afterwards (pulse change = T2 [after experimental paradigm] - T1 [before treatment]). The pulse drop in the metoprolol session is significantly bigger than in the placebo session ($p < 0.001$)

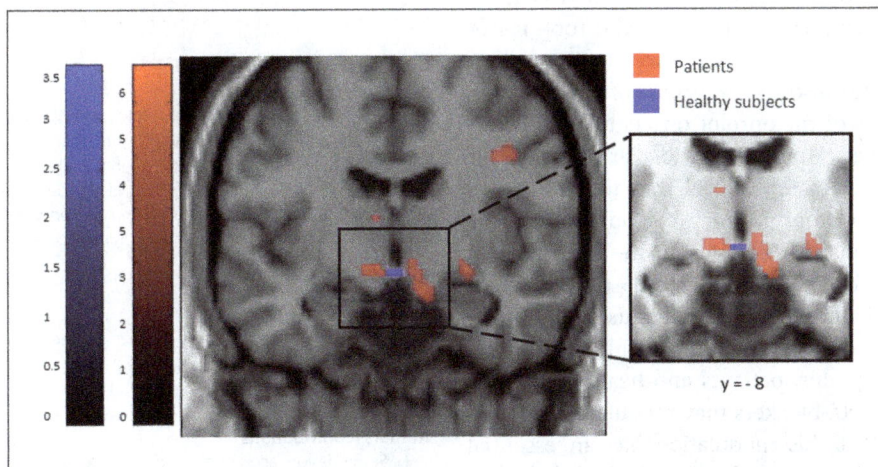

Fig. 4 Increased hypothalamic activation under Metoprolol during pain. At an exploratory threshold of $p < 0.005$ (uncorrected), hypothalamic activity is similarly increased in patients (red) and healthy subjects (blue) under metoprolol during trigeminal stimulation

correlation ($r = -0.44$, $p < 0.05$) between betavalues in the hypothalamus and a reduction of headache days. The bigger the reduction of headache, the fewer hypothalamic activity.

Discussion

Contrary to our hypotheses, we found no significant effect of metoprolol on central trigeminal pain processing, neither in patients, nor in healthy subjects. The healthy subject group showed metoprolol plasma concentrations and a significant drop of heart rate under metoprolol compared to placebo, demonstrating a biological effect of the single dosage. Either, this effect on the vegetative nervous system is not reflected in central neural structures or, more likely, it is due to peripheral activity only.

In either case, the results do not support the notion that beta-blockers act centrally, as suggested by experimental animal studies [16]. However, a purely peripheral site of action of beta-blockers ignores their effect on attack frequency, premonitory symptoms and side effects of central nervous origin [23, 24]. One could argue that the administered dose of 75 mg might have been too low to reach a neural level after a single dose, but this is unlikely given the above mentioned biological effect of the single dosage that we observed. We chose this dosage as this was ethically justifiable and 75 mg per day is the usual dose for migraine prevention. Nonetheless, metoprolol may indeed only exert its central effects leading to a reduction in attack frequency, if taken on a regular basis over several weeks. This was for ethical reasons

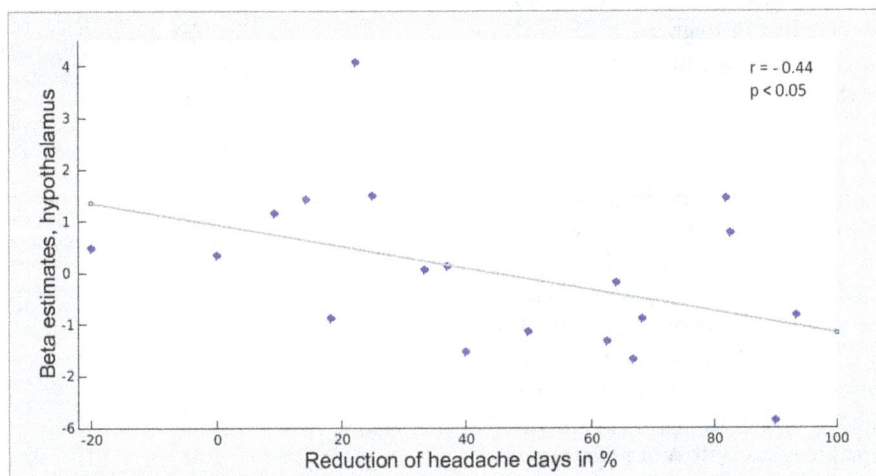

Fig. 5 Relationship of hypothalamic activity and the reduction of headache days in patients under metoprolol treatment. A bigger reduction of headache days in patients, marked by a higher percentage of reduction, is related to lower beta estimates within a cluster in the left hypothalamus (peak: $x = -8$, $y = -8$, $z = -10$)

not feasible in healthy volunteers, for which reason we have also investigated migraine patients who took metoprolol daily over several months before treatment and under treatment. But also in the group of migraineurs, no significant effect of metoprolol on central pain processing was observed. Another possible explanation for the missing effect of metoprolol is that the functional changes caused by metoprolol may be too subtle to be disclosed by functional MRI.Exploring the data further, we used a more lenient threshold of 0.005 (uncorrected) and interestingly found the hypothalamus being more activated following nociceptive input during metoprolol treatment in both groups, patients and healthy subjects. This suggests that beta-blockers may modulate hypothalamic action and that this modulation has an essential role in its preventive effect. Given the hypothalamus' role in the pathophysiology of migraine pain [25] and chronification [26], it would be a conceivable target for preventive migraine medication such as metoprolol. Following this line of investigation, we correlated hypothalamic activity in patients with drug effectiveness and found a negative correlation between hypothalamic activity and reduction of headache days, i.e. the stronger the reduction of headache days, the fewer hypothalamic activity. These speculations have to be seen with caution, as changes in hypothalamic activity were detected only at an exploratory threshold. Nevertheless it is an interesting finding and encourages further investigation of the hypothalamus as a possible target of metoprolol in preventive treatment. An interesting fact of this study is that the hypothalamus already increased after just a single treatment of metoprolol in healthy subjects. It would be interesting to see whether a longer treatment phase would affect physiological phenomenon or (stress) thresholds of healthy participants. However, given that it is still not clear whether central effects of metoprolol determine its therapeutic effect in migraine or if its therapeutic effect is caused by changes in the periphery, the issue merits further studies.

Conclusion

For the first time, the preventive mechanism of metoprolol in migraine treatment is being investigated with the method of pharmacological imaging, which has successfully been applied to enlighten the pharmacodynamics mechanisms of other medications [27–29]. Taken together, our study did not find an effect of systemically administered metoprolol on central pain processing structures, including the thalamus, neither in the healthy system, nor in the pathological system of migraineurs.

Abbreviations

ACC: Anterior cingulate cortex; BOLD: Blood Oxygen Level Dependent;; fMRI: Functional Magnetic Resonance Imaging; FWE: Familywise Error; i.e.: id est.; ITI: Inter-trial interval; MCC: Midcingulate cortex; MR: Magnetic Resonance; SVC: Small volume correction; VAS: Visual analogue scale

Acknowledgements
The authors thank Dr. Inga Kröger and Ludovica Gramegna who completed parts of the data collection in the patients group. Further we thank Prof. Dr. Schwedhelm from the Institute of Experimental Pharmacology and Toxicology (University Medical Center Hamburg-Eppendorf, Germany) for collaboration and analyses of blood plasma concentration of metoprolol. The authors thank Dr. Jan Mehnert for helpful advice with data analyses.

Funding
This work was supported by the German Research Foundation, SFB936/A5 and DFG 1862/12–1 to AM.

Authors' contributions
JMH: Study design, acquisition of data, analysis and interpretation of data, manuscript draft; AM: study concept and design, analysis and interpretation of data, critical revision of manuscript for intellectual content. Both authors read and approved the final manuscript.

Competing interests
Both authors declare that they have no competing interests.

References
1. Diener H-C (2003) Pharmacological approaches to migraine. In: Neuropsychopharmacology. Springer Vienna, Vienna, pp 35–63
2. Silberstein SD, Consortium for the UH (2000) Practice parameter: evidence-based guidelines for migraine headache (an evidence-based review) report of the quality standards Subcommittee of the American Academy of neurology. Neurology 55:754–762. doi: 10.1212/WNL.55.6.754
3. Andersson PG, Dahl S, Hansen JH et al (1983) Prophylactic treatment of classical and non-classical migraine with Metoprolol—a comparison with placebo. Cephalalgia 3:207–212. doi: 10.1046/j.1468-2982.1983.0304207.x
4. Jackson JL, Cogbill E, Santana-Davila R et al (2015) A comparative effectiveness meta-analysis of drugs for the prophylaxis of migraine headache. PLoS One 10:e0130733. doi: 10.1371/journal.pone.0130733
5. Hieble JP (2000) Adrenoceptor subclassification: an approach to improved cardiovascular therapeutics. Pharm Acta Helv 74:163–171
6. Hanbauer I, Kopin IJ, Guidotti A, Costa E (1975) Induction of tyrosine hydroxylase elicited by beta adrenergic receptor agonists in normal and decentralized sympathetic ganglia: role of cyclic 3',5'-adenosine monophosphate. J Pharmacol Exp Ther 193:95–104
7. Maertens de Noordhout A, Timsit-Berthier M, Timsit M, Schoenen J (1987) Effects of beta blockade on contingent negative variation in migraine. Ann Neurol 21:111–112. doi: 10.1002/ana.410210125
8. Diener HC, Scholz E, Dichgans J et al (1989) Central effects of drugs used in migraine prophylaxis evaluated by visual evoked potentials. Ann Neurol 25:125–130. doi: 10.1002/ana.410250204
9. Sandor PS, Afra J, Ambrosini A, Schoenen J (2000) Prophylactic treatment of migraine with beta-blockers and riboflavin: differential effects on the intensity dependence of auditory evoked cortical potentials. Headache J Head Face Pain 40:30–35. doi: 10.1046/j.1526-4610.2000.00005.x
10. Schoenen J (1986) Beta blockers and the central nervous system. Cephalalgia Int J Headache 6(Suppl 5):47–54. doi: 10.1177/03331024860060S506
11. Siniatchkin M, Andrasik F, Kropp P et al (2007) Central mechanisms of controlled-release Metoprolol in migraine: a double-blind, placebo-controlled study. Cephalalgia 27:1024–1032. doi: 10.1111/j.1468-2982.2007.01377.x
12. Schoenen J, Maertens de Noordhout A, Timsit-Berthier M, Timsit M (1986) Contingent negative variation and efficacy of beta-blocking agents in migraine. Cephalalgia 6:229–233. doi: 10.1046/j.1468-2982.1986.0604229.x
13. Coppola G, Iacovelli E, Bracaglia M et al (2013) Electrophysiological correlates of episodic migraine chronification: evidence for thalamic involvement. J Headache Pain 14:76. doi: 10.1186/1129-2377-14-76

14. Coppola G (2005) Somatosensory evoked high-frequency oscillations reflecting thalamo-cortical activity are decreased in migraine patients between attacks. Brain 128:98–103. doi: 10.1093/brain/awh334

15. Coppola G, Tinelli E, Lepre C et al (2014) Dynamic changes in thalamic microstructure of migraine without aura patients: a diffusion tensor magnetic resonance imaging study. Eur J Neurol 21:287–e13. doi: 10.1111/ene.12296

16. Shields KG, Goadsby PJ (2005) Propranolol modulates trigeminovascular responses in thalamic ventroposteromedial nucleus: a role in migraine? Brain 128:86–97. doi: 10.1093/brain/awh298

17. Headache Classification Committee of the International Headache Society (IHS) (2013) The international classification of headache disorders, 3rd edition (beta version). Cephalalgia 33:629–808. doi: 10.1177/0333102413485658

18. Karlson BW, Dellborg M, Gullestad L et al (2014) A pharmacokinetic and Pharmacodynamic comparison of immediate-release Metoprolol and extended-release Metoprolol CR/XL in patients with suspected acute myocardial infarction: a randomized, open-label study. Cardiology 127:73–82. doi: 10.1159/000355003

19. Held PH, Regårdh CG (1986) Metoprolol in acute myocardial infarction. A pharmacokinetic and pharmacodynamic study. Eur J Clin Pharmacol 31:261–265

20. Stankewitz A, Voit H, Bingel U et al (2010) A new trigemino-nociceptive stimulation model for event-related fMRI. Cephalalgia 30:475–485

21. Kröger IL, May A (2014) Central effects of acetylsalicylic acid on trigeminal-nociceptive stimuli. J Headache Pain 15:59

22. Contin M, Riva R, Albani F, Baruzzi A (2001) Simple and rapid liquid chromatographic-turbo ion spray mass spectrometric determination of topiramate in human plasma. J Chromatogr B Biomed Sci App 761:133–137

23. Gleiter C, Deckert J (1996) Adverse CNS-effects of Beta-Adrenoceptor blockers. Pharmacopsychiatry 29:201–211. doi: 10.1055/s-2007-979572

24. Koella WP (1985) CNS-related (side-) effects of beta-blockers with special reference to mechanisms of action. Eur J Clin Pharmacol 28:55–63

25. Denuelle M, Fabre N, Payoux P et al (2007) Hypothalamic activation in spontaneous migraine attacks. Headache 47:1418–1426

26. Schulte LH, Allers A, May A (2017) Hypothalamus as a mediator of chronic migraine: evidence from high-resolution fMRI. Neurology 88:2011–2016. doi: 10.1212/WNL.0000000000003963

27. Kröger IL, May A (2015) Triptan-induced disruption of trigemino-cortical connectivity. Neurology 84:2124–2131. doi: 10.1212/WNL.0000000000001610

28. Scrivani S, Wallin D, Moulton EA et al (2010) A fMRI evaluation of Lamotrigine for the treatment of trigeminal neuropathic pain: pilot study. Pain Med 11:920–941

29. Iannetti GD, Zambreanu L, Wise RG et al (2005) Pharmacological modulation of pain-related brain activity during normal and central sensitization states in humans. Proc Natl Acad Sci 102:18195–18200. doi: 10.1073/pnas.0506624102

16

Non-invasive vagus nerve stimulation for treatment of cluster headache: early UK clinical experience

Juana Marin[1*], Nicola Giffin[2], Elizabeth Consiglio[3], Candace McClure[4], Eric Liebler[5] and Brendan Davies[6]

Abstract

Background: Evidence supports the use of non-invasive vagus nerve stimulation (nVNS; gammaCore®) as a promising therapeutic option for patients with cluster headache (CH). We conducted this audit of real-world data from patients with CH, the majority of whom were treatment refractory, to explore early UK clinical experience with nVNS used acutely, preventively, or both.

Methods: We retrospectively analysed data from 30 patients with CH (29 chronic, 1 episodic) who submitted individual funding requests for nVNS to the National Health Service. All patients had responded to adjunctive nVNS therapy during an evaluation period (typical duration, 3–6 months). Data collected from patient interviews, treatment diaries, and physician notes were summarised with descriptive statistics. Paired t tests were used to examine statistical significance.

Results: The mean (SD) CH attack frequency decreased from 26.6 (17.1) attacks/wk. before initiation of nVNS therapy to 9.5 (11.0) attacks/wk. ($P < 0.01$) afterward. Mean (SD) attack duration decreased from 51.9 (36.7) minutes to 29.4 (28.5) minutes ($P < 0.01$), and mean (SD) attack severity (rated on a 10-point scale) decreased from 7.8 (2.3) to 6.0 (2.6) ($P < 0.01$). Use of abortive treatments also decreased. Favourable changes in the use of preventive medication were also observed. No serious device-related adverse events were reported.

Conclusions: Significant decreases in attack frequency, severity, and duration were observed in these patients with CH who did not respond to or were intolerant of multiple preventive and/or acute treatments. These real-world findings complement evidence from clinical trials demonstrating the efficacy and safety of nVNS in CH.

Keywords: Chronic cluster headache, Refractory, Non-invasive vagus nerve stimulation, Real-world data, Acute treatment, Preventive therapy, Neuromodulation

Background

Cluster headache (CH), a primary headache disorder, is widely regarded as one of the most painful medical conditions and can substantially diminish patients' quality of life by limiting their functional abilities in social, domestic, and work activities [1]. The condition may be classified as episodic (attack periods of 1 week to 1 year separated by 1 month) or chronic (attack periods of 1 year without remission or remission of < 1 month) and has limited available treatment options [2, 3]. A non-invasive vagus nerve stimulation (nVNS) device

(gammaCore®) has demonstrated safety and efficacy for prevention and acute treatment of CH attacks in clinical trials [4–6]. The device is CE marked and indicated for acute and preventive therapy in CH and for treatment of migraine, hemicrania continua, and medication overuse headache in adults. It is also approved in the United States for acute treatment of episodic CH and migraine in adults.

Understanding the practical role of novel treatments such as nVNS in clinical practice is often difficult, despite clinical trial data demonstrating their efficacy. The use of novel treatments in practice can provide data to complement those from clinical trials by documenting qualitative details that are not typically captured during such trials, enabling a real-world view of patient- and

* Correspondence: jcmarin@hotmail.co.uk
[1]Wellcome Foundation Building, King's College Hospital, London SE5 9PJ, UK

health care–centric management. This can provide a broader view of a treatment's risk/benefit profile and of patients' preference and ability to maintain their treatment regimen. To add further insight to the data on nVNS from randomised clinical trials, we conducted this retrospective analysis of data from patients in the United Kingdom with CH who were at various stages in the process of applying for individual funding requests (IFRs) for nVNS from the National Health Service. The IFR process is available to secure financial support for novel therapies that have not been fully evaluated and approved for national reimbursement. The process is reserved for patients with rare conditions that have not responded to available therapies and who are considered exceptional individuals with regard to the treatment of their CH.

Methods

We retrospectively analysed data from patients with CH who previously had an inadequate response and/or intolerable side effects with ≥3 current or previous CH treatments and were offered nVNS therapy for use during an evaluation period. Physicians instructed patients to use nVNS as preventive therapy, acute treatment, or both during this period. Initial nVNS dosing was based on established paradigms and titrated as necessary to achieve maximum benefit. Patients who reported a clinically meaningful decrease in the frequency, severity, or duration of their attacks after ≥3 months of evaluation were considered for inclusion in the IFR process.

Decreases in the use of concomitant medications and clinical assessments of patient quality of life were also considered. The decision to pursue IFR submission for these subjects was at the discretion of physicians and patients, but submission was not encouraged for patients who did not achieve a ≥25% decrease in weekly attack frequency. Patients continued to use nVNS during IFR development, submission, and processing.

All patients provided informed consent for the collection and analysis of their data. Clinical centres provided data on CH attacks and treatments before the nVNS evaluation period, which were obtained from patient diaries and/or medical records, as well as the following data from patient interviews, treatment diaries, and physician notes documented during the nVNS evaluation period (from May 2012 through March 2016): CH type, patient demographics/other characteristics; CH attack frequency, duration, and severity (rated on a 0–10 scale, higher numbers indicating greater severity); number and timing of stimulations administered; concomitant use of preventive and/or abortive treatments; adverse events (AEs); and subjective feedback on nVNS. Data were summarised with descriptive statistics. Within-patient changes from baseline (i.e., during treatment with the standard of care [SoC]

regimen alone) to the end (or latest available point) of the nVNS evaluation period in attack frequency, duration, and severity were assessed via paired t tests. Patients who were no longer experiencing attacks at the time of the analysis were excluded from analyses of attack duration and severity. Data from patients who lacked quantitative information regarding attack duration and severity were included only in qualitative analysis of these variables.

Results

Patient characteristics

Data from 30 patients (Table 1), 29 with chronic CH and 1 with episodic CH, at 10 clinical centres throughout the United Kingdom (see Additional file 1 for list of sites) were analysed.

nVNS use

The mean (range) duration of the evaluation period at the time of analysis was 7.6 (0.9–27.5) months. The most commonly used preventive and acute nVNS regimens are shown in Table 2. Sixteen patients (53%) used nVNS exclusively as preventive therapy, 1 (3%, a patient with episodic CH) used it exclusively as acute treatment, and 13 (43%) used it as both preventive and acute therapy. A single stimulation lasted 120 s, and the mean (range) preventive stimulation frequency was 5.6 (2.0–9.0) stimulations/d. The mean (range) acute stimulation frequency was 4.3 (0.4–18.0) stimulations/d.

Attack frequency, duration, and severity

The mean (range) attack frequency with SoC alone was 26.6 (3.8–77.0) attacks/wk.; this decreased to 9.5 (0–38.5) attacks/wk. with SoC + nVNS ($P < 0.01$; Fig. 1a). Three patients, who averaged 42 to 63 attacks/wk. before the

Table 1 Patient demographics and baseline characteristics

Characteristic	SoC + nVNS ($N = 30$)
Age,[a] mean (range), y	47.9 (16.0–72.0)
Female sex, No. (%)	19 (63)
Diagnosis, No. (%)	
Chronic CH	29 (97)
Episodic CH	1 (3)
Time since CH diagnosis,[a,b] mean (range), y	7.2 (0–22.0)
Failed preventive treatments,[c] mean (range), No.	8.9 (1–16)
Failed acute treatments,[c] mean (range), No.	1.3 (0–4)
Active preventive treatments,[a] mean (range), No.	0.8 (0–2)
Active acute treatments,[a] mean (range), No.	1.8 (1–4)

[a]At the time nVNS therapy was begun
[b]Calculated using the year nVNS was begun minus the year CH was diagnosed
[c]Refers to treatments used and stopped before nVNS therapy was begun
Abbreviations: *CH* cluster headache, *nVNS* non-invasive vagus nerve stimulation, *SoC* standard of care

Table 2 Most commonly used nVNS dosing regimens: preventive and acute treatment

nVNS Dosing Regimen	No. (%)[a] of Patients
Preventive	
2 consecutive stimulations administered 3 × per day	13 (45)
3 consecutive stimulations administered 2 × per day	8 (28)
Acute	
3 consecutive stimulations administered at the onset of each CH attack	10 (71)

[a]Percentages are based on $n = 29$ patients using nVNS as preventive therapy and $n = 14$ patients using nVNS as acute treatment

Abbreviations: *CH* cluster headache, *nVNS* non-invasive vagus nerve stimulation

initiation of nVNS therapy, had no attacks during their nVNS evaluation periods, which ranged from 1.7 to 13.2 months. Among the 25 patients who reported the duration of their attacks, the mean (range) decreased from 51.9 (5.0–140.0) minutes with SoC alone to 29.4 (2.5–152.5) minutes with SoC + nVNS ($P < 0.01$; Fig. 1b). The mean (range) attack severity ($n = 18$) decreased from 7.8 (3.0–10.0) with SoC alone to 6.0 (1.0–10.0) with SoC + nVNS ($P < 0.01$; Fig. 1c). In the qualitative analysis, most patients reported a decrease in attack frequency, duration, and/or severity during the nVNS evaluation period (Table 3).

Concomitant treatment use

Patients used a mean (range) of 0.8 (0–2) preventive treatments before the initiation of nVNS therapy and 0.7 (0–2) preventive treatments afterward. The mean (range) number of acute treatments used was 1.8 (1–4) before the initiation of nVNS therapy and 1.1 (0–2) afterward. Table 4 summarises the use of acute and preventive medications prior and subsequent to the initiation of nVNS therapy, and Table 5 provides details regarding the use of preventive treatments before the initiation of and concomitant with nVNS therapy. Twenty-two patients used triptan injection or nasal spray as acute treatment before the initiation of nVNS therapy. Among these patients, 9 (41%) stopped and 12 (55%) decreased their triptan use during nVNS therapy; triptan use was unchanged in the remaining patient. Twenty-nine patients reported use of high-flow oxygen; 27 (93%) used it as acute treatment before the initiation of nVNS therapy. After treatment with nVNS was initiated, 9 patients (33%) stopped and 17 (63%) decreased high-flow oxygen use; use of this treatment was unchanged in the remaining patient. Overall, after nVNS therapy was established, 3 patients

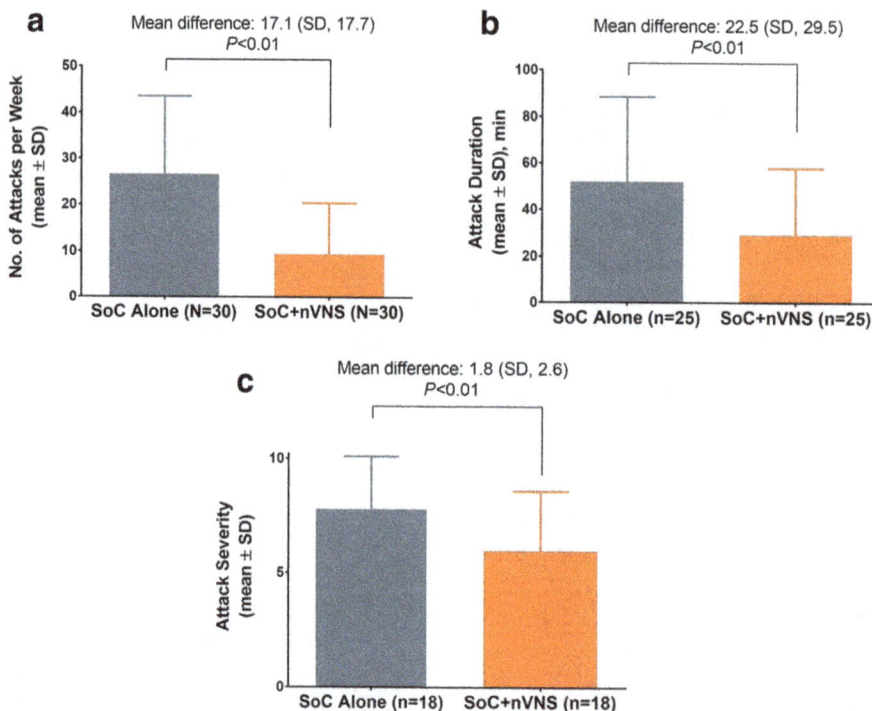

Fig. 1 CH attack frequency (**a**), duration (**b**), and severity (**c**) with SoC alone and with SoC + nVNS. *P* values are from paired *t* tests. Patients who had 0 attacks while using nVNS therapy were excluded from analysis of attack duration and severity. Attack severity was rated on a 0 to 10 scale, with higher scores indicating greater severity. Abbreviations: CH, cluster headache; nVNS, non-invasive vagus nerve stimulation; SD, standard deviation; SoC, standard of care

Table 3 Qualitative analysis of changes in CH attack frequency, duration, and severity with nVNS therapy

	No. (%) of Patients		
	Decrease	No Change	Increase
Frequency	25[a] (83)	5 (17)	0
Duration[b]	17 (65)	7 (27)	2 (8)
Severity[c]	17 (74)	5 (22)	1 (4)

[a]Included 3 patients who had no CH attacks during the evaluation period
[b]26 patients had available qualitative data on attack duration
[c]23 patients had available qualitative data on attack severity
Abbreviations: *CH* cluster headache, *nVNS* non-invasive vagus nerve stimulation

were able to manage their condition with preventive pharmacologic treatment only, and another 4 patients were able to use nVNS as monotherapy.

Safety

No serious device-related AEs were reported during nVNS therapy. Observed AEs in this patient cohort included redness and muscle soreness at the stimulation site, which were also reported in previous randomised clinical trials. Consistent with these previous studies, AEs were mild and transient and were typically reported early in the evaluation period, when the use of nVNS was relatively novel.

Additional observations and outcomes

In addition to the objective findings, some patients spontaneously reported subjective benefits of nVNS that they considered meaningful. These included decreased interictal headache pain ($n = 6$), no longer being housebound ($n = 6$), the ability to return to work or school ($n = 4$), improved sleep ($n = 4$), decreased absenteeism ($n = 4$), avoidance of surgery intended to treat CH ($n = 3$), and improved quality of life ($n = 3$).

Discussion

In these patients with CH, headache burden as measured by attack frequency, duration, and severity significantly improved with nVNS therapy. Three patients (10%), all of

Table 4 Summary of acute and preventive medication use before and after the establishment of nVNS therapy

	No. of Patients	
	Prior to nVNS	Concomitant With nVNS
Using acute treatment only	14	11
Using preventive treatment only	0	3
Using both acute and preventive treatment	16	12
Using neither acute nor preventive treatment	0	4

Abbreviation: *nVNS* non-invasive vagus nerve stimulation

Table 5 Preventive treatment use before and after the establishment of nVNS therapy

Treatment	No. of Patients	
	Prior to nVNS	Concomitant With nVNS
Verapamil	8	6
Topiramate	5	4
Amitriptyline	2	2
Melatonin	2	2
Baclofen	1	1
Bilateral OCS (implanted)	1	1
DBS	1	1
Gabapentin	1	1
Lithium	1	1
Pregabalin	1	0

Abbreviations: *DBS* deep brain stimulation, *nVNS* non-invasive vagus nerve stimulation, *OCS* occipital nerve stimulation

whom had chronic CH, were attack free after beginning nVNS therapy, which constitutes a remission period according to *International Classification of Headache Disorders* (3rd edition) criteria [3]. Most patients were able to decrease or discontinue their use of existing acute treatments during nVNS therapy.

In previous clinical trials, nVNS demonstrated efficacy as preventive therapy in patients with chronic CH [4] and as acute treatment in patients with episodic CH [5, 6], but not as acute treatment in patients with chronic CH [4–6]. In a recent audit from a single centre in the United Kingdom, data from 12 patients with chronic CH suggested that nVNS was not effective as preventive or abortive therapy for most patients [7]. In contrast, patients in this analysis, who predominantly had chronic CH (29/30), reported significant decreases in attack duration and severity, indicating a benefit from nVNS as an acute treatment in chronic CH in this practical setting when the acute use was added to daily preventive use. These conflicting results suggest that further study is warranted, but the idea of a differential response to nVNS among patients with chronic CH and those with episodic CH is well established and has several possible underlying reasons. There appear to be differences in brain anatomy and pharmacology between patients with episodic CH and those with chronic CH [8, 9]. Disparate changes in grey matter volume during attacks in patients with episodic versus chronic CH, as well as apparent impairment of recovery from such changes between attacks in patients with chronic CH, suggest further differences between the 2 CH subtypes [10]. Suboptimal responses to other acute treatments in patients with chronic CH also have been reported [11, 12]. Results from the initial open-label exploratory study of nVNS therapy in CH suggested that several patients with chronic CH had a stable favourable response to nVNS as acute treatment [13]. In that study, unlike in the afore-mentioned clinical trials [4–6], nVNS dosing regimens were adjusted according to individual patient responses to explore optimal treatment approaches [13]. In this study, nVNS dosing regimens were also titrated on an individual basis and, importantly, both acute and preventive uses of nVNS were allowed. Such dosing individualisation, which is common with pharmacologic treatments, could explain why patients with chronic CH benefited from acute nVNS treatment in the current study but not in the acute clin-ical trials, which did not allow for daily preventive use. Further study is needed to determine whether acute treatment regimens in patients with chronic CH might benefit from increased nVNS dosing.

In this report and the initial exploratory study [13], most patients used nVNS as both acute and preventive therapy, which suggests a possible synergy between acute and preventive benefits of nVNS therapy. The pos-sibility that continued or more frequent use of nVNS re-sults in increased efficacy requires further investigation, but some findings suggest this may be the case in CH [6] and migraine [14]. If confirmed, this concept could also help explain the potential synergy between acute and preventive nVNS therapy.

In addition to the clinical benefits of nVNS in CH, an economic benefit of nVNS has also been suggested. Re-sults from a pharmacoeconomic modelling analysis suggested that, compared with SoC alone, SoC + nVNS was associated with 23% lower abortive medication costs and was more effective in patients with CH [15]. Reduc-tions in the use of acute treatments in the current study support the potential cost-effectiveness of nVNS and re-iterate its favourable risk/benefit profile.

During clinical trials, patients are instructed to report any AE they experience, regardless of severity, seriousness, or presumed relationship to the study drug/device. In practice, patients are more likely to report only AEs that they find particularly concerning/bothersome or that they believe to be related to treatment. Patients in the current study reported no serious device-related AEs, which pro-vides valuable information regarding how nVNS therapy is tolerated in real-world conditions and helps confirm the mild side effect profile associated with nVNS in clinical trials [4, 5, 14].

The current study sample comprising 63% women is unusual considering that CH is more common among men [16]. Several factors may have contributed to this discrepancy. Compared with men, women with CH have higher rates of comorbidities such as major depression, migraine, and other conditions that could affect the way CH manifests [16, 17]. Such comorbidities might complicate the treatment of CH to the extent that more women than men pursue the IFR process. Concerns about teratogenicity associated with some medications used to treat CH can also prompt women to seek non-pharmacologic treatment options at greater rates than men do. Finally, in our general clinical experience and in this particular patient sample, women are often more willing than men to rigorously and consistently track the data required to complete IFR applications.

Limitations of this study include its small sample size and inherent inclusion bias. By definition, this was a responder study, and patient responses are not likely representative of the CH population as a whole. Use of an evaluation period appears to be a feasible and prac-tical method for assessing response to nVNS in patients with CH, especially if one considers the mild side effect profile of nVNS and practicality of this therapy.

Conclusions

Treatment with nVNS led to significant decreases in attack frequency, severity, and duration in patients with CH who previously did not benefit from or could not tolerate multiple preventive and/or acute treatments. These findings represent the practical use of this treatment and complement results from clinical trials demonstrating the efficacy and safety of nVNS therapy in patients with CH.

Abbreviations
AE: Adverse event; CH: Cluster headache; IFR: Individual funding request; nVNS: Non-invasive vagus nerve stimulation; SD: Standard deviation; SoC: Standard of care

Acknowledgements
Professional writing and editorial support was provided by Elizabeth Barton, MS, of MedLogix Communications, LLC (Itasca, IL, USA) under the direction of the authors and was funded by electroCore, Inc.

Funding
This study was supported by electroCore, Inc.

Authors' contributions
JM, EC, and EL contributed to study conception and design. BD, NG, and JM contributed to acquisition of data. CMcC, EL, JM, and EC contributed to the analysis or interpretation of data. EL, JM, NG, and BD contributed to drafting the manuscript or revising it critically for important intellectual content. All authors approved the final manuscript for publication. JM agrees to be accountable for all aspects of the work in ensuring that questions related to the accuracy or integrity of any part of the work are appropriately investigated and resolved.

Competing interests
J. Marin has received honoraria and travel grants from electroCore, Inc. E. Consiglio is an employee of Interface Clinical Services. C. McClure is an employee of North American Science Associates, Inc. E. Liebler is an employee of electroCore, Inc., and receives stock ownership. B. Davies and N. Giffin have no competing interests to declare.

Author details

[1]Wellcome Foundation Building, King's College Hospital, London SE5 9PJ, UK. [2]Royal United Hospital, Coombe Park, Bath BA1 3NG, UK. [3]Interface Clinical Services, Gate Way Drive, Yeadon, Leeds LS19 7XY, UK. [4]North American Science Associates, Inc., 400 US-169, Minneapolis, MN 55441, USA. [5]electroCore, Inc., 150 Allen Road, Suite 201, Basking Ridge, NJ 07920, USA. [6]University Hospitals of North Midlands, Newcastle Road, Stoke-on-Trent ST4 6QG, UK.

References

1. D'Amico D, Usai S, Grazzi L, Rigamonti A, Solari A, Leone M, Bussone G (2003) Quality of life and disability in primary chronic daily headaches. Neurol Sci 24(suppl 2):S97–100. https://doi.org/10.1007/s100720300052

2. Ashkenazi A, Schwedt T (2011) Cluster headache--acute and prophylactic therapy. Headache 51(2):272–286. https://doi.org/10.1111/j.1526-4610.2010.01830.x

3. Headache Classification Committee of the International Headache Society (2013) The international classification of headache disorders, 3rd edition (beta version). Cephalalgia 33(9):629–808. https://doi.org/10.1177/0333102413485658

4. Gaul C, Diener HC, Silver N, Magis D, Reuter U, Andersson A, Liebler EJ, Straube A, PREVA Study Group (2016) Non-invasive vagus nerve stimulation for PREVention and acute treatment of chronic cluster headache (PREVA): a randomised controlled study. Cephalalgia 36(6):534–546. https://doi.org/10.1177/0333102415607070

5. Goadsby PJ, de Coo IF, Silver N, Tyagi A, Ahmed F, Gaul C, Jensen RH, Diener HC, Solbach K, Straube A, Liebler E, Marin JC, Ferrari MD, ACT2 Study Group (2018) Non-invasive vagus nerve stimulation for the acute treatment of episodic and chronic cluster headache: a randomized, double-blind, sham-controlled ACT2 study. Cephalalgia 38(5):959–969. https://doi.org/10.1177/0333102417744362

6. Silberstein SD, Mechtler LL, Kudrow DB, Calhoun AH, McClure C, Saper JR, Liebler EJ, Rubenstein Engel E, Tepper SJ, ACT1 Study Group (2016) Non-invasive vagus nerve stimulation for the acute treatment of cluster headache: findings from the randomized, double-blind, sham-controlled ACT1 study. Headache 56(8):1317–1332. https://doi.org/10.1111/head.12896

7. Trimboli M, Al-Kaisy A, Andreou AP, Murphy M, Lambru G (2018) Non-invasive vagus nerve stimulation for the management of refractory primary chronic headaches: a real-world experience. Cephalalgia 38(7):1276–1285. https://doi.org/10.1177/0333102417731349

8. Barloese MC, Jürgens TP, May A, Lainez JM, Schoenen J, Gaul C, Goodman AM, Caparso A, Jensen RH (2016) Cluster headache attack remission with sphenopalatine ganglion stimulation: experiences in chronic cluster headache patients through 24 months. J Headache Pain 17(1):67. https://doi.org/10.1186/s10194-016-0658-1

9. D'Andrea G, Leone M, Bussone G, Fiore PD, Bolner A, Aguggia M, Saracco MG, Perini F, Giordano G, Gucciardi A, Leon A (2017) Abnormal tyrosine metabolism in chronic cluster headache. Cephalalgia 37(2):148–153. https://doi.org/10.1177/0333102416640502

10. Naegel S, Holle D, Desmarattes N, Theysohn N, Diener HC, Katsarava Z, Obermann M (2014) Cortical plasticity in episodic and chronic cluster headache. Neuroimage Clin 6:415–423. https://doi.org/10.1016/j.nicl.2014.10.003

11. Bahra A, Gawel MJ, Hardebo JE, Millson D, Breen SA, Goadsby PJ (2000) Oral zolmitriptan is effective in the acute treatment of cluster headache. Neurology 54(9):1832–1839 https://doi.org/10.1212/WNL.54.9.1832

12. Marmura MJ, Pello SJ, Young WB (2010) Interictal pain in cluster headache. Cephalalgia 30(12):1531–1534. https://doi.org/10.1177/0333102410372423

13. Nesbitt AD, Marin JCA, Tompkins E, Ruttledge MH, Goadsby PJ (2015) Initial use of a novel noninvasive vagus nerve stimulator for cluster headache treatment. Neurology 84(12):1249–1253. https://doi.org/10.1212/WNL.0000000000001394

14. Silberstein SD, Calhoun AH, Lipton RB, Grosberg BM, Cady RK, Dorlas S, Simmons KA, Mullin C, Liebler EJ, Goadsby PJ, Saper JR, EVENT Study Group (2016) Chronic migraine headache prevention with noninvasive vagus nerve stimulation: the EVENT study. Neurology 87(5):529–538. https://doi.org/10.1212/WNL.0000000000002918

15. Morris J, Straube A, Diener HC, Ahmed F, Silver N, Walker S, Liebler E, Gaul C (2016) Cost-effectiveness analysis of non-invasive vagus nerve stimulation for the treatment of chronic cluster headache. J Headache Pain 17:43. https://doi.org/10.1186/s10194-016-0633-x

16. Rozen TD, Fishman RS (2012) Female cluster headache in the United States of America: what are the gender differences? Results from the United States Cluster Headache Survey. J Neurol Sci 317(1–2):17–28. https://doi.org/10.1016/j.jns.2012.03.006

17. Lund N, Barloese M, Petersen A, Haddock B, Jensen R (2017) Chronobiology differs between men and women with cluster headache, clinical phenotype does not. Neurology 88(11):1069–1076. https://doi.org/10.1212/WNL.0000000000003715

17

Use of traditional medicine for primary headache disorders in Kuwait

Jasem Y. Al-Hashel[1,2]* (iD), Samar Farouk Ahmed[1,3], Fatemah J Alshawaf[4] and Raed Alroughani[5]

Abstract

Background: Traditional Medicine (TM) is widely accepted to be used for the treatment headache disorders in Kuwait however, researches remain poorly documented. We aimed to study the frequency of TM use and its impact in the primary headache patients.

Methods: This is a cross sectional self-reported efficacy study, which was conducted in Headache clinic in Kuwait throughout 6 months. Patients who were diagnosed with primary headache disorders of both genders aged from 18 to 65 years were included. Self-reported questionnaires were distributed to patients who used TM in the previous year. It included demographic, and characteristics of headache (headache frequency, duration, number of analgesic used in days per month and severity of headache). TM queried included blood cupping (Hijama), head banding, herbal medicine (sabkha), and diet modification. It assessed characters of headache before and 3 months after the final TM session. Independent sample t test, paired sample t test and Chi-square test were used to compare between different values. $P < 0.05$ is considered significant.

Results: A total of 279 patients were included. The mean age is 40.32 ± 11.75 years; females represented 79.6% of the cohort. Most patients ($n = 195$; 69.9%) reported the use of TM before presentation to headache clinic, mainly Hijama (47.3%). Cultural / religious beliefs were the cause of seeking TM in 51.3% versus 10% used it due to ineffective medical treatment and 8.6% used it because of intolerance of medical treatment. Patients used TM were older at the onset of headache (24.24 ± 10.67 versus 20.38 ± 8.47; $p < 0.003$), and had longer headache disease duration (19.26 ± 13.13 versus 16.12 ± 11.39; $p < 0.044$). All patients with chronic headache (100%) and most of episodic migraine patients (90.4%) sought TM while only (31.5%) of Tension type headache sought TM; $p < 0.047$. Patients who sought TM had more frequent episodes of headache, longer duration of attacks and higher number of days of analgesic-usage respectively over last 3 months before presentation to our side (9.66 ± 7.39 versus 4.14 ± 2.72; $p < 0.001$), (41.23 ± 27.76 versus 32.19 ± 23.29; $p < .0009$), (8.23 ± 7.70 versus 3.18 ± 3.06; $p < 0.001$). At 3 months after the final TM session, there was no significant reduction of frequency of headache days per month (9.19 ± 7.33 versus 8.99 ± 7.59; $p < 0.50$), days of analgesic use per month (7.45 ± 7.43 versus 6.77 ± 6.93; $p < 0.09$) and duration of headache (41.23 ± 27.76 versus 41.59 ± 27.69; $p < 0.78$). However, there was a significant reduction of the severity of headache ($p < 0.02$). Few patients (17.9%) reported adverse events with TM. Most of TM cohorts were not satisfied after receiving this type of medicine.

Conclusion: TM was widely used in Kuwait for primary headache. Patients sought TM before seeking physician because they found them more congruent with their own cultural and religious beliefs. Health care professionals involved in the management of headache should be aware of this and monitor potential benefits or adverse events of TM. The usage of TM was not effective in reducing headache attacks and severity.

Keywords: Migraine, Hijama, Tradional medicine, Kuwai

* Correspondence: jasemkumsa@hotmail.com; dralhashel@hotmail.com
[1]Department of Neurology, Ibn Sina Hospital, P.O. Box 25427, Safat, 13115 Kuwait City, Kuwait
[2]Department of Medicine, Faculty of Medicine, Health Sciences Centre, Kuwait University, Kuwait City, Kuwait
Full list of author information is available at the end of the article

Introduction

Primary headache ranked among the top three diseases contributors to the global burden of disease [1]. The effective treatment of headache disorders is still a moving field and a potential challenge to the neurologist [2] and the approach to its management reflects cultural diversity. Thus, many headache patients seek Traditional medicine (TM) for self-treatment and prevention of headaches. The socioeconomic development and literacy level of a community influences on how headache is perceived and medical treatment sought. Despite the availability of modern medicine, many people may rely more on traditional medical practice because of its cultural acceptability, easy accessibility, and affordability.

The World Health Organization (WHO) defined Traditional medicine (TM) as the sum total of knowledge, skills, and practices based on the theories, beliefs, and experiences indigenous to different cultures that are used to maintain health, as well as to prevent, diagnose, improve, or treat physical and mental illnesses [3]. WHO reported that 80% of the population of developing countries and 65% of the population of developed countries rely on TM for health care [4].

The reasons for people resorting to TM vary widely and include dissatisfaction with modern medicine [5], or congruency with users values and beliefs toward health and life [6]. Popular treatment based on the Qur'an and the Sunna of the Prophet.

Muhammad continues to be practiced in Muslim countries including Kuwait due to religious inspiration [7].

In Kuwait, folk beliefs may play a role in leading patients to try TM. Traditional medicine healers know Farry as an opening or a gap is the skull that would allow air to get inside the skull causing chronic headache. According to TM healers there are several methods to treat this disease. The Arabic word 'hijama' is often translated into English as 'cupping'. Hijama is 'blood cupping which is known as 'wet cupping', in which cups are placed on the surface of the skin, sucking the air out, and creating a vacuum to regulate the flow of blood and to stimulate life-energy, blood-cupping goes one step further, with the practitioner making small incisions on the surface of the skin in order to get rid the patient of blood stasis within the body. This blood is considered unhealthy blood in their beliefs [8]. Wet cupping is known to have also been practiced by many ancient cultures as in ancient Egyptians, India, Greeks, and Romans [8].

Other TM that are used in Kuwait for headache include Sabkha, head massage and diet modification. Sabkha (aka Labkha) is a herbal mixture that includes henna, prepared by specialized person and applied to the head and left for a few days [9]. Head banding or tying the head with a cloth to create pressure around the head to reduce the flow of blood to scalp can help to relieve the pain caused by swollen blood vessels. Application of an ice pack and local scalp pressure are the most commonly used non-pharmacological methods for temporary relief of migraine headache pain [10].

Physicians are often faced with patients who use or ask about TM. They are expected to guide the patient to provide information and give the best options for treatment, but often studies and data are not available to withdraw conclusions about such treatments. The efficacy and safety of many forms of TM are under research as compared to modern medicine [11].

Traditional healers often lack medical training and are not physicians and their limited medical knowledge may put patients at risk [12]. To our knowledge, no study to date has specifically investigated the use of TM in patients suffering from headache in Kuwait. The aim of our study was to assess the rates, reason and efficacy of TM use in patients with primary headache.

Method

This A cross-sectional, questionnaire-based study was conducted in specialized headache clinic in tertiary hospital in Kuwait. Our study included patients aged 18–65 who are diagnosed with primary headaches confirmed by a Neurologist according to International Classification of Headache Disorders III (ICHD-III) [13], and onset of their headache preceded the use of TM for headache. To avoid recall bias, we included only those who reported use of TM for their headache in last year before presentation to headache clinic and completed three months after last TM session.

A questionnaire was distributed to the identified patients. Demographic data such as age, gender and education as well as the characteristics of the headache as number of years with headaches, headache frequency per month, duration of headache in hours, number of analgesics use days per month, headache pain intensity [14], and use of acute and prophylactic medication over last three month before presenting to headache clinic were collected. Headache pain intensity was measured on a four-point scale where 0 = no headache; 1 = mild headache; 2 = moderate headache; 3 = severe headache. This scale is recommended for use in research by the International Headache Society [14].

To avoid recall bias, we included only those who reported use of TM in last year before presentation to headache clinic and completed three months after last TM session. Also, we collected data of headache days, duration and number of analgesics used over the last three months before seeking clinical headache.

The self-reported efficacy questionnaire queried history of TM before presentation to headache clinic. It queried TM and its efficacy. The questions were: "Have you ever tried TM for headache?" "Which type of TM?" TM queried included blood cupping (Hijama), head banding, herbal medicine (sabkha), and diet modification which are known to be the most common used TM for headache in Kuwait. "Did you experience any efficacy in terms of reduction of headache frequency, duration, use of analgesics and/or intensity?" The questionnaire assessed characters of headache before and 3 months after the final TM session to assess the efficacy of TM. Participants were reported if they are satisfied or not satisfied with TM for headache. They were also asked to report any adverse events related to TM use.

Statistical analysis

Statistical analyses were performed using SPSS 20.00 (SPSS Inc., Chicago, IL, USA). Simple descriptive statistical tests (mean and standard deviation) are used to describe the numerical values of the sample and the number and percentage of the non-numerical values. The significance of the differences between patients who used TM and others who did not used was determined using independent t test. Paired t-test was used to compare the frequency, duration of headache and number of analgesics use days, 3 months before and 3 months after the end of TM. A chi-squared test was used to compare between nonparametric variables. A probability of (P) ≤0.05 is accepted as significant.

All participants gave informed consents.

Result

Out of 317 participants presented to headache clinic throughout the six months of study duration, 279 patients completed the questionnaires. The socio demographic characteristics of participants and characters of primary headache were outlined in Table 1. Most of them 79.6% were female. The mean age was 40.32 ± 11.75 and mean age at headache onset was 23.06 ± 10.19. In the cohort 44.4% had completed high school education.

Episodic migraine was the most presented headache in our cohort 44.8% followed by tension-type headache 31.9%, chronic migraine 12.5%, and other types of primary headache disorders 10.8% including cluster headache, paroxysmal hemicranias and other trigeminal autonomic cephalgias.

Most of our patients 69.5% tried TM in the last year before presentation to headache clinic. Table 1 compare the Socio demographic data and Characters of primary headache in those who used TM and those who do not use it over last three month before presentation to headache clinic to avoid recall bias. No significant differences were found in seeking TM depending on gender ($p < 0.79$). However, those who sought TM are significantly older at onset of headache ($p < 0.003$) and have longer disease duration ($p < 0.044$). There was no statistically significant difference between education status and use of TM ($p < 0.54$), (Table 1).

All participants with chronic headache, 90.4% participants with episodic migraine versus only 31.5% of Tension Type Headache (TTH) Tried TM ($p < 0.047$), (Table 1). Those who used TM when presented to headache clinic had significant frequent headache attacks ($p < 0.001$), longer duration of headache attacks ($p < 0.009$) and more frequent use of analgesic compared to those who did not use TM. The use of TM was significantly higher among those who do not use medical treatment compared to those who used it (p < 0.001). (Table 1).

The frequency, reasons and satisfaction of TM were shown in Table 2. Most of the participants used Hijama 65.6% either alone 47.3% or with Sobakh 18.3%, followed with those who were treated with Sobkh and few of our cohort used other modalities of TM as head banding, head massage and diet modifications. Culture/religion beliefs were the cause of seeking TM in 51.3% versus 10% used it due to ineffective medical treatment and 8.6% used it because of intolerance/fear of medical treatment. Most of participants 69.9% used TM before seeking neurologist. Only 26.2% reported that they are satisfied with TM. Few of them 17.9% reported adverse events as allergy, pain or trauma.

Self-reported efficacy of TM was outlined in Table 3. At 3 months after the final TM session, there was no significant reduction of frequency of headache days per month ($P < 0.50$), days of analgesic use per month ($P < 0.09$) and duration of headache ($P < 0.78$). However, there is significant reduction of the severity of headache for 3 months ($P < 0.02$).

Discussion

TM is widely used for primary headache disorder in Kuwait, however efficacy has not been proven. We aimed to highlight the frequent use of traditional medicine in our community. TM, is sometimes used instead of conventional medicine and may lead to delay the diagnosis and prober management. We did not study its efficacy or its procedures. We included the patients who finished the course of TM according to their traditional healers. To us Hijama, head banding, sabkha, and diet modification all are non-conventional medicine that interfere with proper management in our community. Evidence indicated that traditional medicine was not only used for the healthcare of the poor; its prevalence increased in countries where allopathic medicine is predominant in the healthcare system [3]. The prevalence rate of TM use in Gulf is high. It is 67% in a United Arab Emirates [15] and 42% in Saudi Arabia [12]. To our knowledge, this is the first study of TM use by headache patients in Kuwait. We reported that 69.5% of patients who attended headache clinics used TM. When comparing our result with other western studies of non-conventional medicine use our figure of 69.5% headache clinic patients using TM is higher than the 31%, 40%

Table 1 Comparison between patient who used TM and who did not use 3 months before presentation to headache clinic

Socio demographic data and Characters of primary headache	Total Sample (n = 279) Mean (SD)/No (%)	Patients Used TM (n = 194) Mean (SD)/No (%)	Patients did not use TM* (n = 85) Mean (SD)/No (%)	P
Mean Age	40.32 ± 11.75	40.42 ± 11.17	40.09 ± 11.75	0.83
Mean Age at onset	23.06 ± 10.19	24.24 + 10.67	20.38 ± 8.47	0.003*
Mean disease duration	17.08 ± 12.01	19.26 + 13.13	16.12 ± 11.39	0.044*
Gender				
Female	222 (79.6)	156 (70.3)	66 (29.7)	0.79
Male	75 (20.4)	39 (86.4)	18 (31.6)	
Education				
University	77 (27.6)	24 (28.6)	53 (27.2)	
High school	123 (44.1)	40 (47.6)	83 (42.6)	0.54
Primary school	79 (28.3)	20 (23.8)	59 (30.3)	
Diagnosis				
Episodic Migraine	125 (44.8)	113 (90.4)	12 (9.6)	
Tension Type	89 (31.9)	28 (31.5)	61 (68.5)	0.047*
Headache	35(12.5)	35 (100)	0	
Chronic Headache	30 (10.8)	19 (63.3)	11 (36.7)	
Others as TAC				
Frequency of headache/month	7.99 + 6.83	9.66 + 7.39	4.14 + 2.72	0.001*
Mean Duration of headache in hours	38.51 + 26.78	41.23 + 27.76	32.19 + 23.29	.0009*
Mean Number of analgesics/Month	7.71 + 7.04	8.23 + 7.70	3.18 + 3.06	0.001*
Severity of headache				
Mild	32(11.5)	0	32 (100)	
Moderate	165(59.1)	117 (70.9)	48 (29.1)	0.001*
Severe	82(29.4)	78 (95.1)	4 (4.9)	
Used treatment for headache	76 (27.2)	72 (36.9)	4 (4.8)	
No drugs	72 (25.8	48 (24.6)	24 (28.6)	0.001*
Prophylactic treatment	131 (47)	75 (38.5)	56 (66.7)	
Symptomatic treatment				

TM: Traditional Medicine
TAC: Trigeminal autonomic cephalgia

and 29% shown in Italian migraine, chronic tension type headache and cluster headache patients respectively [16–18], 32% of headache clinic in United Kingdom [19] 44.4% [20], 41.3% [21] in United state of America but less than the 81—85%reported in Austrian and German [22] and United state of America [23] headache clinic patients. This might reflect cultural and regional differences on how and by whom complementary and alternative medicine therapies were provided.

In our study, TM users were older than TM non-users. There was no significant difference between both groups regarding gender or education level. It was surprising that highly educated subjects used TM which is of unknown mechanism of action. They preferred the tradional medicine because of its spiritual origin.

In the last three months before presentation to headache clinic, were more likely to suffer from more frequent attacks, more intense headaches for a longer period of time, when compared to non-TM used; which is consistent with previous studies [17, 19, 22, 24, 25]. Worse headache may be the cause of seeking TM since more than 50% of our participants sought TM because of their religion beliefs. We think that the headache get worse in TM users who did not received the required adequate conventional

Table 2 Analysis of frequency, reasons and satisfaction of TM (N = 194)

Variables	Number (%)	P value
TM		
Cupping (Hijama)	132 (47.3)	
Sobakh	81(29.1)	0.001*
Cupping (Hijama) and Sobakh	51 (18.3)	
Others (Head banding, head massage, special diet)	33 (11.8)	
Cause of asking for TM		
Cultural/ Religious	143 (51.3)	0.001*
Ineffective medicine	28 (10)	
Intolerance to/fear of medicine	24 (8.6)	
Time of TM		
Before seeking Neurologist	105 (69.9)	0.001*
After seeking Neurologist	90 (30.1)	
Satisfaction		
Satisfied	51 (26.2)	.001*
Not satisfied	144 (73.8)	
Adverse events		
Yes	35 (17.94)	0.001*
No	160 (82.05)	

TM: Traditional Medicine

medicine when compare to TM non-users. We noticed also that all chronic headache patients who were presented to headache clinic tried TM and TM users have significant long disease duration.

This study reported that 70% of participants used TM before seeking help from neurologist which is the reverse of previous western studies, around 2/3 cases in headache clinic in Italy [16, 17], 67% [19] in headache clinic in UK and 62% of general population in UK [26] sought conventional treatment before non-conventional medicine. The majority of participants in western studies gave the reason for using non-conventional medicine that they believed it

would effectively treat headache _after ineffective conventional treatment. However most of the participants in our study, 69.5% used TM before conventional treatment because it is in congruent with their culture and religion believes. TM healers are usually trusted members of the community [27].

Hijama was the most common used TM for primary headache, in 65.6% of our cohort. The religious roots of hijama is that the Prophet Muhammad advocated its practice. It is taken from Prophetic tradition. The prophet Mohammed (peace be upon him) referred to hijamah for curing an illness [28]. It is noted in al-Buhary and Muslim, the two most authoritative Sunni compilations of the Prophet's sayings, that Muhammad reportedly said that healing is "in the incision of a cupper" [29]. Prophet mohammed didn't specify which disease hijama will heal, moreover, he didn't stop people from seeking medical advice at first, so doing it has some blessing since following a practice of the prophet but in view of advanced medicine the prophet didn't stop any person from seeking a doctor. However, few of our patients tried TM because they were not satisfied by efficacy of conventional fear of or intolerance to side effects.

TM use has the potential to be harmful if patients use it with non-educated personnel (especially when using instruments with poor hygiene resulting in infections) or if they stop effective conventional therapies while using a TM therapy. Physicians need to be understanding, supportive and open minded when interacting with patients use TM. Healthcare providers should educate patients about their TM use, monitor potential benefits or adverse events and educate patients about conventional medicine. Physicians and TM practitioners need better communication and coordination of care in order to provide the best available patient benefit. TM unfortunately used by some unprofessional healers just to gain money which is totally misuse of the healthcare system and using the illness of the people solely for financial reasoning. Also, some of those healers they don't know how to deal with vasovagal attacks or loss of consciousness that some patients can have especially during hijama.

Table 3 self-reported efficacy of TM (N = 195)

Variables	Before TM use	3 month after TM use	P
Frequency of headache/month	9.66 ± 7.39	9.44 ± 7.70	0.47
Mean Duration of headache in hours	41.23 ± 27.76	41.59 ± 27.69	0.78
Mean Number of analgesics days /Month	8.04 ± 7.62	7.34 ± 7.20	0.09
Severity of headache			
Moderate	117(60)	144(73.8)	
Severe	78 (40)	51 (22.2)	0.03*

TM: Traditional Medicine

Although the self-reported efficacy of TM is modest, the use of TM is high in this study. Conventional medicine may not always improve the headache, and some patients do not tolerate acute and/or prophylactic medicine due to side effects or contraindications. Similar to other studies [16, 17] some patients may wish to avoid medication due to possible side effects or risk for medication tolerance.

Limitations of the study

The study includes patients attending clinic who are a special subset of primary headache sufferers. They may have refractory or disabling headaches, so the results of this study might not reflect the majority headache patients.

The efficacy of TM are based on self-reports and therefore subjected to recall bias. We tried to minimize recall bias by including the patients who used TM only in the last year before enrolment in the study and collecting data headache days, duration and number of analgesics used over the last three months before seeking clinical headache.

Personal causality, individual perception and understanding of pain in addition to belief in TM modalities could affect the subjective judgment.

of headache relief and satisfaction of TM.

Conclusion

The frequent use of TM for primary headache in our community is a major concern. Health care professionals involved in the management of headache patients should be aware of this. There is a need for evaluation of the benefits and safety of TM therapies for headache. Community awareness for medical headache treatment should be improved. Healthcare providers should educate the patients about TM use, monitor potential benefits or adverse events. Most of our patients, at some point, seek some or all traditional medicine because of their cultural and religious believes. Conventional healthcare providers and TM practitioners need better communication and coordination of care in order to provide the best available patient care and safety. Those healers should have also some sort of license in order to practice TM this may protect safety of the patients.

For future research, it will be interesting to conduct a general population survey to see if rates of TM use in treating headache are similar to those attending headache clinics. TM may be helpful as a complementary medicine so we need to study its efficacy and safety in details and we recommend to coordinate with traditional healers to avoid hazards of TM and keep this type of treatment under our observation.

Abbreviations
CH: Chronic headache; TAC: Trigeminal autonomic cephalgia; TM: Trational medicine; TTH: Tension type headache

Acknowledgments
We would like to thank the study participants and the nurses in Ibn Sina Hospital for actively participating in the study.

Funding
This study was not funded.

Disclosure
RA received honoraria as a speaker and for serving in scientific advisory boards from Bayer, Biogen, Biologix, Genzyme, Genpharm, Novartis, GSK, Merck-Serono. SA, WA, FA and JA have nothing to disclose.

Authors' contributions
JA contributed to research design. SA: contributed to project design and development of the methodology, data acquisition and statistical analysis and drafted the manuscript. FA: contributed to data acquisition. RA revised the manuscript critically. All authors read and approved the final manuscript.

Competing interest
The authors declare that they have no competing interests.

Author details
[1]Department of Neurology, Ibn Sina Hospital, P.O. Box 25427, Safat, 13115 Kuwait City, Kuwait. [2]Department of Medicine, Faculty of Medicine, Health Sciences Centre, Kuwait University, Kuwait City, Kuwait. [3]Department of Neurology and Psychiatry, Al-Minia University, Minia, Egypt. [4]Mubarak Al-Kabeer Hospital, Jabriya, Hawalli, Kuwait. [5]Division of Neurology, Amiri Hospital, P.O. Box 1661, Qurtoba, 73767 Kuwait City, Kuwait.

References
1. Steiner TJ, Birbeck GL, Jensen RH, Katsarava Z, Stovner LJ, Martelletti Pet. (2015). Headache disorders are third cause of disability worldwide. J Headache Pain 16:58. doi: 10.1186/s
2. Sinclair AJ, Sturrock A, Davies B, Matharu M (2015) Headache management: pharmacological approaches. Pract Neurol 15:411–423. https://doi.org/10.1136/practneurol-2015-001167
3. WHO (2000) In: WHO Traditional Medicine Strategy 2002-2005 (ed) General guidelines for methodologies on research and evaluation of traditional medicine. World Health Organization, Geneva, pp 1–71
4. Zulfakar, R. S. (2013). Pendakwaan Jenayah Sihir: Prinsip-Prinsip Pembuktian dan Akta Keterangan Mahkamah Syariah" (kertas kerja, Muzakarah Pakar: Pendakwaan Pesalah Sihir di Mahkamah Syariah. Shah Alam, Malaysia: Jabatan Mufti Negeri Selangor dengan kerjasama PISANG.Şeker N: [Prophet and preventive medicine: The case of bloodletting.] The University of Kahramanmaras Sutcu Imam Review of the Faculty of Theology,:21:157–87 [in Turkish]
5. Astin JA (1998) Why patients use alternative medicine: results of a national survey. JAMA 279:1548–1553
6. Siapush M (1998) Post-modern values, dissatisfaction with conventional medicine and popularity of alternative therapies. J Social 34:58–70
7. Qur'an, Surah An-Nahl 16:69, http://www.searchtruth.com/chapter_display.php?chapter=16&translator=2&mac=&show_arabic=1
8. El-Wakil A (2011) Observations of the popularity and religious significance of blood-cupping (al-hijama) as an Islamic medicine. Contemporary Islamic Studies 2011:2. https://doi.org/10.5339/cis.2011.2
9. El-Hag AG, Al-Jabri AA, Habbal OA (2007) Antimicrobial properties of Lawsonia inermis (henna): a review. Australian Journal of Medical Herbalism 19(3):114
10. Vijayan N (1993) Head band for migraine headache relief. Headache 33(1):40–42
11. Ernst E, Cohen MH, Stone J (2004) Ethical problems arising in evidence-based complementary and alternative medicine. J Med Ethics. 30:156–159
12. Al-Rowais N, Al-Faris E, Mohammad AG, Al-Rukban M, Abdulghani HN (2010) Traditional healers in Riyadh region: reasons and health problems for seeking their advice. A household survey. J Altern Complement Med 16(2):199–204
13. Headache Classification Committee of the International Headache Society (2013) The international classification of headache disorders, 3rd edition (beta version). Cephalalgia 33:629–808

14. Tfelt-Hansen P, Pascual J, Ramadan N, Dahlof C, Diener HC, Hansen JM, Lanteri Minet M, Loder E, McCrory D, Plancade S, Schwedt T, International Headache Society Clinical Trials Subcommittee (2012) Guidelines for controlled trials of drugs in migraine: third edition. A guide for investigators. Cephalalgia. 32:6–38

15. AlBraik FA, Rutter PM, Brown DA (2008) Cross- sectional survey of herbal remedy taking by united Arab emirate (UAE) citizens in Abu Dhabi. Pharmacoepidemiol Drug Saf 17:725–732

16. Rossi P, Di Lorenzo G, Malpezzi MG, Faroni J, Cesarino F, Di Lorenzo C, Nappi G (2005) Prevalence, pattern and predictors of use of complementary and alternative medicine (CAM) in migraine patientsatt ending a headache clinic in Italy. Cephalalgia 25:493–506

17. Rossi P, Di Lorenzo G, Faroni J, Malpezzi MG, Cesarino F, Nappi G (2006) Use of complementary and alternative medicine by patients with chronictension-type headache: results of a headache clinic survey. Headache 46:622–631

18. Rossi P, Torelli P, Di Lorenzo C et al (2008) Use of complementary and alternative medicine by patients with cluster headache: results of a multi-Centre headache clinic survey. Complement Ther Med 16:220–227

19. Lamberta TD, Morrisona KE, Edwardsc J, Clarkea CE (2010) The use of complementary and alternative medicine by patients attending a UK headache clinic. Complement Ther Med. 18:128–134

20. Rhee TG, Harris IM (2017) Gender differences in the use of complementary and alternative medicine and their association with moderate mental distress in U. S. adults with migraines/severe headaches. Headache 57(1):97e108

21. Rhee TG, Harris IM (2018) Reasons for and perceived benefits of utilizing complementary and alternative medicine in U.S. adults with migraines/severe headaches. Complement Ther Clin Pract 30:44e49

22. Gaul C, Eismann R, Schmidt T, Ma A, Leinisch E, Wiesse T, Ever S, Henkel K, Franz G, Zierz S (2009) Use of complementary and alternative medicine in patients suffering from primary headache disorders. Cephalalgia 29:1069–1078

23. Von Peter S, Ting W, Scrivani S et al (2002) Survey on the use of complementary and alternative medicine among patients with headache syndromes. Cephalalgia 22:395–400

24. Adams J, Barbery G, Lui CW (2013) Complementary and alternative medicine use for headache and migraine: a critical review of the literature. J Head Face Pain 53(3):459–473

25. Wachholtz A, Malone C, Bhowmick A (2015) The chronic migraineur and health services: national survey results. Pain Manag Med 1(1):1–7

26. Thomas K, Coleman P (2004) Use of complementary or alternative medicine in a general population in Great Britain. Results from the National Omnibus survey. J PublicHealth 26:152–157

27. World Health Organization (2012) Traditional and complementary medicine policy. In: Policy and economic issues

28. Albinali H (2004) Traditional medicine among gulf Arabs. Heart Views 5(2):1–11

29. Abu 'Abdullah Muhammad bin Isma'il al-Buhary, Sahh, Kita b al-Tib (2011). 71:587, 603, 605

Preventive effects of galcanezumab in adult patients with episodic or chronic migraine are persistent: data from the phase 3, randomized, double-blind, placebo-controlled EVOLVE-1, EVOLVE-2, and REGAIN studies

Stefanie Förderreuther[1], Qi Zhang[2], Virginia L. Stauffer[3*], Sheena K. Aurora[3] and Miguel J. A. Láinez[4]

Abstract

Background: Maintenance of effect following treatment with galcanezumab compared to placebo in adult patients with episodic or chronic migraine was evaluated.

Methods: In 2 similarly designed studies of patients with episodic migraine (6 months) and 1 study of patients with chronic migraine (3 months), patients randomized in a 1:1:2 ratio received a subcutaneous injection of galcanezumab 120 mg/month (after an initial loading dose of 240 mg) or 240 mg/month or placebo. Maintenance of effect during the double-blind phase was evaluated based on a comparison of the percentages of galcanezumab- and placebo-treated patients with maintenance of 30, 50, 75, and 100% response (defined as ≥30, ≥50, ≥75, and 100% reduction from baseline in monthly migraine headache days [MHD]) at an individual patient level. Logistic regression analyses were used for between treatment comparisons.

Results: A total of 1773 adult patients with episodic migraine ($n = 444$ for galcanezumab 120 mg; $n = 435$ for galcanezumab 240 mg; $n = 894$ for placebo for 2 studies pooled) and 1113 patients with chronic migraine ($n = 278$ for galcanezumab 120 mg; $n = 277$ for galcanezumab 240 mg; $n = 558$ for placebo) were evaluated. In patients with episodic migraine, ≥50% response was maintained in 41.5 and 41.1% of galcanezumab-treated patients (120 mg and 240 mg, respectively) for ≥3 consecutive months (until patient's endpoint) and 19.0 and 20.5%, respectively, for 6 consecutive months and was significantly greater than the 21.4 and 8.0% of placebo-treated patients at ≥3 and 6 months consecutively ($P < 0.001$). Approximately 6% of galcanezumab-treated patients maintained ≥75% response all 6 months versus 2% of placebo-treated patients. Few galcanezumab-treated patients maintained 100% response. In patients with chronic migraine, 29% of galcanezumab-treated patients maintained ≥30% response all 3 months compared to 16% of placebo patients while ≥50% response was maintained in 16.8 and 14.6% of galcanezumab-treated patients (120 mg and 240 mg) and was greater than placebo (6.3%; $p < 0.001$). Few patients maintained ≥75% response.

Conclusions: Treatment with galcanezumab 120 mg or 240 mg demonstrated statistically significant and clinically meaningful persistence of effect in patients with episodic migraine (≥3 and 6 consecutive months) and in patients with chronic migraine (for 3 months).

(Continued on next page)

* Correspondence: vstauffer@lilly.com
[3]Eli Lilly and Company, Lilly Corporate Center, Indianapolis, IN 46285, USA
Full list of author information is available at the end of the article

(Continued from previous page)
Study identification and trial registration: Study Identification: EVOLVE-1 (I5Q-MC-CGAG); EVOLVE-2 (I5Q-MC-CGAH); REGAIN (I5Q-MC-CGAI)
Keywords: Galcanezumab, Migraine, Preventive, Persistence, Maintenance

Background

Galcanezumab is a humanized monoclonal antibody, indicated for the prevention of migraine, that binds to calcitonin gene-related peptide (CGRP) and prevents its biological activity without blocking the CGRP receptor [1]. The efficacy of galcanezumab was examined in 3 randomized, double-blind, placebo-controlled, Phase 3 studies of galcanezumab (120 and 240 mg/month) in patients with episodic (EVOLVE-1 and EVOLVE-2 6-month studies) or chronic (REGAIN 3-month study) migraine [2–4]. The mean monthly percentages of galcanezumab-treated patients with episodic migraine or chronic migraine that achieved ≥50% reduction in MHD was greater than the percentages of placebo-treated patients (60% versus 36% to 39% and 27% versus 15%, respectively) [2–4]. For patients with episodic migraine, galcanezumab-treated patients experienced approximately 4 fewer MHD/month (versus 2 with placebo) and patients with chronic migraine had approximately 5 fewer MHD/month (versus 3 with placebo) with a similar effect in both galcanezumab dose groups [2–4].

Data on current treatments for migraine prevention support that patients on recently approved and older treatments for migraine prevention do achieve a ≥ 50% level of response [5–7]. However, the important question of whether a ≥ 50% reduction in monthly MHD is maintained over time has not been sufficiently addressed for both episodic and chronic migraine [5, 8–10]. Further, can the additional responses of ≥30, ≥75, and 100% reduction in monthly MHD, also recognized to be clinically meaningful, be maintained [11–13]? For patients on a preventive treatment, this is a particularly important aspect since patients seek a medication with a consistent efficacy profile over time. Clinically, tachyphylaxis has been reported frequently by patients and physicians.

The current study evaluated data from the placebo-controlled EVOLVE-1 and EVOLVE-2 episodic migraine trials and the REGAIN chronic migraine trial and compared galcanezumab treatment to placebo in the maintenance of ≥30% (chronic only), ≥50, ≥75, and 100% (episodic only) response in the reduction of MHD from baseline.

Methods
Study design

Detailed descriptions of the study design for the 2 episodic migraine (6-month) and 1 chronic migraine

(3-month) double-blind studies, have been reported separately (ClinicalTrials.gov NCT02614183, NCT02614196, and NCT02614261) [2–4]. Briefly, adult patients were randomized 1:1:2 and received subcutaneous injections of galcanezumab 120 mg/month (after a 240 mg initial loading dose) or 240 mg/month or placebo. Episodic migraine was defined as having between 4 and 14 MHD and at least 2 migraine attacks per month [2, 3, 14]. Chronic migraine was defined as having headache ≥15 days per month for ≥3 months and having features of migraine headache ≥8 days per month [4, 14]. The continuation or start of any additional migraine preventive treatments was not permitted; the exception for patients with chronic migraine was the use of topiramate or propranolol provided they entered trial on a stable dose. The ≥50, ≥75, and ≥ 100% response rates during the 6-month (episodic) or 3-month (chronic) study periods were key secondary objectives (adjusted for multiple testing) and response rates at each month (episodic and chronic studies) were secondary outcomes (not adjusted for multiple testing). The study protocols were reviewed and approved by the appropriate institutional review board for each of the study sites. The studies were conducted according to Good Clinical Practice and the Declaration of Helsinki guidelines. Patients provided written informed consent before undergoing study procedures. The trials are registered with ClinicalTrials.gov (NCT02614183, NCT02614196, and NCT02614261).

Statistical method

Data from the 2 episodic migraine trials combined and 1 chronic migraine trial were included in the analysis. In these trials, a 30, 50, 75, and 100% response rate at each month was defined as the percentage of patients meeting a defined threshold (≥30, ≥50, ≥75, and 100%) in the reduction of the number of monthly MHD during the double-blind treatment period. Only patients with both a baseline and ≥ 1 month of non-missing post-baseline MHD values were included in the analysis. The evaluation of maintenance of effect during the double-blind treatment period was a comparison of the percentages of galcanezumab- and placebo-treated patients with maintenance of ≥30, ≥50, ≥75, and 100% response at the individual patient level. In the episodic studies, maintenance of response was calculated for those with at least 3 months (until patient's endpoint) and 6 consecutive months and 3 consecutive months for chronic migraine. A

Preventive effects of galcanezumab in adult patients with episodic or chronic migraine are persistent: data...

157

logistic regression analysis was used for between-treatment group comparisons. At each month, a cumulative 50% maintenance of response was also calculated and defined as patients with ≥50% response at a specific month (or before) and all subsequent months. For repeated binary data of monthly ≥50% response and cumulative ≥50% sustained response, a categorical, pseudolikelihood-based repeated measures model was implemented with SAS PROC GLIM-MIX [15]. Two-sided p-values were calculated and compared with significance level of 0.05.

Results

Patient disposition

Data from the episodic migraine trials were from 1773 adult patients with episodic migraine treated with 120 mg galcanezumab ($n = 444$), 240 mg galcanezumab ($n = 435$), or placebo ($n = 894$). Data from the chronic migraine trial were from 1113 patients with chronic migraine treated with 120 mg galcanezumab ($n = 278$), 240 mg galcanezumab ($n = 277$), or placebo ($n = 558$). Baseline demographics and disease characteristics of the episodic and chronic migraine populations show that over 80% were female, over 74% were white, had a mean age of 40 years, and had migraine disease duration of 20 years. As permitted by protocol for the chronic migraine trial, concomitant use of topiramate or propranolol during the double-blind phase, across all treatment groups, occurred in 10.3 and 3.6% of patients, respectively. At baseline, the mean MHD/month was 9.1 for episodic migraine and 19.3 for chronic migraine. The mean baseline Migraine Disability Assessment score for patients treated with galcanezumab or placebo was 33.1 for episodic migraine and 65.8 (galcanezumab) and 68.7 (placebo) for chronic migraine and was reflective of severe (episodic) and very severe (chronic) migraine disability. The mean baseline Migraine-Specific Quality of Life Questionnaire Role Function-Restrictive subdomain score for patients treated with galcanezumab or placebo with episodic migraine was 51.1 and 52.1, respectively, and with chronic migraine was 39.1 and 38.4, respectively. Patients with chronic migraine had greater functional impairment than patients with episodic migraine (Table 1).

Proportions of patients with ≥50% response

The model-estimated proportions of patients with episodic migraine achieving ≥50% response were significantly greater for both galcanezumab dose groups compared to placebo starting at Month 1 ($p < 0.001$) and at each month after ($p < 0.001$), as well as overall across 6 months ($p < 0.001$) (Table 2). For patients with chronic migraine, the model-estimated proportions of patients achieving ≥50% response was significantly greater for both dose groups compared to placebo starting at Month 1 ($p < 0.001$) and at each month after ($p \leq 0.004$),

as well as overall across 3 months ($p < 0.001$) (Table 2). The absolute values for the proportions of patients with episodic or chronic migraine that achieved ≥50% response were very similar to the estimated values proportions and are shown in Additional file 1: Table S1.

Maintenance of response

Significantly more patients with episodic migraine treated with galcanezumab in both dose groups (approximately 41%) maintained response of ≥50% fewer MHD for ≥3 consecutive months until patient's endpoint compared to placebo (21%). Over Month 1 to Month 6, approximately 20% of galcanezumab-treated patients in both dose groups maintained a response of ≥50% fewer MHD that was significantly greater than placebo (8%) (Fig. 1).

In patients with chronic migraine, significantly more patients in both the 120 mg (17%) and 240 mg (15%) galcanezumab dose groups maintained a response of ≥50% fewer MHD for 3 consecutive months compared to placebo (6%) (Fig. 2). The difference between dose groups for either episodic or chronic migraine in the proportions of patients with maintenance of response was not significant.

The model-estimated proportions of patients with episodic migraine who maintained a response of ≥75 and 100% and those patients with chronic migraine who maintained a response of ≥30 and ≥75% are shown in (Table 3). The proportions of galcanezumab-treated patients with episodic migraine who maintained a response of ≥75% fewer MHD for 3 consecutive months until patient's endpoint (19.7 and 21.3%) was significantly greater than placebo (8.5%; $p < 0.001$). While fewer, 6% of galcanezumab-treated patients maintained a response of ≥75% fewer MHD for all 6 months compared with 1.8% of placebo-treated patients. A small percentage of patients maintained 100% response for 3 consecutive months and very few maintained 100% response for all 6 months. The proportions of galcanezumab-treated patients with chronic migraine who maintained a response of ≥30% fewer MHD for all 3 months (29%) was significantly greater than placebo (16.4%; $p < 0.001$). The proportions of patients who maintained ≥75% fewer MHD for all 3 months was not different between the galcanezumab and placebo groups.

Characterization of patients with episodic migraine with ≥50% response at month 1

Among the 50.9 and 47.2% of galcanezumab 120 mg- and 240 mg-treated patients with episodic migraine who met ≥50% response at Month 1, the average reduction in MHD over the remaining 5 months of the double-blind phase was 66.6 and 71.5%. Of the 23.8% of placebo-treated patients

Table 1 Patient demographics and disease characteristics of galcanezumab -treated patients from episodic and chronic migraine trials

Variables	Episodic Migraine Studies[a]		Chronic Migraine Study[b]	
	Galanezumab[a] N = 879	Placebo N = 894	Galcanezumab[b] N = 555	Placebo N = 558
Age, years, mean (SD)	40.7 (11.4)	41.9 (11.4)	40.4 (12.2)	41.6 (12.1)
Female, n (%)	744 (84.6)	755 (84.5)	463 (83.4)	483 (86.6)
Race white, n (%)	652 (74.2)	681 (76.2)	447 (80.7)	432 (77.4)
Ethnicity not Hispanic or Latino[c], n (%)	664 (78.4)	677 (79.4)	387 (74.0)	401 (76.7)
Geographic region, n (%)				
North America	647 (73.6)	657 (73.5)	320 (57.7)	321 (57.5)
Europe	119 (13.5)	122 (13.7)	138 (24.9)	140 (25.1)
Other	113 (12.9)	115 (12.9)	97 (17.5)	97 (17.4)
Body mass index, kg/m^2 mean (SD)	27.6 (5.5)	27.6 (5.5)	26.5 (5.4)	26.9 (5.6)
Migraine disease duration, years, mean (SD)	20.1 (12.2)	20.5 (12.5)	20.2 (12.7)	21.9 (12.9)
Migraine headache days/month, mean (SD)	9.1 (2.9)	9.1 (3.0)	19.3 (4.4)	19.6 (4.6)
MHD/month with acute medication use, mean (SD)	7.4 (3.4)	7.5 (3.4)	14.8 (6.3)	15.5 (6.6)
Headache days/month, mean (SD)	10.7 (3.7)	10.6 (3.4)	21.3 (4.0)	21.5 (4.1)
Migraine with aura, n (%)	467 (53.1)	471 (52.7)	294 (53.0)	310 (55.6)
Prior preventive treatment in past 5 years, n (%)	559 (63.6)	555 (62.1)	431 (77.7)	435 (78.0)
Failed ≥ 2 preventives in past 5 years, n (%)	88 (10.0)	85 (9.5)	165 (29.7)	163 (29.2)
MIDAS total, mean (SD)	33.1 (28.2)	33.1 (29.3)	65.8 (57.3)	68.7 (57.4)
MSQ RF-R, mean (SD)	51.1 (16.1)	52.1 (15.6)	39.1 (17.3)	38.4 (17.2)
PGI-S, mean (SD)	4.3 (1.2)	4.3 (1.2)	4.8 (1.3)	4.9 (1.2)

Abbreviations: *MHD* migraine headache days, *MIDAS* Migraine Disability Assessment, *MSQ* Migraine-Specific Quality of Life Questionnaire version 2.1, *PGI-S* Patient Global Impression of Severity, *RF-R* Role Function-Restrictive, *SD* standard deviation
[a]Pooled data from two parallel 6-month trials in patients with episodic migraine
[b]3-month trial
[c]Not all patients reported ethnicity data

with ≥50% response at Month 1, the average reduction in MHD was 63.2%. Further, among only those with ≥50% response at Month 1, 85.4 and 92.4% of patients in the 2 galcanezumab dose groups and 80.7% in the placebo group averaged at least a 40% response over the remaining 5 months. Moreover, 80.8 and 85.4% of patients in the 2 galcanezumab groups respectively and 71.1% of patients in the placebo group averaged at least ≥50% response over the remaining 5 months.

Cumulative and onset of maintenance of response

The cumulative maintenance of response is defined as individual patients who met ≥50% response starting at a given month (or before) and then all the months subsequent. The proportions of patients with episodic migraine in the galcanezumab 120 mg and 240 mg groups achieving cumulative maintenance of ≥50% response was superior to placebo at every month of the 6-month double-blind phase ($p < 0.001$) (Fig. 3). For example, 31% of patients with episodic migraine treated with galcanezumab 120 mg reached ≥50% at or before Month 3 and maintained that response in the subsequent months (Month 4 to Month 6). The difference

between the galcanezumab dose groups for cumulative maintenance of response was not significant.

The onset of ≥50% maintenance of response and the percentage of patients with episodic or chronic migraine who reached ≥50% response at the specific month (but not before) and then maintained that response in the subsequent months of treatment is shown in Table 4. To illustrate the onset for patients with episodic migraine, 19, 6, and 6% of patients treated with galcanezumab 120 mg reached ≥50% response at Months 1, 2, and 3, respectively, and maintained that response in the subsequent months of treatment (Months 2 to 6, Months 3 to 6, and Month 4 to 6, respectively). Across the 6-month double-blind phase, onset of maintenance of response occurred for approximately 4 to 21% of galcanezumab-treated patients with highest rate occurring in Month 1. In all but one time point, the proportions of patients were greater in the galcanezumab treatment groups than the placebo group at each month. The exception was at 6 months where the proportions of patients were similar between the galcanezumab 120 mg (10.6%) and placebo (10.9%) groups.

Table 2 Model-estimated proportion of patients with episodic and chronic migraine with ≥ 50% response

Response rate	Galcanezumab 120 mg (N = 436)	Galcanezumab 240 mg (N = 428)	Placebo (N = 875)
Episodic migraine			
Overall 6 months	60.8%	58.7%	37.2%
Odds ratio (95% CI)	2.6 (2.2, 3.1)*	2.4 (2.0, 2.8)*	
Month 1, %	50.9%	47.2%	23.8%
Odds ratio (95% CI)	3.3 (2.6, 4.2)*	2.9 (2.2, 3.7)*	
Month 6, %	65.7%	63.2%	44.3%
Odds ratio (95% CI)	2.4 (1.9, 3.1)*	2.2 (1.7, 2.8)*	
Chronic migraine	Galcanezumab 120 mg (N = 273)	Galcanezumab 240 mg (N = 274)	Placebo (N = 538)
Overall 3 months	27.6%	27.5%	15.4%
Odds ratio (95% CI)	2.1 (1.6, 2.8)*	2.1 (1.6, 2.8)*	
Month 1, %	23.7%	21.2%	9.9%
Odds ratio (95% CI)	2.8 (1.9, 4.2)*	2.5 (1.7, 3.6)*	
Month 3, %	31.9%	34.0%	22.4%
Odds ratio (95% CI)	1.6 (1.2, 2.3)†	1.8 (1.3, 2.5)*	

Abbreviations: CI confidence interval
* $p < 0.001$ versus placebo
† $p \leq 0.004$ versus placebo

In patients with chronic migraine, the proportions of patients treated with galcanezumab 120 mg or 240 mg achieving cumulative maintenance of ≥50% response was superior to placebo at every month of the 3-month double-blind phase ($p < 0.001$). At Month 3 or before, approximately 30% of patients in the galcanezumab treatment groups achieved and maintained ≥50% response (Fig. 4). The difference between the galcanezumab dose groups for cumulative maintenance of response was not significant. To illustrate the onset of the maintenance of ≥50% response for patients with chronic migraine (Table 4), 15, 5, and 11% of patients treated with galcanezumab 120 mg reached ≥50% response at Month 1, 2, and 3, respectively.

Safety and tolerability
The most commonly reported treatment-emergent adverse events (TEAE) were injection site-related pain, reaction, erythema, pruritus, and swelling. Discontinuation due to an injection site-related TEAE was low (< 0.5% across all 3 trials). There were no significant differences between galcanezumab and placebo in changes in vital signs and blood pressure. The safety

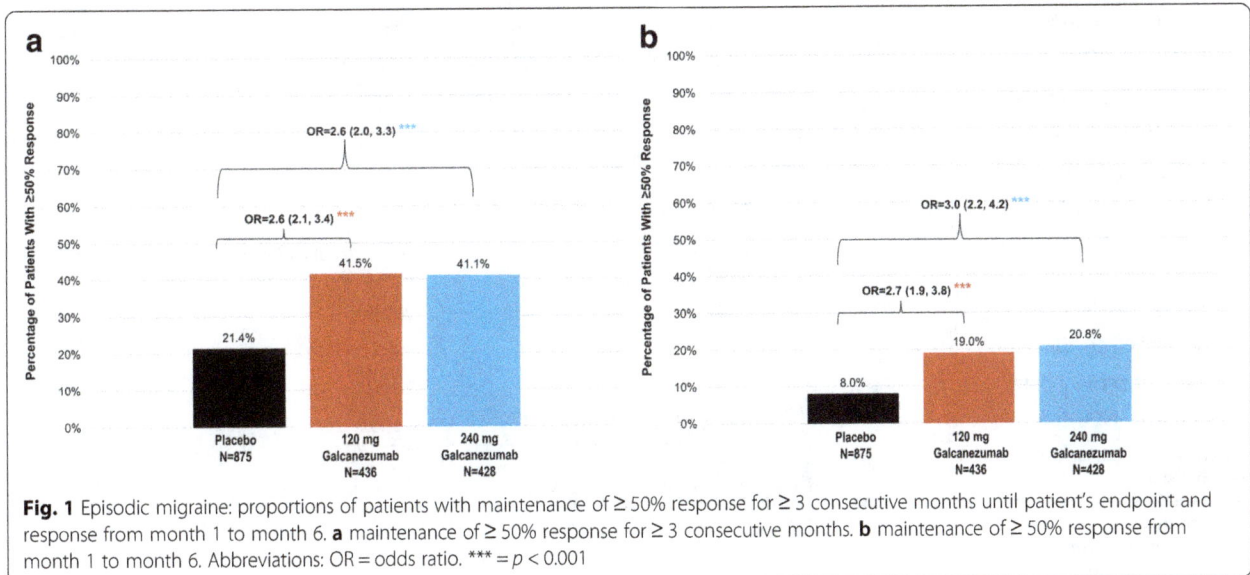

Fig. 1 Episodic migraine: proportions of patients with maintenance of ≥ 50% response for ≥ 3 consecutive months until patient's endpoint and response from month 1 to month 6. **a** maintenance of ≥ 50% response for ≥ 3 consecutive months. **b** maintenance of ≥ 50% response from month 1 to month 6. Abbreviations: OR = odds ratio. *** = $p < 0.001$

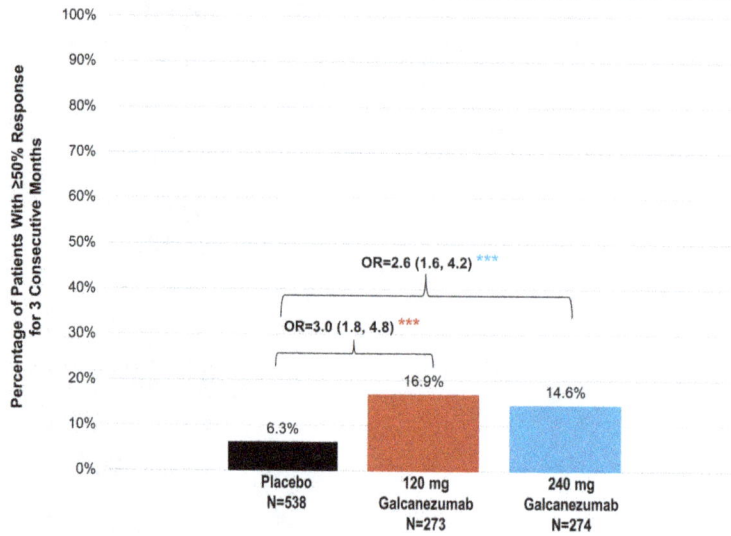

Fig. 2 Chronic migraine: proportions of patients with maintenance of ≥ 50% response for 3 consecutive months. Abbreviations: OR = odds ratio. *** = p < 0.001

profile between the 120 mg and 240 mg doses were similar [2–4].

Discussion

Treatment with galcanezumab 120 mg or 240 mg demonstrated statistically significant and clinically meaningful maintenance of effect in patients with episodic migraine (≥3 consecutive months until patient's endpoint and 6 consecutive months) or chronic migraine (3 months). Starting at Month 1, about 20% of galcanezumab-treated patients (either dose group) with episodic migraine had a sustained response of ≥50% reduction of MHD over 6 months; about 41% of patients maintained ≥50% response over ≥3 months. Among only

Table 3 Model-estimated proportion of patients with episodic and chronic migraine with maintained response

Response rate	Galcanezumab 120 mg (N = 436)	Galcanezumab 240 mg (N = 428)	Placebo (N = 875)
Episodic migraine[a]			
75% Response ≥3 consecutive months[b]	19.7%	21.3%	8.5%
Odds ratio (95% CI)	2.7 (1.9, 3.7)*	2.9 (2.1, 4.1)*	
75% Response all 6 months	6.2%	6.8%	1.8%
Odds ratio (95% CI)	3.5 (1.9, 6.3)*	3.9 (2.1, 6.9)*	
100% Response ≥3 consecutive months[b]	3.7%	6.5%	2.7%
Odds ratio (95% CI)	1.4 (0.7, 2.5)	2.5 (1.4, 4.2)*	
100% Response all 6 months	0.7%	1.4%	0.2%
Odds ratio (95% CI)	2.9 (0.8, 10.4)	5.3 (1.6, 17.1)[†]	
Chronic migraine[c]	Galcanezumab 120 mg (N = 273)	Galcanezumab 240 mg (N = 274)	Placebo (N = 538)
30% Response all 3 months	29.3%	29.2%	16.4%
Odds ratio (95% CI)	2.1 (1.5, 3.0)*	2.1 (1.5, 3.1)*	
75% Response all 3 months	2.6%	2.9%	2.0%
Odds ratio (95% CI)	1.3 (0.6, 3.1)	1.5 (0.6, 3.4)	

Abbreviations: CI confidence interval
[a]6-month study
[b]Maintained response until patient's endpoint of the 6-month, double-blind period
[c]3-month study
*p < 0.001 versus placebo
[†] p = 0.006 versus placebo

Preventive effects of galcanezumab in adult patients with episodic or chronic migraine are persistent: data...

161

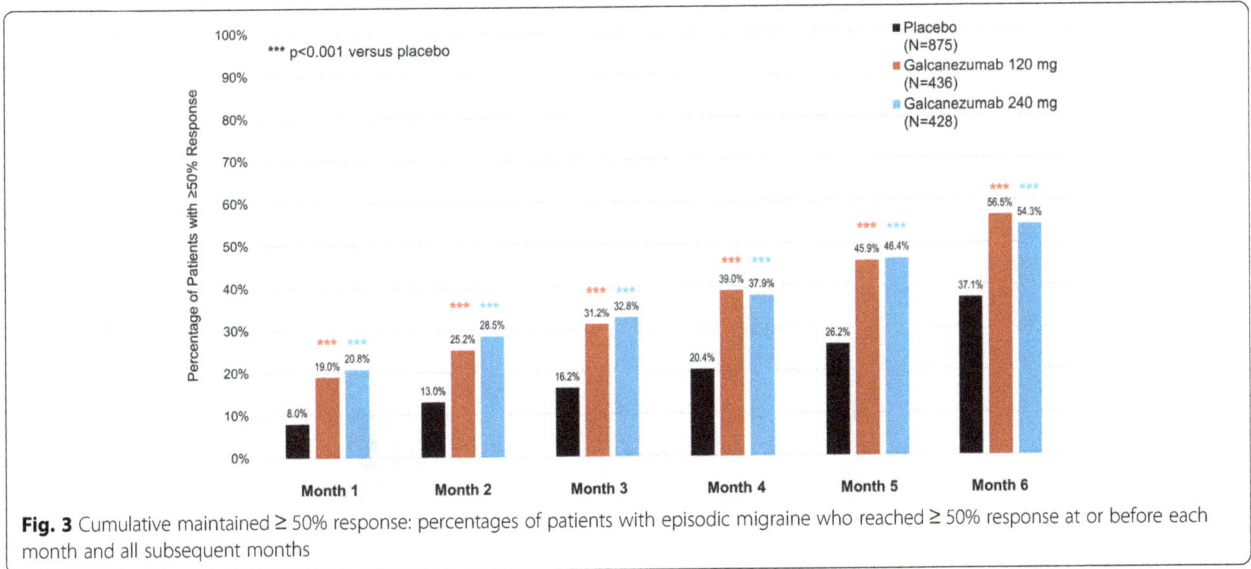

Fig. 3 Cumulative maintained ≥ 50% response: percentages of patients with episodic migraine who reached ≥ 50% response at or before each month and all subsequent months

the galcanezumab-treated patients who had a ≥ 50% reduction of MHD in Month 1, an average reduction of MHD of ≥40 and ≥ 50%, was achieved by 89 and 83% of patients, respectively, in the remaining 5 months of treatment suggesting minimal loss of efficacy among Month 1 responders. In galcanezumab-treated patients with chronic migraine, about 15% showed a ≥ 50% reduction of MHD over 3 consecutive months. Sustained efficacy was also observed in the placebo groups of patients with episodic and with chronic migraine; however, the placebo response was always significantly inferior to galcanezumab treatment. For example, galcanezumab-treated patients with episodic migraine were well over 2 times more likely than placebo-treated patients to achieve a sustained ≥50% response at 6 months and overall. Similarly, galcanezumab-treated patients with chronic migraine were twice as likely than placebo-treated patients to achieve a sustained ≥50% response at 3 months and overall. Several studies have shown the importance of expectation for the size of the placebo response and so a relatively high placebo response, typical for controlled

treatment studies in migraine, was not an unexpected observation in our analysis [16–18]. The placebo response rate is likely a result of intensive patient care within the setting of a study. Regardless, the importance of this analysis is based on the fact that responders do not develop tachyphylaxis, for example, by up-regulation of other mediators of neurovascular inflammation.

Studies with monoclonal antibodies have shown sustained levels of 50% as well as 75 and 100% response in patients with episodic or chronic migraine [10]. Based on pre-specified analyses for our study, about 41% of galcanezuamb-treated patients with episodic migraine maintained ≥50% response for ≥3 consecutive months until patient's endpoint and is a clinically relevant finding. In the additional post-hoc analysis of assessing the cumulative and onset of maintenance of ≥50% response, most patients reach ≥50% response and all subsequent months starting at Month 1, with approximately similar percentages of patients reaching ≥50% response and all subsequent months starting at Month 2, 3, 4, 5, and 6. These findings were generally consistent in the chronic

Table 4 Onset of 50% maintenance of response in patients with episodic and chronic migraine: percentage of patients reach 50% response at each month and all the subsequent months

	Episodic migraine			Chronic migraine		
	Galcanezumab 120 mg (N = 436)	Galcanezumab 240 mg (N = 428)	Placebo (N = 875)	Galcanezumab 120 mg (N = 273)	Galcanezumab 240 mg (N = 274)	Placebo (N = 538)
Month 1	19.0%	20.8%	8.0%	14.8%	12.7%	5.6%
Month 2	6.2%	7.7%	5.0%	4.5%	6.6%	6.2%
Month 3	6.0%	4.3%	3.2%	10.9%	13.1%	9.0%
Month 4	7.8%	5.1%	4.2%	N/A	N/A	N/A
Month 5	6.9%	8.5%	5.8%	N/A	N/A	N/A
Month 6	10.6%	7.9%	10.9%	N/A	N/A	N/A

Abbreviations: *N/A* not applicable

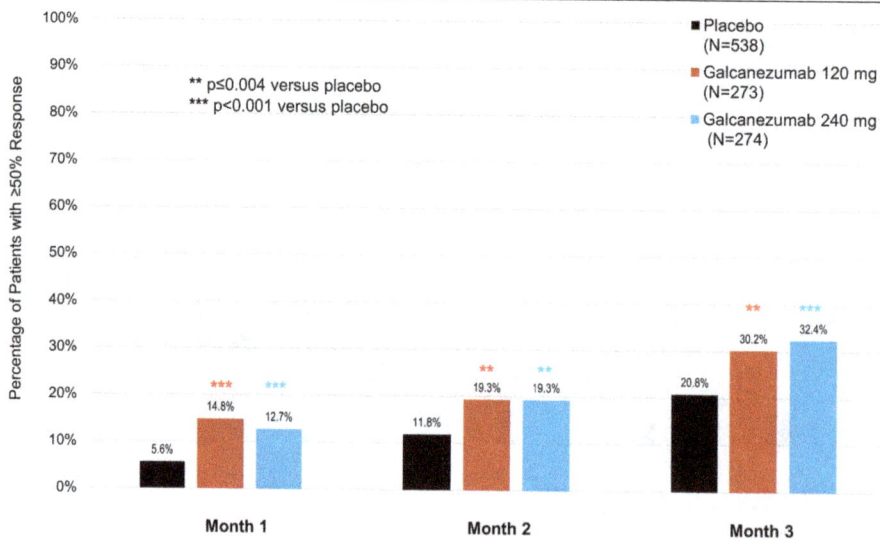

Fig. 4 Cumulative maintained ≥ 50% response: percentages of patients with chronic migraine who reached ≥ 50% response at or before each month and all subsequent months

migraine study although the percentages of patients with maintenance of response were generally lower given the higher baseline number of MHD. The 50% responder rate has been used as a secondary end-point in other trials, for example, with topiramate and botulinum toxin, in episodic and chronic migraine [5, 7, 19]. Comparison of those results to our data are difficult because only the 50% responder rate at the end of the double-blind period or at the end of cycle with botulinum toxin without any monthly and maintenance of response analysis was published.

Early and sustained response to preventive treatment is of special relevance. There is some evidence that improvement with preventive treatment at 3 months might be a predictor of persistent remission [20]. In addition, there is emerging evidence that more severely affected patients with a history of medication overuse, a high frequency of migraine attacks, and previously ineffective preventive treatments require long-term preventive treatment to maintain a reduced attack frequency, even after withdrawal of the preventive medication [21–23].

The maintenance of effect in patients with episodic or chronic migraine were similar between the galcanezumab 120 mg and 240 mg dose. This finding is consistent with previous reports in which there were no meaningful differences in efficacy measures between the galcanezumab doses and as such, the recommended dose is 120 mg after an initial loading dose of galcanezumab 240 mg (given as two 120 mg injections) [2–4].

One of the limitations of this paper is that the response rate was defined based on the primary efficacy measure, reduction in the number of MHD only.

Additional analyses could be conducted in further publications to assess the response rate based on other efficacy measures, such as days of acute medication use, and measures of function and disability.

Conclusions

Treatment with galcanezumab 120 mg or 240 mg demonstrated statistically significant and clinically meaningful maintenance of effect in patients with episodic migraine (at least 3 and 6 consecutive months) and in patients with chronic migraine (for 3 months).

Abbreviations
CGRP: Calcitonin gene-related peptide; MHD: Migraine headache days

Acknowledgements
Medical writing support was provided by Millie Hollandbeck and editorial support by Stephanie Bruns (Synchrogenix) which was funded by Eli Lilly and Company, Indianapolis, Indiana, USA. The authors thank Mallikarjuna Rettiganti, PhD (Eli Lilly and Company) for additional statistical review.

Funding
This study was funded by Eli Lilly and Company, Indianapolis, Indiana, USA.

Prior data disclosures
Data were presented in part at the American Headache Society 60th Annual Meeting, June 28–July 1, 2018, San Francisco, CA, USA; the 17th Biennial Migraine Trust International Symposium, September 6–9, 2018, London,

England, UK; and the 12th European Headache Federation, September 28–30, 2018, Florence, Italy.

Authors' contributions

SF, QZ, VLS, SKA, and MJAL participated in the conception, design and acquisition. QZ performed all statistics and analyses of the data and SF, QZ, VLS, SKA, and MJAL participated in the interpretation of the data. SF, QZ, VLS, and MJAL were major contributors for the drafting of the manuscript and revision for intellectual content. All authors read and approved the final manuscript.

Competing interests

Stefanie Förderreuther, MD Steffi.Foerderreuther@med.uni-muenchen.de
Ludwig-Maximilians-University of Munich, Department of Neurology
Speaker's Bureau: Novartis, Sanofi
Consultation: Sanofi
Honoraria: Allergan, Hormosan Pharma, AstraZeneca
Advisory Boards: Novartis, Eli Lilly
Qi Zhang, PhD qi.zhang@sanofi.com
Employee of Sanofi, Bridgewater, NJ, USA
Former employee of Eli Lilly and Company, and/or one of its subsidiaries, Indianapolis, IN, USA
Virginia L. Stauffer, PharmD vstauffer@lilly.com
Employee of Eli Lilly and Company, and/or one of its subsidiaries, Indianapolis, IN, USA
Sheena K. Aurora, MD sheena.aurora@lilly.com
Employee of Eli Lilly and Company, and/or one of its subsidiaries, Indianapolis, IN, USA
Miguel JA Láinez, MD, PhD miguel.lainez@sen.es
Hospital Clínico Universitario, Universidad Católica de Valencia, Spain
Research Grants: Allergan, Amgen, ATI, Bayer, Boehringer, electroCore, Eli Lilly, Medtronic, Novartis, Otsuka, Roche, Teva and UCB
Consultation: Allergan, Amgen, ATI, Bayer, Boehringer, electroCore, Eli Lilly, Medtronic, Novartis, Otsuka, Roche, Teva and UCB
Honoraria: Allergan, Amgen, ATI, Bayer, Boehringer, electroCore, Eli Lilly, Medtronic, Novartis, Otsuka, Roche, Teva and UCB

Author details

[1]Department of Neurology, Ludwig Maximilian University, Munich, Bavaria, Germany. [2]Sanofi, Bridgewater, NJ, USA. [3]Eli Lilly and Company, Lilly Corporate Center, Indianapolis, IN 46285, USA. [4]Hospital Clínico Universitario, Universidad Católica de Valencia, Valencia, Spain.

References

1. Benschop RJ, Collins EC, Darling RJ, Allan BW, Leung D, Conner EM et al (2014) Development of a novel antibody to calcitonin gene-related peptide for the treatment of osteoarthritis-related pain. Osteoarthr Cartil 22:578–585
2. Stauffer VL, Dodick DW, Zhang Q, Carter JN, Ailani J, Conley RR (2018) Evaluation of galcanezumab for the prevention of episodic migraine: the EVOLVE-1 randomized clinical trial. JAMA Neurology 75:1080–1088
3. Skljarevski V, Matharu M, Millen BA, Ossipov MH, Kim BK, Yang JY (2018) Efficacy and safety of galcanezumab for the prevention of episodic migraine: results of the EVOLVE-2 phase 3 randomized controlled clinical trial. Cephalalgia 38:1442–1454
4. Detke HC, Goadsby PJ, Wang S, Friedman DI, Selzler KJ, Aurora SK (2018) Galcanezumab in chronic migraine: the randomized, double-blind, placebo-controlled REGAIN study. Neurology [Epub ahead of print, November 16]
5. Diener HC, Bussone G, Van Oene JC, Lahaye M, Schwalen S, Goadsby PJ, TOPMAT-MIG-201(TOP-CHROME) study group (2007) Topiramate reduces headache days in chronic migraine: a randomized, double-blind, placebo-controlled study. Cephalalgia 27:814–823
6. Tepper S, Ashina M, Reuter U, Brandes JL, Doležil D, Silberstein S et al (2017) Safety and efficacy of erenumab for preventive treatment of chronic migraine: a randomised, double-blind, placebo-controlled phase 2 trial. Lancet Neurol 16:425–434
7. Dodick DW, Ashina M, Brandes JL, Kudrow D, Lanteri-Minet M, Osipova V et al (2018) ARISE: a phase 3 randomized trial of erenumab for episodic migraine. Cephalalgia 38:1026–1037
8. Brandes JL, Saper JR, Diamond M, Couch JR, Lewis DW, Schmitt J et al (2004) Topiramate for migraine prevention a randomized controlled trial. JAMA 291:965–973
9. Dodick DW, Turkel CC, DeGryse RE, Aurora SK, Silberstein SD, Lipton RB et al (2010) OnabotulinumtoxinA for treatment of chronic migraine: pooled results from the double-blind, randomized, placebo-controlled phases of the PREEMPT clinical program. Headache 50:921–936
10. Halker Singh RB, Aycardi E, Bigal ME, Loupe PS, McDonald M et al (2018) Sustained reductions in migraine days, moderate-to-severe headache days and days with acute medication use for HFEM and CM patients taking fremanezumab: post-hoc analyses from phase 2 trials. Cephalalgia: 333102418772585 [Epub ahead of print]
11. Tfelt-Hansen P, Pascual J, Ramadan N, Dahlöf C, D'Amico D, Diener HC et al (2012) Guidelines for controlled trials of drugs in migraine: third edition. A guide for investigators. Cephalalgia 32:6–38
12. Silberstein S, Tfelt-Hansen P, Dodick DW, Limmroth V, Lipton RB, Pascual J et al (2008) Guidelines for controlled trials of prophylactic treatment of chronic migraine in adults. Cephalalgia 28:484–495
13. Tassorelli C, Diener HC, Dodick DW, Silberstein SD, Lipton RB, Ashina M et al (2018) Guidelines of the international headache society for controlled trials of preventive treatment of chronic migraine in adults. Cephalalgia 38:815–832
14. [ICHD-3] Headache Classification Committee of the International Headache Society (IHS). The International Classification of Headache Disorders, 3rd edition (beta version). Cephalalgia. 2013;33:629-808.
15. SAS Institute Inc (2017) SAS/STAT® 14.3 User's Guide. SAS Institute Inc, Cary
16. Diener HC, Schorn CF, Bingel U, Dodick DW (2008) The importance of placebo in headache research. Cephalalgia 28(10):1003–1011
17. Diener HC (2010) Placebo effects in treating migraine and other headaches. Curr Opin Investig Drugs 11(7):735–739
18. Meissner K, Fässler M, Rücker G, Kleijnen J, Hróbjartsson A, Schneider A et al (2013) Differential effectiveness of placebo treatments: a systematic review of migraine prophylaxis. JAMA Intern Med 173:1941–1951
19. Silberstein SD, Dodick DW, Aurora SK, Diener HC, DeGryse RE, Lipton RB et al (2015) Percent of patients with chronic migraine who responded per onabotulinumtoxinA treatment cycle: PREEMPT. J Neurol Neurosurg Psychiatry 86:996–1001
20. Bhoi SK, Kalita J, Misra UK (2013) Is 6 months of migraine prophylaxis adequate? Neurol Res 35:1009–1014
21. Wöber C, Wöber-Bingöl C, Koch G, Wessely P (1991) Long-term results of migraine prophylaxis with flunarizine and beta-blockers. Cephalalgia 11(6):251–256
22. Pascual J, El Berdei Y, Gómez-Sánchez JC (2007) How many migraine patients need prolonged (>1 year) preventive treatment? Experience with topiramate. J Headache Pain 8(2):90–93
23. Silva-Néto RP, Almeida KJ, Bernardino SN (2014) Analysis of the duration of migraine prophylaxis. J Neurol Sci 337(1–2):38–41

19

Treatment of chronic migraine with transcutaneous stimulation of the auricular branch of the vagal nerve (auricular t-VNS): a randomized, monocentric clinical trial

Andreas Straube[1*], J. Ellrich[2,3], O. Eren[1], B. Blum[1] and R. Ruscheweyh[1]

Abstract

Background: Aim of the study was assessment of efficacy and safety of transcutaneous stimulation of the auricular branch of the vagal nerve (t-VNS) in the treatment of chronic migraine.

Methods: A monocentric, randomized, controlled, double-blind study was conducted. After one month of baseline, chronic migraine patients were randomized to receive 25 Hz or 1 Hz stimulation of the sensory vagal area at the left ear by a handhold battery driven stimulator for 4 h/day during 3 months. Headache days per 28 days were compared between baseline and the last month of treatment and the number of days with acute medication was recorded The Headache Impact Test (HIT-6) and the Migraine Disability Assessment (MIDAS) questionnaires were used to assess headache-related disability.

Results: Of 46 randomized patients, 40 finished the study (per protocol). In the per protocol analysis, patients in the 1 Hz group had a significantly larger reduction in headache days per 28 days than patients in the 25 Hz group (-7.0 ± 4.6 vs. -3.3 ± 5.4 days, $p = 0.035$). 29.4 % of the patients in the 1 Hz group had a ≥ 50 % reduction in headache days vs. 13.3 % in the 25 Hz group. HIT-6 and MIDAS scores were significantly improved in both groups, without group differences. There were no serious treatment-related adverse events.

Conclusion: Treatment of chronic migraine by t-VNS at 1 Hz was safe and effective. The mean reduction of headache days after 12 weeks of treatment exceeded that reported for other nerve stimulating procedures.

Keywords: Sensory nerve; Neuromodulation; Clinical study; Chronic headache; Electrical pulses

Background

Migraine is a frequent neurological disorder. In some patients, episodic migraine (with < 15 headache days per month) evolves towards chronic migraine, which is characterized by ≥ 15 headache days per month of which ≥ 8 have migraine-like features [1], see also: http://ihs-classification.org/de/0_downloads/. Chronic migraine affects approximately 1.3 to 2.4 % of the general population [2]. It is associated with significant disability and reduced health-related quality of life and often complicated by

* Correspondence: Andreas.Straube@med.uni-muenchen.de
[1]Klinik und Poliklinik für Neurologie, Oberbayerisches Kopfschmerzzentrum, Klinikum Großhadern, Ludwig-Maximilians-Universität München, Marchioninistr. 15, 81377 Munich, Germany

overuse of acute pain medications [3, 4]. Up to now, randomized controlled trials showing a significant effect in the treatment specifically of chronic migraine have been published only for topiramate and onabotulinumtoxin A [5, 6]. Treatment of chronic migraine is often difficult, with significant numbers of patients not responding to pharmacological management.

In recent years, neuromodulation was introduced in the treatment of headache [7]. Invasive occipital nerve stimulation (ONS) has been investigated for the treatment of chronic migraine, with inconsistent results [8–10]. Significant reduction in headache days was demonstrated in only one of the three studies, which however did not meet its primary endpoint (a 50 % reduction of mean daily pain ratings) [10]. A major disadvantage of ONS is the safety profile with frequent adverse events such as infections, lead migration or lead disconnection [8, 10]. This is also the reason why in some health markets the reimbursement of ONS was stopped by the regulatory administration. Thus, less invasive forms of neuromodulation such as transcutaneous electrical nerve stimulation are under investigation. For example, supraorbital transcutaneous stimulation for 3 months has been shown to be effective for the preventive treatment of episodic migraine (active treatment: 38 % responders, sham: 12 % responders, p < 0.05) [11].

Vagal nerve stimulation using implanted electrodes is used as a treatment option in otherwise therapy-refractory epilepsy and depression [12]. Case reports and small series of patients who received an implanted vagal nerve stimulator for treatment of epilepsy and had comorbid migraine suggest that VNS may have a preventive effect in migraine [13–16]. A recently developed medical device (NEMOS®, cerbomed, Erlangen, Germany) allows for non-invasive, transcutaneous stimulation of the auricular branch of the vagus nerve (auricular t-VNS) using a special ear electrode. Auricular t-VNS excites thick myelinated sensory Aβ-fiber afferents in the vagal nerve, activating the nucleus of the solitary tract [17, 18]. Effects on autonomous activity have been demonstrated in healthy subjects where auricular t-VNS increases heart rate variability [19]. Anticonvulsive effects in rodents are similar to those achieved with invasive VNS [18]. Functional imaging during auricular t-VNS has shown a pattern consistent with afferent vagal stimulation [20, 21]. Both invasive VNS and auricular t-VNS reduce pinprick and pressure pain in humans [22, 23]. In addition, a recent observational study has suggested that t-VNS to the right cervical branch of the vagus nerve (cervical t-VNS) may be effective for acute migraine treatment [24]. In the present study, we investigated the effect of auricular t-VNS on chronic migraine.

Methods

This was a monocentric, prospective, double-blind, randomized, parallel-group, controlled trial analyzed both on intention-to-treat basis (ITT), and on per protocol basis (PP). The trial was conducted in a German tertiary headache outpatient clinic (Department of Neurology, University of Munich). The study was approved by the ethics committee of the medical faculty of the University of Munich and written informed consent was obtained from all participants. The study is registered in the German Clinical Trials Register (DRKS00003681).

Study participants

Men or women between 18 and 70 years with a diagnosis of chronic migraine according to the ICHD-IIR (code A1.5.1.) (http://ihs-classification.org/de/0_downloads/), duration of ≥ 6 months, no migraine-prophylactic medication or stable migraine-prophylactic medication for ≥1 month, and stable acute medication were eligible, medication overuse was not an exclusion criterion.

Patients were excluded if they suffered from other primary or secondary headaches, severe neurologic or psychiatric disorders including opioid- or tranquilizer-dependency, cranio-mandibulary dysfunction, fibromyalgia, had a Beck's Depression Inventory (BDI [25]) score >25 at the screening visit, anatomic or pathologic changes at the left outer ear, currently participated in another clinical trial, or were unable to keep a headache diary. Pregnant or breast-feeding women were also excluded. A pregnancy test was performed at the screening visit in women of childbearing potential and they were required to use a reliable means of contraception. In addition, patients who had less than 15 headache days per 28 days during the 4-week baseline period were excluded.

Study design (Fig. 1)

The study consisted of a 4-week screening period ("baseline") followed by a 12-week randomized, double-blind, parallel-group treatment period with either 1 Hz or 25 Hz tVNS with the NEMOS® device (Fig. 2). Adverse events were recorded at visits 2 to 6. Compliance with stimulation was checked at visits 3 to 6 by reading out the NEMOS® device and quantified in percent of the

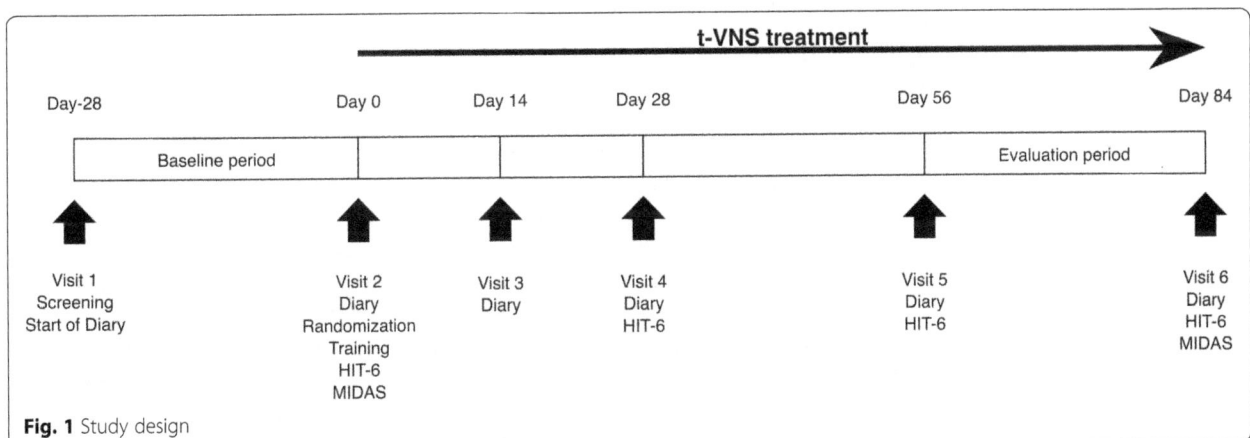

Fig. 1 Study design

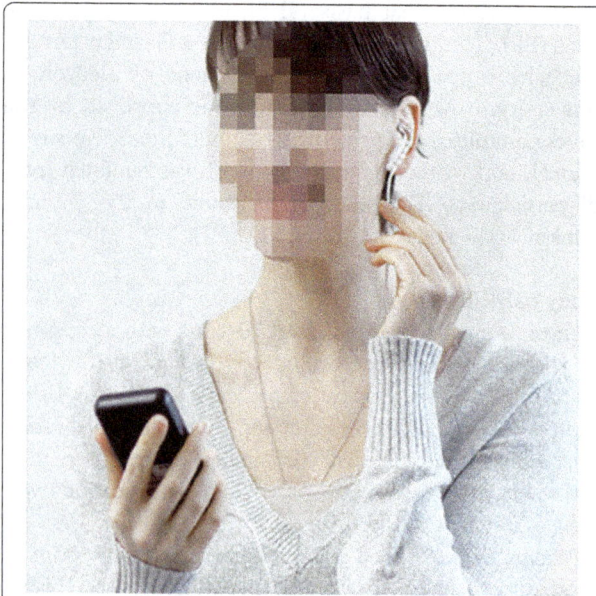

Fig. 2 NEMOS® device and positioning of the electrode for stimulation of the vagus afferents at the concha

intended daily stimulation time (4 h). Re-training was administered during visits 3 to 6 as necessary. The Migraine Disability Assessment (MIDAS [26]) and the Headache Impact Test (HIT-6 [27]) were filled in by the patient as indicated in Fig. 1. Patients kept a paper-and-pencil headache diary during the entire period, handing in their diaries and receiving a fresh sheet at each visit. In the diary, patients indicated for every day (1) headache duration in hours, (2) headache intensity (on a 0 to 10 numerical rating scale: 0, no pain; 10, strongest pain imaginable), and (3) intake of acute headache medication (analgesics, triptans).

Sample size calculations were based on published studies on successful pharmacological treatment of chronic migraine (mean effect size: –4,68 headache days/month after removal of the placebo effect) [5, 6, 28, 29]. To detect an effect of this size with an α error of 0.05 and a power of 0.80, a group size of 49 patients per treatment group was estimated, including 10 % drop-out. An interims analysis after 46 patients was planned. Since patient recruitment was slower than expected, the sponsor decided to terminate the study at the interims analysis, and no further patients were enrolled.

Neurostimulation

The NEMOS® t-VNS device (Cerbomed, Erlangen, Germany) is a transcutaneous vagus nerve stimulator designed for electrical stimulation at the concha of the outer ear, which receives sensory innervation from the auricular branch of the vagal nerve (Fig. 2). The NEMOS® device has received the CE mark for treatment of pain (CE0408) and is registered in the European Databank on Medical Devices (EUDAMED, CIV-11-09-002381). It consists of a handheld, battery driven electrical stimulator connected to an ear electrode placed in contact with the skin of the concha. Impedance is measured automatically and insufficient electrode contact with the skin evokes an alarm. During stimulation, series of electrical pulses (pulse width: 250 μs, frequency: 1 Hz or 25 Hz, duty cycle: 30s on, 30 s off, to avoid habituation) are applied to the skin of the concha. Stimulus intensity was individually fitted during visit 2 to elicit a tingling but not painful sensation, and could later be adjusted by the patient as needed. Patients were asked to stimulate for a total of 4 h per day (in sessions of 1 to 4 h, a specific distribution over the day or interval between sessions was not required), and were free to stimulate for an additional hour if they thought this was useful, e.g. for treatment of acute headache. The effect of such acute treatment was not recorded. Stimulation parameters of the 25 Hz group were chosen so that with 4 h of daily stimulation, the number of electrical stimuli per day would be similar to those normally used for invasive vagal nerve stimulation in patients with epilepsy. The 1 Hz stimulation was intended as an active control. The active control was chosen in order to avoid un-blinding of the subjects.

Primary and secondary outcome parameters

All outcome measures refer to change from baseline (the 4-week period between visits 1 and 2) to the evaluation period (the 4-week period between visits 5 and 6, Fig. 1). The primary outcome measure was mean change in *headache days per 28 days*. A headache day was defined as a calendar day with headache of ≥ 4 h duration or headache successfully aborted by acute headache medication or any other treatment known to be typically effective in the specific patient (e.g. sleep, progressive relaxation exercises).

Secondary outcome parameters were: (1) percentage of "responders" (subjects having at least 50 % reduction of headache days per 28 days from baseline to evaluation); (2) change in mean headache intensity on days with headache; (3) change in days with acute headache medication intake per 28 days; (4) change in headache-related disability, as assessed by the MIDAS and HIT-6 questionnaires; (5) number and type of adverse events.

Statistical analysis

Mean ± standard deviation (SD) is reported unless stated otherwise. The threshold for significance of statistical comparisons was set at $p < 0.05$. Statistical analysis was performed both on ITT and on per protocol basis (PP). For the ITT analysis, a last observation carried forward approach was used for patients who dropped out during the course of the study.

Group comparisons at baseline, of duration of the treatment period, compliance or number of patients affected by adverse events were done using Mann–Whitney U-Test or Fisher's exact test as appropriate. Analysis of the primary endpoint was done using an analysis of covariance (ANCOVA) model with the factors treatment group (1 Hz vs. 25 Hz) and sex as categorical variables and baseline values as covariate. The same type of ANCOVA was used for the analysis of the following secondary outcome parameters: change in mean headache intensity, change in days with acute headache medication intake per 28 days and change in MIDAS and HIT-6 scores. The number of responders was compared between groups using a logistic regression model that included treatment group and sex as factor and the number of headache days per 28 days at baseline as covariate. An estimate of the treatment odds ratio (Wald method) was derived from this model.

Results

The study was conducted between March 2012 and July 2014. A total of 46 patients were randomized to the 1 Hz group ($n = 22$) or the 25 Hz group ($n = 24$, ITT). 6 patients dropped out during the study. Reasons for dropouts were: adverse events in 4 patients (treatment-related stimulation site ulcer in 3 patients, gastrectomy not related to treatment in 1 patient), insufficient compliance in 1 patient, patient's request in 1 patient. One additional patient was excluded from the per protocol (PP) analysis after the end of the study because of violation of inclusion criteria (<15 headache days per 28 days in the screening period). This left 17 patients in the 1 Hz group and 22 patients in the 25 Hz group for the PP analysis (Fig. 3) Demographic and headache characteristics of the population are shown in Table 1. There were no significant differences between both groups.

Primary outcome measure

PP-analysis indicated a significant decrease in headache days per 28 days from baseline to evaluation, which was significantly larger in the 1 Hz group than in the 25 Hz group ($F[35] = 4.82$, $p = 0.035$, Table 2). In the 1 Hz group, the reduction amounted to −7.0 days per 28 days (36.4 % reduction from baseline), while the 25 Hz group reached only −3.3 days (17.4 % reduction from baseline). In the ITT analysis, there also was a significant decrease in headache days per 28 days in both groups, but no significant group difference ($F[42] = 2.94$, $p = 0.094$, Table 2). Visual inspection of headache days per 28 days over the treatment period revealed a continuous decrease in the 1 Hz group, while a steady state was reached after 14 days in the 25 Hz group (Fig. 4).

Secondary outcome measures

Results of secondary outcome measures and the corresponding statistics are summarized in Table 2. The number of responders (>50 % improvement in headache days) was in the 1 Hz group (PP) 29.4 % and in the 25 Hz group (PP) 13.6 %. Headache intensity was not significantly changed by t-VNS in either treatment group, and there were no group differences. The number of days with intake of acute headache medication as well as the MIDAS and HIT-6 scores were significantly reduced in both treatment groups, there were no group differences.

Treatment duration and compliance

Results and statistics are listed in Table 3. Duration of the treatment period was similar between groups. The average number of stimulated hours per day during the treatment period was around 3.4 in all groups, corresponding to around 85 % of the requested 4 h of daily

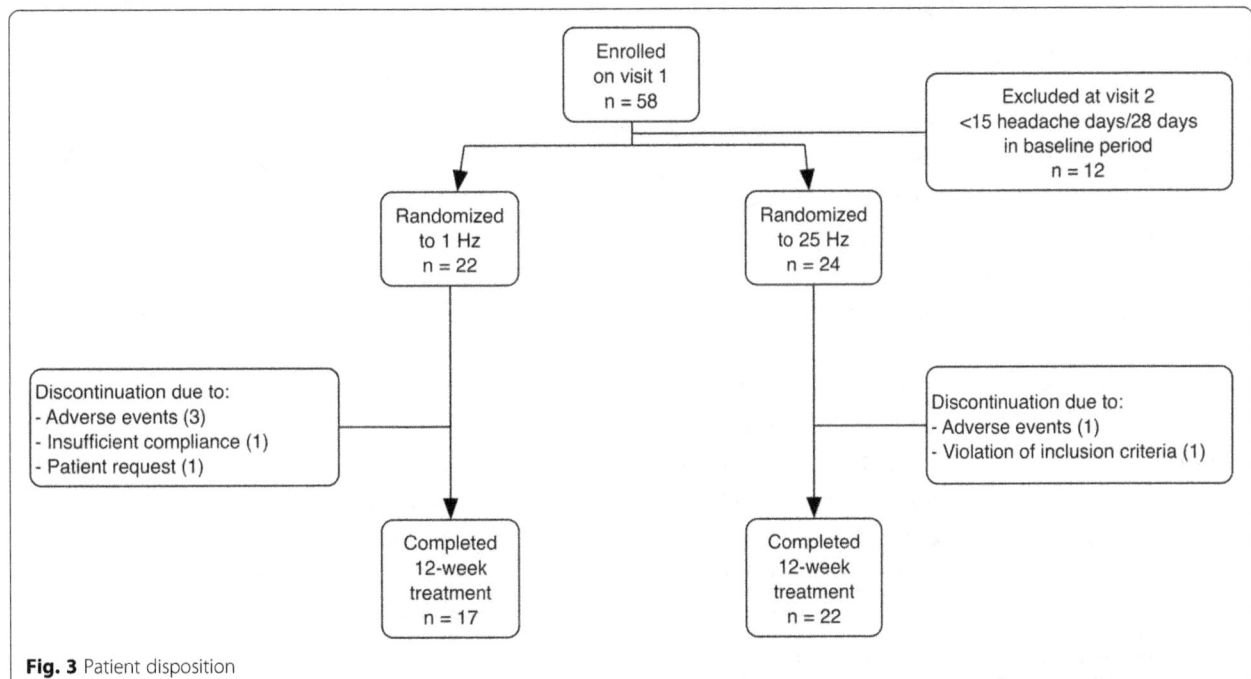

Fig. 3 Patient disposition

Table 1 Baseline characteristics of the cohort

	Intention-to-treat analysis			Per protocol analysis		
	1 Hz (n = 22)	25 Hz (n = 24)	Group comparison	1 Hz (n = 17)	25 Hz (n = 22)	Group comparison
Age	43.8 ± 11.5	39.3 ± 12.4	$p = 0.21$	44.1 ± 11.4	39.0 ± 12.5	$p = 0.21$
Females	18	21	$p = 0.69$	13	19	$p = 0.68$
Headache days/28 days	19.4 ± 4.0	18.9 ± 5.1	$p = 0.47$	19.1 ± 3.7	19.2 ± 4.7	$p = 0.66$
Headache intensity (NRS: 0–10)	5.2 ± 1.5	5.0 ± 1.5	$p = 0.73$	5.0 ± 1.5	5.0 ± 1.5	$p = 0.98$
Migraine history (years)	27.1 ± 13.0	20.4 ± 12.1	$p = 0.08$	27.8 ± 11.5	21.4 ± 12.1	$p = 0.11$
Days with acute headache medication/28 days	10.3 ± 6.4	8.2 ± 4.9	$p = 0.24$	11.1 ± 6.6	8.6 ± 4.8	$p = 0.17$
MIDAS score	76.8 ± 64.8	83.6 ± 56.0	$p = 0.55$	77.2 ± 70.1	82.1 ± 58.0	$p = 0.71$
HIT-6 score	64.3 ± 4.7	66.0 ± 4.1	$p = 0.25$	64.8 ± 5.0	66.0 ± 4.2	$p = 0.55$
BDI	6.9 ± 5.7	7.9 ± 5.6	$p = 0.59$	6.9 ± 5.9	7.2 ± 5.0	$p = 0.95$

Demographic and headache characteristics assessed at the first visit or during the baseline period (4 weeks) are given. Values are mean ± SD or numbers of subjects. Results of Mann–Whitney U test or Fisher's Exact test are given. Headache intensity (NRS: numerical rating scale 0–10)
MIDAS migraine disability assessment, *HIT* headache impact test, *BDI* beck's depression inventory

stimulation, indicating good compliance with treatment. There were no significant group differences.

Safety and tolerability
Adverse events (AEs) were analysed in the full analysis set (safety set) and summarized in Table 4. The number of treatment emergent AEs (AEs occurring after initiation of treatment) was higher in the 25 Hz group (112 events, 76 treatment-related events) as compared to the 1 Hz group (67 events, 39 treatment-related events, Table 4),. Most AEs were mild or moderate in severity and resolved without sequelae. The most frequent treatment-related AE were local problems at the stimulation site, such as mild or moderate pain, paresthesia, or pruritus during or after stimulation, and erythema, ulcer or scab (31 events in 10 patients in the 1 Hz group, 70 events in 17 patients in the

25 Hz group, $p = 0.14$). Treatment-related AEs leading to discontinuation of the study were stimulation site ulcer (accompanied by pain, paresthesia, or pruritus) in 2 patients of the 1 Hz group and in 1 patient of the 25 Hz group. These three cases of application site ulcer occurred early during the study. After that, patients were asked to specially care for the skin of their ear after each use of the NEMOS® device, using a custom rich skin cream, and no more cases of application site ulcer occurred. There were no treatment-related SAEs. Three SAEs, leading to hospitalization of the patient, were recorded during the whole study (infectious mononucleosis, gastrectomy, intervertebral disc protrusion).

Discussion
The present monocentric, randomized, controlled, double-blind, parallel-group clinical trial provides evidence that

Table 2 Results of primary and secondary treatment outcome measures

	Intention-t-treat analysis			Per protocol analysis		
	1 Hz (n = 22)	25 Hz (n = 24)	Group comparison	1 Hz (n = 17)	25 Hz (n = 22)	Group comparison
Change in headache days/28 days	**−5.6 ± 5.0**	**−3.0 ± 5.3**	F[42] = 2.94	**−7.0 ± 4.6**	**−3.3 ± 5.4**	**F[35] = 4.82**
	(−5.9; −0.5)	**(−8.5; −3.2)**	$p = 0.094$	**(−9.6; −4.1)**	**(−5.9; −0.4)**	**$p = 0.035$**
Responder (50 % reduction in headache days)	5 (22.7 %)	3 (12.5 %)	OR = 2.44	5 (29.4 %)	3 (13.6 %)	OR = 3.21
			$p = 0.29$			$p = 0.18$
Change in headache intensity (NRS 0 – 10)	−0.1 ± 1.1 (n = 20)	0.2 ± 1.0	F[40] = 0.30	0.02 ± 1.2 (n = 15)	0.2 ± 1.0	F[33] = 0.28
	(−0.2; 0.9)	(−0.4; 0.7)	$p = 0.58$	(−0.4; 0.8)	(−0.2; 0.9)	$p = 0.60$
Change in days with acute headache medication in 28 days	**−2.0 ± 4.2**	**−1.3 ± 4.4**	F[42] = 0.01	**−2.7 ± 4.5**	**−1.6 ± 4.1**	F[35] < 0.01
	(−4.2; −0.3)	**(−4.4; −0.3)**	$p = 0.91$	**(−4.7; −0.4)**	**(−4.7; −0.3)**	$p = 0.96$
Change in MIDAS score	**−18.7 ± 28.0**	**−21.8 ± 54.5**	F[42] < 0.01	**−24.2 ± 29.8**	**−26.5 ± 53.9**	F[35] < 0.01
	(−38.6; −0.9)	**(−39.2; −0.8)**	$p = 0.98$	**(−43.2; −4.0)**	**(−42.1; −3.7)**	$p = 0.96$
Change in HIT-6 score	**−2.5 ± 6.8**	**−3.8 ± 5.5**	F[42] = 0.12	**−3.8 ± 7.1**	**−3.9 ± 5.69**	F[35] = 0.01
	(−6.7; −0.7)	**(−7.3; −1.2)**	$p = 0.73$	**(−7.8; −1.1)**	**(−7.6; −1.0)**	$p = 0.93$

Change refers to change from the 4-week baseline period to the last 4 weeks of the 12-week treatment period. Means, SDs and 95 % confidence intervals are given. For the responder analysis, numbers of subjects and percent of the total group are given. Significant differences are marked in bold. Number of subjects is given in parentheses, where different from the total group. Primary outcome parameter: change in headache days/28 days
MIDAS migraine disability assessment, *HIT* headache impact test, *NRS* numerical rating scale 0–10

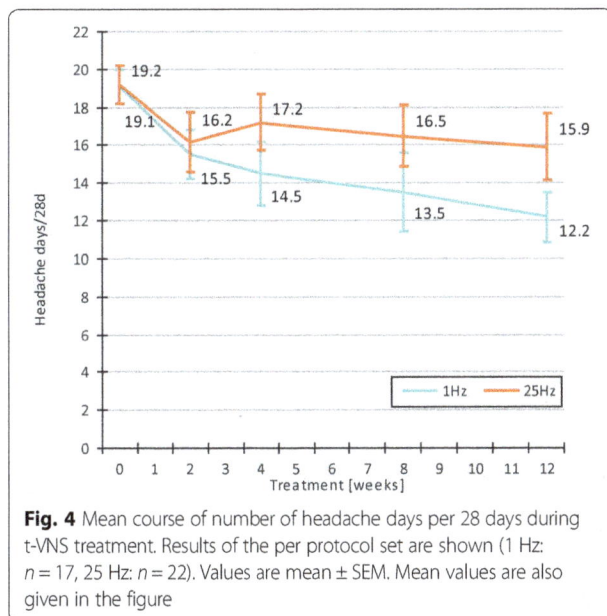

Fig. 4 Mean course of number of headache days per 28 days during t-VNS treatment. Results of the per protocol set are shown (1 Hz: $n = 17$, 25 Hz: $n = 22$). Values are mean ± SEM. Mean values are also given in the figure

daily treatment with auricular t-VNS is effective in chronic migraine.

Both in the 1 Hz and the 25 Hz group the number of headache days per 28 days decreased significantly by 7.0 and 3.3 days, respectively (PP-analysis, Table 2), with a significantly larger reduction in the 1 Hz compared to the 25 Hz group ($p = 0.035$). 29.4 % of the patients in the 1 Hz group and 13.6 % of the patients in the 25 Hz group achieved a reduction of more than 50 % in headache days ("responder"). With an absolute reduction in headache days per 28 days by 7.0 in the 1 Hz group and a mean group difference of 2.7 headache days, the effect of auricular t-VNS was comparable to the effects of topiramate and onabotulinumtoxin A versus placebo. Previous trials in chronic migraine with topiramate for 4 months have shown a reduction in headache days per month of 3.5 and 6.4 days in the verum group, which exceeded the effect in the placebo group by 3.7 and 1.7 days, respectively [6, 30]. In the large PREEMPT trials onabotulinumtoxin A was able to reduce the number of headache days per month in chronic migraine patients by 9.0 and 7.8 days after 6 months, which exceeded the placebo effect by 2.3 and 1.4 days, respectively [5, 31]. Compared to previous trials investigating neurostimulation devices the results are

favorable. In the ONS trials for chronic migraine, reduction of headache days after 3 months was by 6.7, 5.5 and 6.1 days in the verum group, which exceeded the sham group by 5.2, 1.6 and 3.1 days, respectively [8–10]. However, none of these studies reached significance for its primary end point. Transcutaneous supraorbital neurostimulation has so far only been tested in episodic migraine, achieving a reduction by 2.5 headache days from a baseline of 7.8 headache days, which was 2.3 days more than placebo [11].

It has to be mentioned that the study was planned as a trial with an active comparator in order to be sure that the patients were blinded and that we expected that the 25 Hz stimulation would be more effective than the 1 Hz stimulation, corresponding to the results from the use of invasive VNS in epilepsy [32, 33]. This means that it is very unlikely that partial unblinding may have affected the results, as the local sensation is more intense with 25 Hz stimulation, and the study physicians expected the 25 Hz stimulation to be more effective. However, it is not clear why the 1 Hz stimulation was more effective than the 25 Hz stimulation. The mechanisms by which VNS influences chronic migraine may be different from those in epilepsy. In addition, activation of central nervous system structures by stimulation of thickly myelinated sensory fibers in the auricular branch of the vagus nerve may require different stimulation patterns than the cervical branch, which is a mixed nerve with myelinated and non-myelinated efferent as well as afferent fibers. As no dose–response or frequency-response data are available for any neurostimulation method in migraine treatment, the question whether frequency or total number of stimuli influence the result remains open.

Analgesic effects of electrical low-frequency stimulation (LFS) in various pain models have been demonstrated in man and rodents [34]. Electrical pulse series with optimum frequency of 1 Hz for 20 min significantly suppressed nociceptive signaling and pain perception by approximately 40 % for hours [35, 36]. This phenomenon of long-term depression (LTD) has been shown in the spinal system [37–41] and in the craniofacial area [42–44]. Stimulation parameter of t-VNS in the present study resemble electrical LFS and could have provoked LTD of nociceptive processing in the spinal trigeminal nucleus that plays a critical role in migraine pain [45]. Actually, the auriculotemporal nerve, a branch of the trigeminal nerve, supplies the outer ear and could, therefore, mediate access of electrically evoked neural

Table 3 Duration of treatment period and compliance with stimulation during the treatment period

	Intention-to-treat analysis			Per protocol analysis		
	1 Hz ($n = 22$)	25 Hz ($n = 24$)	Group comparison	1 Hz ($n = 17$)	25 Hz ($n = 23$)	Group comparison
Treatment period (days)	77.9 ± 25.8	85.7 ± 11.4	$p = 0.22$	89.0 ± 8.4	87.5 ± 7.5	$p = 0.67$
Average number of stimulated hours per day	3.42 ± 0.59	3.44 ± 0.61	$p = 0.69$	3.34 ± 0.62	3.44 ± 0.62	$p = 0.51$

Mean ± SD values are given. Treatment period indicates the number of days between visits 2 and 6. The average number of stimulated hours per day of the treatment period is given. Patients were requested to stimulate 4 h per day during the treatment period. The real average stimulation time per day was slightly lower

Table 4 Overview of adverse events (safety set)

	1 Hz (n = 22)		25 Hz (n = 24)	
	Number of events	Number of patients (%)	Number of events	Number of patients (%)
Treatment emergent AEs	67	17 (77.3 %)	112	19 (79.2 %)
Treatment-related AEs	39	11 (50.0 %)	76	17 (70.8 %)
Stimulation site treatment-related TEAEs	31	10 (45.5 %)	70	17 (70.8 %)
All serious AEs (including pre-treatment SAEs)	2	2 (9.1 %)	0	0
Serious treatment emergent AEs	2	2 (9.1 %)	0	0
Serious treatment-related AEs	0	0	0	0
Treatment-related AEs leading to discontinuation of study	8	4 (18.2 %)	4	1 (4.2 %)
Death	0	0	0	0

signals to brainstem nuclei of the trigeminal nerve [46]. Thus, LTD could be a mechanism that might, at least, contribute to the analgesic effect of t-VNS in the present study.

In fact, other stimulation parameters might be even more effective than the 1 Hz stimulation, and the 25 Hz stimulation might have been partially active in the present study, possibly reducing the effect in the group comparison. Indeed, 25–30 Hz stimulation has been shown to significantly reduce experimental pain in humans [23] and seizures in rodents [18]. In addition, in the present study both groups significantly improved in headache-related disability measures (MIDAS and HIT-6), and reduced their intake of acute headache medication, although it cannot be determined if this is due to the placebo effect or due to stimulation effects in both groups. The missing significant difference in the reduction of the MIDAS and HIT6 between the 1Hz and the 25Hz group is probably due to the too small sensitivity of these tests in detecting differences in quality of life. Furthermore, it is unclear if 25 Hz stimulation also have a mood stabilizing effect which influences the ratings in the used tests.

Furthermore, it is still not clear how vagus nerve stimulation interferes with migraine generation. One possibility is a direct or indirect inhibition of nociceptive trigeminal neurons by vagal activation. Indeed, animal data show that afferent vagal stimulation can reduce the activation of nociceptive neurons in the caudal trigeminal nucleus in response to noxious stimulation of the face or dura [47–49]. This might be due to the existence of dense reciprocal connections between the spinal trigeminal nucleus and the nucleus tractus solitarii (NTS) which is the major target of vagal afferents [50]. Responses of spinal trigeminal neurons might also be reduced by activation of the descending pain inhibitory systems. Although this has not been shown directly for the trigeminal area, animal studies showed that vagal nerve stimulation can activate descending pain inhibitory systems, probably involving projections from the NTS to the nucleus raphe magnus and the locus coeruleus, which are at the origin of serotonergic and noradrenergic

descending pain inhibitory pathways [51]. Alternatively, VNS might exert migraine prophylactic actions by modifying cortical excitability. Altered cortical excitability in chronic migraine has been demonstrated in various electrophysiological measurements is thought to contribute to its pathogenesis [52]. Several lines of evidence indicate that the cortical excitability is increased in chronic migraine patients: 1) There is a reduced habituation of the blink reflex interictally [53]. 2) The magnetic suppression of perceptual accuracy was decreased in patients with chronic migraine compared to episodic migraine and controls which may indicate also a higher cortical excitability [54]. 3) Analysis of the high frequency somatosensory evoked potentials showed early response sensitization and late habituation, most probably due an increased coupling between thalamus and cortex in chronic migraine [55]. Afferent vagal information is relayed via the NTS and the parabrachial nucleus to several subcortical and cortical regions, including thalamus, insula and lateral prefrontal cortex. In addition, the NTS has strong projections to the locus coeruleus and the nucleus raphe magnus which provide widespread noradrenergic and serotonergic innervation of the cortex [56]. Modulation of cortical excitability via these pathways is thought to be important for the anticonvulsant effects of VNS [33]. Increased GABA levels have been found in the cerebrospinal fluid of epilepsy patients treated with VNS, suggesting an increase in inhibitory neurotransmission [57]. Auricular t-VNS increases parasympathetic activity and/or reduces sympathetic activity [19], which might also affect cortical excitability, maybe by mechanisms similar to those assumed for the migraine preventive effects of beta-blocking agents [58]. In summary, VNS is well positioned to alter cortical excitability, especially to reduce cortical hyperexcitability. Direct evidence that this interferes with pain processing or migraine generation is currently lacking. It would be interesting to repeat the above described experiments which showed an increased cortical excitability in chronic migraine under t-VNS stimulation. A third possibility is that the antimigraine action of VNS relies on modification of transmitter release from efferent parasympathetic fibers innervating dural vessels, e.g. fibers stemming from the spheno-palatine ganglion. The release of neurotransmitters, especially calcitonin-gene related peptide (CGRP), at dural vessels with subsequent neurogenic inflammation and sensitization of primary afferents is thought to play an important role in migraine pathophysiology [59]. Parasympathetic fibres innervating the dura mater release vasoactive intestinal polypeptide (VIP) and pituitary adenylate cyclase-activating polypeptide (PACAP), which are potent vasodilatators and thought to contribute to sensitization of nociceptive trigeminal primary afferents. Increased peripheral blood VIP levels have been detected in chronic migraine [60], and intravenous administration of PACAP has been shown to induce migrainous headache in migraine patients [61], suggesting that both transmitters are related to migraine pathophysiology. Although auricular t-VNS stimulates only vagal afferents, there are close connections between afferent and efferent parasympathetic brainstem centers, making an influence of VNS on dural efferents likely.

A major practical advantage of auricular t-VNS is good tolerability and safety. For comparison, in the pooled topiramate trial analysis, 1 out of 4 patients (25 %) dropped out because of intolerable adverse effects [62]. In our study only 3 of 46 patients (7 %) dropped out due to side effects of t-VNS. All three cases occurred early in the study and were due to stimulation site ulcer which later in the study could be prevented by appropriate skin care. Another advantage of t-VNS therapy is that it can be combined with any other drug treatment without risking cumulative adverse effects or pharmacodynamic interactions. In addition, auricular t-VNS allows patients to continue routine activities, leading to a high compliance with stimulation times (around 85 % on average). However, long-term effects and sustainability of efficacy of t-VNS are still unknown and need to be demonstrated in appropriate open-label trials.

Conclusions

In conclusion, the present parallel-group randomized controlled trial, provides evidence that auricular t-VNS at 1 Hz for 4 h daily is effective for chronic migraine prevention over 3 months. The absolute reduction in headache days (7.0) and the difference between groups (2.7 headache days) is comparable to the effects of topiramate and onabotulinum toxin A in chronic migraine prevention. The t-VNS treatment also results in a meaningful improvement in the quality of life as assessed by MIDAS and HIT 6. The safety profile was favourable and compliance with daily stimulation was high.

Competing interests
Cerbomed funded the study.
A. Straube has received honoraries by Pharm Allergan, Boehringer Ingelheim, Hormosan, electroCore, CerboMed. Grants from the German Science foundation, German Minister of Research and Education and the Kröner-Fresenius foundation.

J. Ellrich was employed as Chief Medical Officer by the company cerbomed GmbH.
O. Eren has nothing to disclose
B. Blum has nothing to disclose
R. Ruscheweyh has received honaries by Pharm Allergan, MSD, Mundipharma, Pfizer and grants from the Else Kröner Fresenius Stiftung.

Authors' contributions
The study was planned by JE and AS. AS, RR, OE, BB recruited the patients and collected the data. Statistical analysis was performed by Metronomia Clinical Research GmbH (Munich, Germany). Cerbomed supported the preparation of the figures and the layout. The paper was written by the authors and all authors participated in the decision to publish the paper and had full access to all study data. All authors read and approved the final manuscript.

Acknowledgement
The authors thank Nadine Wolf, PhD for her contribution to the clinical investigation plan and A. Hartlep, PhD and V. Koepke for their help in the preparation of the manuscript.

Author details
[1]Klinik und Poliklinik für Neurologie, Oberbayerisches Kopfschmerzzentrum, Klinikum Großhadern, Ludwig-Maximilians-Universität München, Marchioninistr. 15, 81377 Munich, Germany. [2]Department of Health Science and Technology, Professor Dr. med. Jens Ellrich, Aalborg University, Fredrik Bajers Vej 7D2, DK-9220 Aalborg, Denmark. [3]Cerbomed GmbH, Medical Valley Center, Henkestr. 91, 91052 Erlangen, Germany.

References
1. Headache Classification Subcommittee of the International Headache Society (2013) The International Classification of Headache Disorders, 3rd edition (beta version). Cephalalgia 33:629–808
2. Bigal ME, Serrano D, Reed M, Lipton RB (2008) Chronic migraine in the population: burden, diagnosis, and satisfaction with treatment. Neurology 71:559–566
3. Dodick DW (2006) Clinical practice. Chronic daily headache. N Engl J Med 354:158–165
4. Lipton RB, Bigal ME (2003) Chronic daily headache: is analgesic overuse a cause or a consequence? Neurology 61:154–155
5. Diener HC, Dodick DW, Aurora SK, Turkel CC, DeGryse RE, Lipton RB, Silberstein SD, Brin MF (2010) OnabotulinumtoxinA for treatment of chronic migraine: results from the double-blind, randomized, placebo-controlled phase of the PREEMPT 2 trial. Cephalalgia 30:804–814
6. Silberstein SD, Lipton RB, Dodick DW, Freitag FG, Ramadan N, Mathew N, Brandes JL, Bigal M, Saper J, Ascher S, Jordan DM, Greenberg SJ, Hulihan J (2007) Efficacy and safety of topiramate for the treatment of chronic migraine: a randomized, double-blind, placebo-controlled trial. Headache 47:170–180
7. Martelletti P, Jensen RH, Antal A, Arcioni R, Brighina F, de Tommaso M, Franzini A, Fontaine D, Heiland M, Jurgens TP, Leone M, Magis D, Paemeleire K, Palmisani S, Paulus W, May A (2013) Neuromodulation of chronic headaches: position statement from the European Headache Federation. J Headache Pain 14:86
8. Saper JR, Dodick DW, Silberstein SD, McCarville S, Sun M, Goadsby PJ (2011) Occipital nerve stimulation for the treatment of intractable chronic migraine headache: ONSTIM feasibility study. Cephalalgia 31:271–285
9. Lipton RB, Goadsby PJ, Cady RK, Aurora SK, Grosberg BM, Freitag FG, Silberstein SD, Whiten DM, Jaax KN (2009) PRISM study: occipital nerve stimulation for treatment-refractory migraine. Cephalalgia 29:30
10. Silberstein SD, Dodick DW, Saper J, Huh B, Slavin KV, Sharan A, Reed K, Narouze S, Mogilner A, Goldstein J, Trentman T, Vaisman J, Ordia J, Weber P, Deer T, Levy R, Diaz RL, Washburn SN, Mekhail N (2012) Safety and efficacy of peripheral nerve stimulation of the occipital nerves for the management of chronic migraine: results from a randomized, multicenter, double-blinded, controlled study. Cephalalgia 32:1165–1179
11. Schoenen J, Vandersmissen B, Jeangette S, Herroelen L, Vandenheede M, Gerard P, Magis D (2013) Migraine prevention with a supraorbital

transcutaneous stimulator: a randomized controlled trial. Neurology 80:697–704

12. Beekwilder JP, Beems T (2010) Overview of the clinical applications of vagus nerve stimulation. J Clin Neurophysiol 27:130–138

13. Hord ED, Evans MS, Mueed S, Adamolekun B, Naritoku DK (2003) The effect of vagus nerve stimulation on migraines. J Pain 4:530–534

14. Sadler RM, Purdy RA, Rahey S (2002) Vagal nerve stimulation aborts migraine in patient with intractable epilepsy. Cephalalgia 22:482–484

15. Mauskop A (2005) Vagus nerve stimulation relieves chronic refractory migraine and cluster headaches. Cephalalgia 25:82–86

16. Lenaerts ME, Oommen KJ, Couch JR, Skaggs V (2008) Can vagus nerve stimulation help migraine? Cephalalgia 28:392–395

17. Ellrich J (2011) Transcutaneous vagus nerve stimulation. Eur Neurol Rev 6:254–256

18. He W, Jing XH, Zhu B, Zhu XL, Li L, Bai WZ, Ben H (2013) The auriculo-vagal afferent pathway and its role in seizure suppression in rats. BMC Neurosci 14:85

19. Clancy JA, Mary DA, Witte KK, Greenwood JP, Deuchars SA, Deuchars J (2014) Non-invasive vagus nerve stimulation in healthy humans reduces sympathetic nerve activity. Brain Stimul 7:871–877

20. Kraus T, Kiess O, Hosl K, Terekhin P, Kornhuber J, Forster C (2013) CNS BOLD fMRI effects of sham-controlled transcutaneous electrical nerve stimulation in the left outer auditory canal - a pilot study. Brain Stimul 6:798–804

21. Frangos E, Ellrich J, Komisaruk BR (2015) Non-invasive access to the vagus nerve central projections via electrical stimulation of the external Ear: fMRI evidence in humans. Brain Stimul 8:624–636

22. Kirchner A, Birklein F, Stefan H, Handwerker HO (2000) Left vagus nerve stimulation suppresses experimentally induced pain. Neurology 55:1167–1171

23. Busch V, Zeman F, Heckel A, Menne F, Ellrich J, Eichhammer P (2013) The effect of transcutaneous vagus nerve stimulation on pain perception–an experimental study. Brain Stimul 6:202–209

24. Goadsby PJ, Grosberg BM, Mauskop A, Cady R, Simmons KA (2014) Effect of noninvasive vagus nerve stimulation on acute migraine: an open-label pilot study. Cephalalgia 34:986–993

25. Beck AT, Erbaugh J, Ward CH, Mock J, Mendelsohn M (1961) An inventory for measuring depression. Arch Gen Psychiatry 4:561–571

26. Stewart WF, Lipton RB, Dowson AJ, Sawyer J (2001) Development and testing of the Migraine Disability Assessment (MIDAS) questionnaire to assess headache-related disability. Neurology 56:S20–S28

27. Kosinski M, Bayliss MS, Bjorner JB, Ware JE Jr, Garber WH, Batenhorst A, Cady R, Dahlof CG, Dowson A, Tepper S (2003) A six-item short-form survey for measuring headache impact: the HIT-6. Qual Life Res 12:963–974

28. Freitag FG, Diamond S, Diamond M, Urban G (2008) Botulinum toxin type A in the treatment of chronic migraine without medication overuse. Headache 48:201–209

29. Silvestrini M, Bartolini M, Coccia M, Baruffaldi R, Taffi R, Provinciali L (2003) Topiramate in the treatment of chronic migraine. Cephalalgia 23:820–824

30. Diener HC, Bussone G, Van Oene JC, Lahaye M, Schwalen S, Goadsby PJ (2007) Topiramate reduces headache days in chronic migraine: a randomized, double-blind, placebo-controlled study. Cephalalgia 27:814–823

31. Aurora SK, Dodick DW, Turkel CC, DeGryse RE, Silberstein SD, Lipton RB, Diener HC, Brin MF (2010) OnabotulinumtoxinA for treatment of chronic migraine: results from the double-blind, randomized, placebo-controlled phase of the PREEMPT 1 trial. Cephalalgia 30:793–803

32. The Vagus Nerve Stimulation Study Group (1995) A randomized controlled trial of chronic vagus nerve stimulation for treatment of medically intractable seizures. Neurology 45:224–230

33. Milby AH, Halpern CH, Baltuch GH (2008) Vagus nerve stimulation for epilepsy and depression. Neurotherapeutics 5:75–85

34. Ellrich J (2006) Long-term depression of orofacial somatosensory processing. Suppl Clin Neurophysiol 58:195–208

35. Ellrich J (2004) Electric low-frequency stimulation of the tongue induces long-term depression of the jaw-opening reflex in anesthetized mice. J Neurophysiol 92:3332–3337

36. Jung K, Rottmann S, Ellrich J (2009) Long-term depression of spinal nociception and pain in man: influence of varying stimulation parameters. Eur J Pain 13:161–170

37. Rottmann S, Jung K, Vohn R, Ellrich J (2010) Long-term depression of pain-related cerebral activation in healthy man: an fMRI study. Eur J Pain 14:615–624

38. Rottmann S, Jung K, Ellrich J (2010) Electrical low-frequency stimulation induces long-term depression of sensory and affective components of pain in healthy man. Eur J Pain 14:359–365

39. Jung K, Larsen LE, Rottmann S, Ellrich J (2011) Heterotopic low-frequency stimulation induces nociceptive LTD within the same central receptive field in man. Exp Brain Res 212:189–198

40. Jung K, Lelic D, Rottmann S, Drewes AM, Petrini L, Ellrich J (2012) Electrical low-frequency stimulation induces central neuroplastic changes of pain processing in man. Eur J Pain 16:509–521

41. Rottmann S, Jung K, Ellrich J (2008) Electrical low-frequency stimulation induces homotopic long-term depression of nociception and pain from hand in man. Clin Neurophysiol 119:1895–1904

42. Aymanns M, Yekta SS, Ellrich J (2009) Homotopic long-term depression of trigeminal pain and blink reflex within one side of the human face. Clin Neurophysiol 120:2093–2099

43. Yekta SS, Lamp S, Ellrich J (2006) Heterosynaptic long-term depression of craniofacial nociception: divergent effects on pain perception and blink reflex in man. Exp Brain Res 170:414–422

44. Ellrich J, Schorr A (2004) Low-frequency stimulation of trigeminal afferents induces long-term depression of human sensory processing. Brain Res 996:255–258

45. Noseda R, Burstein R (2013) Migraine pathophysiology: anatomy of the trigeminovascular pathway and associated neurological symptoms, CSD, sensitization and modulation of pain. Pain. 154 Suppl 1.

46. Peuker ET, Filler TJ (2002) The nerve supply of the human auricle. Clin Anat 15:35–37

47. Lyubashina OA, Sokolov AY, Panteleev SS (2012) Vagal afferent modulation of spinal trigeminal neuronal responses to dural electrical stimulation in rats. Neuroscience 222:29–37

48. Multon S, Schoenen J (2005) Pain control by vagus nerve stimulation: from animal to man…and back. Acta Neurol Belg 105:62–67

49. Bossut DF, Maixner W (1996) Effects of cardiac vagal afferent electrostimulation on the responses of trigeminal and trigeminothalamic neurons to noxious orofacial stimulation. Pain 65:101–109

50. Zerari-Mailly F, Buisseret P, Buisseret-Delmas C, Nosjean A (2005) Trigemino-solitarii-facial pathway in rats. J Comp Neurol 487:176–189

51. Randich A, Gebhart GF (1992) Vagal afferent modulation of nociception. Brain Res Brain Res Rev 17:77–99

52. Coppola G, Pierelli F, Schoenen J (2009) Habituation and migraine. Neurobiol Learn Mem 92:249–259

53. De Marinis M, Pujia A, Colaizzo E, Accornero N (2007) The blink reflex in "chronic migraine". Clin Neurophysiol 118:457–463

54. Aurora SK, Barrodale PM, Tipton RL, Khodavirdi A (2007) Brainstem dysfunction in chronic migraine as evidenced by neurophysiological and positron emission tomography studies. Headache 47:996–1003

55. Coppola G, Iacovelli E, Bracaglia M, Serrao M, Di LC, Pierelli F (2013) Electrophysiological correlates of episodic migraine chronification: evidence for thalamic involvement. J Headache Pain 14:76

56. Henry TR (2002) Therapeutic mechanisms of vagus nerve stimulation. Neurology 59:S3–S14

57. Ben-Menachem E, Hamberger A, Hedner T, Hammond EJ, Uthman BM, Slater J, Treig T, Stefan H, Ramsay RE, Wernicke JF (1995) Effects of vagus nerve stimulation on amino acids and other metabolites in the CSF of patients with partial seizures. Epilepsy Res 20:221–227

58. Richter F, Mikulik O, Ebersberger A, Schaible HG (2005) Noradrenergic agonists and antagonists influence migration of cortical spreading depression in rat-a possible mechanism of migraine prophylaxis and prevention of postischemic neuronal damage. J Cereb Blood Flow Metab 25:1225–1235

59. Pietrobon D, Striessnig J (2003) Neurobiology of migraine. Nat Rev Neurosci 4:386–398

60. Cernuda-Morollon E, Martinez-Camblor P, Alvarez R, Larrosa D, Ramon C, Pascual J (2015) Increased VIP levels in peripheral blood outside migraine attacks as a potential biomarker of cranial parasympathetic activation in chronic migraine. Cephalalgia 35:310–316

61. Schytz HW, Birk S, Wienecke T, Kruuse C, Olesen J, Ashina M (2009) PACAP38 induces migraine-like attacks in patients with migraine without aura. Brain 132:16–25

62. Bussone G, Diener HC, Pfeil J, Schwalen S (2005) Topiramate 100 mg/day in migraine prevention: a pooled analysis of double-blind randomised controlled trials. Int J Clin Pract 59:961–968

20

Positive effects of the progestin desogestrel 75 μg on migraine frequency and use of acute medication are sustained over a treatment period of 180 days

Gabriele S Merki-Feld[1*], Bruno Imthurn[1], Ronald Langner[2], Burkhardt Seifert[3] and Andreas R Gantenbein[4]

Abstract

Background: Premenopausal migraines frequently are associated with fluctuations of estrogen levels. Both, migraine and combined hormonal contraceptives (CHC) increase the risk of vascular events. Therefore progestagen-only contraceptives (POC) are a safer alternative. A previous short-term study demonstrated a positive impact of the oral POC desogestrel on migraine frequency. To study the effect of the POC desogestrel 75 μg on migraine frequency, intensity, use of acute medication and quality of life in a clinical setting over the period of 180 days.

Methods: Patients' charts were screened for women with migraine, who had decided to use desogestrel for contraception. Charts were included, if routinely conducted headache diaries were complete for 90 days before treatment (baseline) and over a treatment period of 180 days. We also report about starters who stopped treatment early, because of adverse events. Baseline data (day 1–90 before treatment) were compared with first and second treatment period (treatment days 1–90 and days 91–180). Quality of life was evaluated using MIDAS questionnaires.

Results: Days with migraine (5.8 vs 3.6), with any kind of headache (9.4 vs 6.6), headache intensity (15.7 vs 10.7), days with severe headache (5.4 vs 2.4) and use of triptans (12.3 vs7.8) were significantly reduced after 180 days. MIDAS score and grade improved significantly.

Conclusion: Contraception with desogestrel 75 μg resulted in a significantly improved quality of life and a reduction of migraine days over the observation period of 180 days. A clinically meaningful 30% reduction in pain was observed in 25/42 (60%) participants. For counselling reasons it is of importance, that the major reduction in migraine frequency occured during the initial 90 days, however further improvement occurs with longer duration of use. Prospective studies are needed to confirm these results.

Keywords: Hormonal migraine; Contraception; Progestagen-only pill; Desogestrel; Migraine without aura; Headache; Migraine with aura; Cardiovascular risk; Triptans

Background

Epidemiological data suggest that combined hormonal contraceptives (CHC) initiate or worsen migraine and headache in predisposed women [1-5]. The incidence of migraine is highest during the reproductive years and more than 50% of women report an association between migraine attacks and their menstrual cycle [6,7]. The reproductive phase is also the life span in which most women need efficient contraception. Migraine with aura (MA) and to a lesser extent migraine without aura (MO) increase the risk for cardiovascular events, especially for stroke [8-11]. There is a substantial elevation of these risks in migraineurs using CHC [11-14]. The cardiovascular risk associated with CHC, has been mainly attributed to the estrogen component which exerts a strong effect on the coagulation system. Finding a well-tolerated estrogen-free form of contraception for headache patients therefore is an important issue.

* Correspondence: gabriele.merki@usz.ch
[1]Department of Reproductive Endocrinology, University Hospital Zürich, Rämistrasse 100, CH - 8091 Zürich, Switzerland

Progestagen-only pills (POP) have so far not been found to be associated with an increased risk for thromboembolic or ischemic events [15]. Most guidelines recommend progestagen-only contraception as a safer option [16]. The POP desogestrel 75 μg (Cerazette®; MSD Merck Sharp & Dohme AG, Luzern, Switzerland) is used continuously and combines efficient inhibition of ovulation with maintenance of low estrogen levels [17,18]. Avoidance of estrogen peaks and withdrawal could contribute to good tolerability of this contraceptive in migraineurs. Recently we reported a benefit of desogestrel 75 μg on migraine and quality of life over a 3 month period of use [19,20]. The effect on frequency and quality of life was comparable to improvements observed with prophylactic agents. However, the observation interval was short. In the present study, we report effects of 6 cycles desogestrel contraception on headache frequency, intensity and use of pain medication.

Methods

This study was performed at the divison for family planning, unit of the Department of Reproductive Endocrinology, University Hospital Zürich, Switzerland where one of the authors (GM) runs an outpatient clinic for migraine patients with need for hormonal therapy. Migraine is diagnosed according to the IHS (International Headache Society) criteria by the referring neurologists from headache centres in Zürich, Bad Zurzach or by the author [21]. Reasons for referral were need for contraception in women with migraine, menstrual migraine or any form of hormonal therapy of headaches. To allow an exact diagnosis of the headache type and frequency according to the IHS our patients are principally instructed to conduct headache diaries for 3 cycles before their first visit and to continue after any intervention. MIDAS questionnaires are used before interventions and in intervals of 90 days thereafter. The majority of our premenopausal patients have a need for efficient contraception. In the context of the discussions around the elevated risks for cardiovascular disease and stroke we advise against combined hormonal contraceptives as a first choice contraception in migraineurs and in women aged 35 years or more. Before starting a hormonal treatment women are informed about risks and potential side effects which include information about irregular bleeding and acne with the use of desogestrel.

For the present study patients' charts were screened for women with migraine, who had decided to use the POP desogestrel 75 μg and had conducted headache diaries 90 days before initiation and over 180 days of use of this medication. We included patients suffering from all types of migraine. The observation period was defined from July 2009 to December 2013. In a previous study we already reported 90 day treatment data of 16 included patients. Women had to be premenopausal and had to need effective contraception. We report about all adverse events causing discontinuation earlier than 180 days. Exclusion criteria were: incomplete diaries, less than 10 headache episodes during the pretreatment period, initiation or change of prophylactic medications during the observation and postmenopause. This resulted in a drop-out rate of 26 out of 68 charts.

The diaries include information on the number of migraine and headache days, the severity of headache, the use of triptans and other pain medication, the use of hormones and days with vaginal bleeding. Days of bleeding were assessed to allow an exact diagnosis of the migraine type according to the IHS criteria. Headache severity was rated in the diaries according to a 4-point scale (0 = no pain, 3 = severe pain). This score is easy to understand and has been proven to be useful in daily work with migraineurs. For ethical reasons all diaries were anonymised before data evaluation. The evaluation of anonymised data in our setting was accepted by the ethical committee of the Kanton Zürich.

Primary efficacy variables were the differences in number of migraine and headache days, the difference in pain score as well as MIDAS score and grade. Secondary outcomes included differences in the number of all pain medications and triptans used as well as differences in days with pain score three. In population-based studies of migraine- and headache sufferers in the US and UK the MIDAS questionnaire and the MIDAS summary scores proved to be a highly reliable means of assessment of the impact of the ailment on daily life [22,23]. The total MIDAS score strongly correlates with both the clinical evaluation of the severity of a patient's headache problem, and the frequency of the episodes, determined from daily-based headache diaries [23].

Statistical analyses

Data were compared between baseline (BL) (day 1–90 before treatment) and treatment periods (TP): TP1 (day 1–90) TP2 (day 91–180). In addition all variables were compared between TP1 and TP2. Statistical analyses were done using IBM SPSS Statistics, version 22 (Armonk, New York, IBM Corp). Data are presented as mean (SD). Pain intensity score was calculated as the sum of headache intensities for baseline and each treatment period according to the above mentioned 4-point scale. For each period this sum was divided by three to obtain a mean monthly pain score. To calculate monthly frequencies, the numbers for each observational episode was divided by three. Numbers of monthly migraine days, headache days, headache intensity, days with use of pain medication and questions of the MIDAS questionnaire were compared with Friedman's test. Post-hoc comparisons between single time points were performed using Wilcoxon's signed rank test with Bonferroni correction.

Results

A total of 68 women with migraine initiated contraception with desogestrel 75 µg. Headache diaries of 42 subjects were complete and eligible for analysis. Six patients had stopped desogestrel because of side effects within 42 or less days and were excluded (prolonged bleeding n = 3, increase of headache n = 2, acne = 1) (Figure 1). Demographics and characteristics of eligible women and drop-outs did not differ significantly (Table 1). Hormonal contraception was used by 50% (n = 21) of the included patients and 61% (n = 16) in the drop-out (p > 0.05). One included woman had used a copper-device (drop-outs: n = 0). Chronic headaches (>15 /month) were found in 6 included patients and more than 8 triptans were used monthly by 9 included patients. Mean age of migraine onset was 22.4 years (SD 5.2). Two women suffered from endometriosis. Frequency of migraine, headache intensity, days with use of pain medication and triptans were significantly reduced during TP2 in comparison with BL (Table 2). Days with severe pain declined from 5.4 (SD 4.2) to 2.4 (SD 3.5) (p < 0.001) (Table 2). The improvements were in large parts visible during TP1 and persisted during further follow-up. A according to the IHS clinically meaningful 30% reduction in pain was observed in 25/42 (60%) participants, whereas another 28% (12/42) experienced even a 50% reduction [24,25]. We found a 255 reduction in the sum of headache and migraine days in 55% (23/42) of the included migraineurs. Seven of 42 patients (16%) experienced 1–5 more headache/migraine days during TP2 in comparison to BL. Interestingly, however, quality of life improved in five of these seven women. Further analyses to explain this seemingly contradictory result revealed a decrease in days with pain score 3 and a decrease in overall pain intensity in all these five patients. Two women with more migraine attacks and without improvement in the MIDAS score, decided to change to a non-hormonal contraception after 180 days.

Table 3 demonstrates the changes in quality of life. All MIDAS items improved significantly during 180 days of desogestrel use (TP2). Again significant improvement was already observed after TP1. Separate analyses for MO and MA women revealed no differences with regard to demographic parameters between the groups. In MO patients significant improvements of all features (except headache days) days were observed (Table 4). The very small group of subjects with MA experienced significant reductions in the number of pain medications and triptans, MIDAS score and MIDAS grade.

Discussion

In the present study we report the effects of 180 days of contraception with the progestin-only pill desogestrel 75 µg on headache and migraine. We observed a significant reduction in migraine frequency, migraine intensity, use of triptans and pain score. Quality of life measured by the MIDAS score improved by more than 50%. Mean MIDAS grades were diminished by point (Table 3). The majority of positive effects were apparent after 90 days and small further improvements were noted up to 180 days of use (Table 2). To our knowledge, we report for the first time that hormonal treatment can reduce the use of triptans significantly. This might be of relevance for women at the boarder of medication overuse headaches. As different pathophysiologies underlie MA and MO, we performed subanalyses for both types of headaches. In women with MO, significant improvements for all variables except headache days were observed. In the group of patients suffering from MA (n = 10) migraine days decreased by two/month, what possibly as a result of the small group size

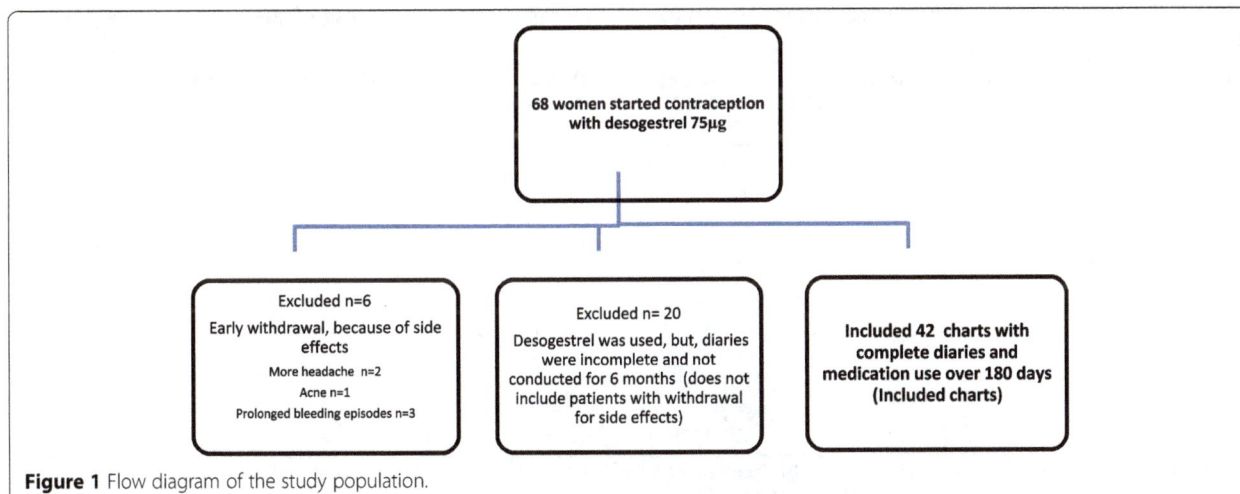

Figure 1 Flow diagram of the study population.

Table 1 Demographic and baseline characteristics of included charts (n = 42) and excluded charts (n = 26)

Demographics	Included patients n = 42 Mean (SD)	Drop-out group n = 26 Mean (SD)	P - value
Age (years)	35.1 (8.9)	31.1 (9.8)	0.64
Height (cm)	165.7 (6.5)	166.2 (5.7)	0.78
Weight (kg)	60.6 (8.4)	61.6 (9.0)	0.37
Systolic blood pressure (mmHG)	119.9 (12.6)	114.7 (26.1)	0.19
Diastolic blood pressure (mmHG)	73.7 (9.9)	75.7 (9.6)	0.91
Baseline characteristics			
Migraine days per month	5.8 (4.3)	6.6 (3.6)	0.62
Headache Intensity /month	15.7 (7.6)	20.3 (9.5)	0.28
Age of migraine onset	22.4 (5.2)	24.2 (7.2)	0.42
Triptan users	12.3 (15.0)	12.1 (11.7)	0.71
MIDAS: Headache days	25.2 (17.2)	23.0 (12.8)	0.37
MIDAS: (Pain intensity)	6.4 (1.7)	6.7 (1.6)	0.57
MIDAS: Grade	3.5 (0.7)	3.3 (0.8)	0.38
	Number (%)	Number (%)	
Migraine with aura	10 (24)	10 (38)	0.19
Migraine without aura	32 (76)	16 (61.1)	

was not significant. Significant bettermends were observed with regard to use of pain medications, use of triptans and MIDAS score and grade.

Migraine is a typical disorder with a high response rate to placebo in controlled trials. For ethical reasons placebo-controlled studies in the area of contraception are not acceptable. An important strength of the present study is the long run-in period and the evaluation not only of migraine frequency but also of additional parameters, like pain intensity, use of pain medications and quality of life. The combination of these data is a better reflection of the overall well-being as demonstrated in the detailed data analysis of the patients developing more migraine in our study. The run in period of 90

days allowed a balanced overview with regard to migraine frequencies which can vary markedly from month to month. However, even if the headache diaries had been conducted prospectively our analyses could have generated selection or information bias. In particular, we assume that a prospective design might have resulted in a higher continuation rate and exclusion of less charts with incomplete diaries. A control group of women using other hormonal contraceptive methods would have been of advantage.

Our findings for MO patients are in accordance with a very recent retrospective diary-based study, demonstrating a significant reduction in migraine frequency, pain intensity and use of pain medication with 6 months use

Table 2 Changes in migraine, frequency, intensity and use of pain medication during use of the contraceptive pill desogestrel 75 μg over 180 days of use

Days/month	Mean baseline (SD)	Mean treatment TP 1(SD)	Mean treatment TP 2 (SD)	Overall P-value	P-value baseline vs. TP 1	Posthoc* P-value baseline vs. TP2	P-value TP 1 vs TP 2
Headache days	4.1 (4.5)	3.8 (4.1)	3.0 (4.1)	0.051	0.867	0.050	0.062
Migraine days	5.8 (4.3)	3.7 (3.4)	3.6 (4.0)	<0.001	<0.001	0.001	0.701
Sum headache and migraine	9.4 (5.1)	7.6 (5.5)	6.6 (5.4)	0.002	0.008	<0.001	0.130
Headache intensity	15.7 (7.6)	11.4 (7.5)	10.7 (8.0)	<0.001	<0.001	<0.001	0.312
Days with headache score 3 in 3 months	5.4 (4.2)	2.2 (2.7)	2.4 (3.5)	<0.001	<0.001	<0.001	0.776
Pain medication	7.2 (5.9)	5.0 (3.3)	5.0 (4.0)	0.044	<0.001	0.015	0.751
Triptan use in 3 months	12.3 (15.0)	8.1 (9.4)	7.8 (10.2)	0.035	0.010	0.041	0.599

Baseline: 90 days before treatment; TP = treatment period. TP1: Treatment period days 1–90; TP2: Treatment period days 91–180.
*after Bonferroni correction, post-hoc p-values are significant at p < 0.017.

Table 3 Changes in quality of life measured with the MIDAS after 90 days and 180 days contraception with desogestrel 75 µg

N = 42	Mean (SD) Baseline	Mean (SD) TP 1	Mean (SD) TP 2	Overall p-value	P-value baseline vs. TP1	Posthoc* P-value baseline vs. TP2	P-value TP1 vs. TP2
MIDAS SCORE	36.3 (41.9)	18.3 (38.8)	16.0 (32.8)	<0.001	<0.001	<0.001	0.176
MIDAS 1: days missed at work	7.0 (15.2)	3.8 (13.6)	2.6 (10.9)	<0.001	<0.001	0.002	0.093
MIDAS 2: days with >50% reduced productivity at work	7.6 (5.4)	4.2 (4.6)	3.9 (4.9)	0.001	0.002	0.001	0.650
MIDAS 3: days without household work	6.3 (9.7)	3.6 (8.1)	2.6 (4.4)	<0.001	0.002	<0.001	0.161
MIDAS 4: days with >50% reduced productivity in household work	5.8 (6.8)	3.9 (7.0)	3.9 (8.2)	0.006	<0.009	0.046	0.766
MIDAS 5: days when family, social or leisure activities are missed	9.8 (15.3)	3.7 (9.9)	3.1 (7.2)	<0.001	<0.001	<0.001	0.481
MIDAS: Headache days	26.4 (19.3)	17.0 (15.5)	17.0 (18.1)	<0.001	0.002	<0.001	0.487
MIDAS: Pain intensity (scale 0–10)	6.1 (1.7)	4.8 (1.5)	4.5 (2.0)	<0.001	<0.001	<0.001	0.078
MIDAS: Grade	3.6 (0.7)	2.4 (1.0)	2.2 (1.2)	<0.001	<0.001	<0.001	0.295

Baseline: before treatment, TP1: 1–90 days use of desogestrel; TP2: 91–180 days desogestrel use.
*after Bonferroni correction, post-hoc p-values are significant at p < 0.017.

of desogestrel [26]. Triptan use did not decline, which contrasts with our result and might be related to the lower number of included patients. The comparison with a control group of users of a combined pill (COC) in a long-cycle in this study is of great interest, because both forms of contraception prevent hormone withdrawal [26]. While migraine attacks and pain intensity decreased significantly with the POP, headache frequency declined with the COC regimen only. Desogestrel use failed to exert a significant effect on non-migrainous-headache in our sample and the comparative trial. This can be explained, by our earlier reported findings showing in an individual follow-up of both headache and migraine, that a temporary transformation of migraines to headaches occurs in some women [19]. Our present study with a longer observation period however indicates that, on the long-term, these headaches might decline as well (p = 0.05). Although our study includes only few women with MA, the findings are backed by Nappi et al. who reported a significant

reduction in migraine frequency in MA patients, but did not investigate pain intensity and quality of life [27].

Even if there is still a lack of prospective controlled trials several diary-based studies indicate a positive impact of desogestrel on migraine without aura [19,26,27]. Continuous use of COCs exerts a positive impact on headaches and hormone-withdrawal migraines, however POP are much safer with regard to the cardiovascular and thromboembolic risks [26,28-32]. The benefit of desogestrel on migraine with aura, which is not typically associated with estrogen withdrawal, has to be confirmed in future studies. Many migraineurs are reluctant to use hormones as a consequence of previous bad experience. During counselling it is helpful to know that major improvements can be expected during 90 days of desogestrel use. Furthermore, two trials indicate that migraines and pain tend to improve further beyond 3 months [19,26,27]. On the other hand, patients have to be informed that migraine rarely worsens. The clinically meaningful 30% reduction in pain (considered by the

Table 4 Changes in migraine and headache frequency during use of the progestin-only pill desogestrel 75 µg, comparison between MO (n=32) and MA (10) patients

	MO Mean (SD) baseline	MA Mean (SD) baseline	MO Mean (SD) TP 2	MA Mean (SD) TP 2	p-value MO baseline vs. TP 2	p-value MA baseline vs. TP 2
Headache days/month	4.1 (4.3)	3.8 (5.2)	3.4 (4.6)	1.9 (2.0)	0.06	0.60
Migraine days/month	5.4 (4.1)	6.8 (4.8)	3.2 (3.8)	4.6 (4.3)	0.007	0.09
Sum headache and migraine/month	9.5 (5.6)	8.8 (3.6)	6.6 (4.4)	6.6 (4.4)	<0.001	0.11
Headache intensity/month	16.0 (8.3)	14.4 (5.4)	11.4(8.4)	8.5 (6.4)	<0.001	0.24
Pain medication	6.2 (3.6)	9.8 (9.5)	4.7 (3.6)	5.8 (4.8)	0.03	0.03
Triptan use in 3 months	11.9 (11.8)	13.1 (22.2)	8.4 (10.7)	6.2 (8.6)	0.005	0.02

MO = migraine without aura, MA = Migraine with aura, baseline : days 1–90 before treatment; TP 2: days 91–180 of treatment.

IHS as clinically meaningful) in 60% of our patients is another argument to prefer this contraceptive method in women with migraine [24,25]. Reduction in use of triptans and other pain medications might contribute of the prevention of medication-overuse headaches.

In daily life the degree to which a reduction in headache frequency translates to decreased disability and improved quality of life is highly relevant. The MIDAS demonstrated highly reduced disability and significantly improved quality of life in our patients.

Use of POP can cause a variety of bleeding patterns including amenorrhoea, infrequent bleeding, frequent bleeding and prolonged bleeding episodes. Unfavorable bleeding patterns such as frequent bleeding and prolonged bleeding occur as result of the continuous progestin effect on the endometrium and can be a reason for withdrawal from this form of contraception [33]. Prolonged and frequent bleedings usually stop with longer duration of use and can be treated if not.

Unanswered questions

New insights in the hormonal effects on the brain allow speculations about mechanisms underlying our observations. Avoidance of hormone withdrawal can only explain the decline of cycle-related headaches. In contrast to estrogens, progesterone seems to attenuate trigeminovascular nociception and reduces dural plasma protein extravasation following stimulation of the trigeminal ganglion [34-36]. Thus direct or receptor-mediated effects of the desogestrel on the trigeminovascular system can be postulated. The variety of responses on desogestrel treatment could be a result of the genetic variability of estrogen receptors in women, with some polymorphisms being a significant risk factor for migraine [37]. The neurological basis of migraine auras has not yet been established, increasing evidence indicates that they are a clinical manifestation of a cortical spreading depression (CSD).

In mice the thresholds for cortical spreading depression (CSD) is lower in cycling females than in males. This would allow to hypothesise that maintenance of low estrogen levels induced by desogestrel might upregulate the threshold for CSD thus reduce MA attacks. A further mechanism could be that desogestrel or its metabolite etonogestrel, like progesterone and allopregnanolone decrease cortical excitability via the GABA -receptor [38-40].

At the moment we have no means to predict how an individual migraineur will react on desogestrel. Outside the study we achieved positive effects with higher dosages. However, this is off-label use and cannot be generally recommended before prospective trials have been conducted. Several trials highlight a positive effect of desogestrel on migraine. Among neurologists it is well known that headaches may be cycle-related, but they rarely consider to search advice for a hormonal treatment. Vice versa gynaecologists are not always aware of the fact that hormonal treatment affects headache frequency in predisposed women. A closer collaboration between gynaecologic endocrinologists and headache specialists might provide better care and safety for young women, suffering from migraine during use of any hormones or in association with their natural cycle.

Conclusion

In conclusion our data indicate a positive impact of desogestrel 75 µg on migraine frequency, intensity, use of pain medication and quality of life. The major improvement was observed during the initial 90 days of use, which might be important for patients' counselling. Randomised controlled trials are needed to substantiate our results.

Competing interests

Gabriele S Merki-Feld and Bruno Imthurn had financial relationship (lecturer, member of advisory boards and// or consultant) with Bayer-Schering Pharma and MSD AG.
RL and AG declared no conflicts of interest.

Authors' contributions

GM: participated in the design of the study, the acquisition and analysis of data and the drafting of the manuscript. BI: has been involved in drafting the manuscript and revising it critically. RL participated in the acquisition and interpretation of data and revision of the manuscript. BS has been involved in the analysis and interpretation of data and revision of the manuscript. AG participated in the design of the study, acquisition of data and drafting the manuscript. All authors read and approved the final version of the manuscript.

Acknowledgements

The authors declare that they received not any funding for the study or for preparing the manuscript with the exception of the salaries from their institutions.

Funding

This research received no specific grant from any funding agency in the public, commercial or for non-profit sectors.

Author details

[1]Department of Reproductive Endocrinology, University Hospital Zürich, Rämistrasse 100, CH - 8091 Zürich, Switzerland. [2]Headache Clinic Hirslanden Zürich, Zurich, Switzerland. [3]Epidemiology, Biostatistics and Prevention Institute, Department of Biostatistics, University of Zürich, Zurich, Switzerland. [4]Neurorehabilitation, RehaClinic, Bad Zurzach, Switzerland.

References

1. Aegidius K, Zwart JA, Hagen K, Schei B, Stovner LJ (2006) Oral contraceptives and increased headache prevalence: the Head-HUNT Study. Neurology 66(3):349–353
2. Allais G, Gabellari IC, Airola G, Borgogno P, Schiapparelli P, Benedetto C (2009) Headache induced by the use of combined oral contraceptives. Neurol Sci 30(Suppl 1):S15–S17
3. Teepker M, Peters M, Kundermann B, Vedder H, Schepelmann K, Lautenbacher S (2011) The effects of oral contraceptives on detection and pain thresholds as well as headache intensity during menstrual cycle in migraine. Headache 51(1):92–104

4. Loder EW, Buse DC, Golub JR (2005) Headache as a side effect of combination estrogen-progestin oral contraceptives: a systematic review. Am J Obstet Gynecol 193(3 Pt 1):636–649

5. Archer DF, Jensen JT, Johnson JV, Borisute H, Grubb GS, Constantine GD (2006) Evaluation of a continuous regimen of levonorgestrel/ethinyl estradiol: phase 3 study results. Contraception 74(6):439–445

6. Macgregor EA (2007) Menstrual migraine: a clinical review. J Fam Plann Reprod Health Care 33(1):36–47

7. Macgregor EA, Rosenberg JD, Kurth T (2011) Sex-related differences in epidemiological and clinic-based headache studies. Headache 51(6):843–859

8. Chang CL, Donaghy M, Poulter N (1999) Migraine and stroke in young women: case–control study. The World Health Organisation Collaborative Study of Cardiovascular Disease and Steroid Hormone Contraception. BMJ 318(7175):13–18

9. Bigal ME, Kurth T, Santanello N, Buse D, Golden W, Robbins M, Lipton RB (2010) Migraine and cardiovascular disease: a population-based study. Neurology 74(8):628–635

10. Tzourio C, Tehindrazanarivelo A, Iglesias S, Alperovitch A, Chedru F, D'Anglejan-Chatillon J, Bouser MG (1995) Case–control study of migraine and risk of ischaemic stroke in young women. BMJ 310(6983):830–833

11. Schurks M, Buring JE, Kurth T (2010) Migraine, migraine features, and cardiovascular disease. Headache 50(6):1031–1040

12. Tzourio C, Iglesias S, Hubert JB, Visy JM, Alperovitch A, Tehindrazanarivelo A, Biousse V, Woimant F, Bousser MG (1993) Migraine and risk of ischaemic stroke: a case–control study. BMJ 307(6899):289–292

13. Gillum LA, Mamidipudi SK, Johnston SC (2000) Ischemic stroke risk with oral contraceptives: A meta-analysis. JAMA 284(1):72–78

14. Sacco S, Ricci S, Degan D, Carolei A (2012) Migraine in women: the role of hormones and their impact on vascular diseases. J Headache Pain 13(3):177–189

15. Lidegaard O, Lokkegaard E, Svendsen AL, Agger C (2009) Hormonal contraception and risk of venous thromboembolism: national follow-up study. BMJ 339:b2890

16. Nappi RE, Merki-Feld GS, Terreno E, Pellegrinelli A, Viana M (2013) Hormonal contraception in women with migraine: is progestogen-only contraception a better choice? J Headache Pain 14:66

17. Barkfeldt J, Virkkunen A, Dieben T (2001) The effects of two progestogen-only pills containing either desogestrel (75 microg/day) or levonorgestrel (30 microg/day) on lipid metabolism. Contraception 64(5):295–299

18. Kivela A, Ruuskanen M, Agren U, Dieben T (2001) The effects of two progestogen-only pills containing either desogestrel (75 microgram/day) or levonorgestrel (30 microgram/day) on carbohydrate metabolism and adrenal and thyroid function. Eur J Contracept Reprod Health Care 6(2):71–77

19. Merki-Feld GS, Imthurn B, Langner R, Sandor PS, Gantenbein AR (2013) Headache frequency and intensity in female migraineurs using desogestrel-only contraception: a retrospective pilot diary study. Cephalalgia 33(5):340–346

20. Merki-Feld GS, Imthurn B, Seifert B, Merki LL, Agosti R, Gantenbein AR (2013) Desogestrel-only contraception reduces headache frequency and improves quality of life in female migraineurs. Eur J Contracept Reprod Health Care 18:394–400

21. IHS International Headache Society (2004) The International Classification of Headache Disorders: 2nd edition. Cephalalgia 24 Suppl 1:9–160

22. Stewart WF, Lipton RB, Kolodner KB, Sawyer J, Lee C, Liberman JN (2000) Validity of the Migraine Disability Assessment (MIDAS) score in comparison to a diary-based measure in a population sample of migraine sufferers. Pain 88(1):41–52

23. Lipton RB, Stewart WF, Sawyer J, Edmeads JG (2001) Clinical utility of an instrument assessing migraine disability: the Migraine Disability Assessment (MIDAS) questionnaire. Headache 41(9):854–861

24. Silberstein S, Tfelt-Hansen P, Dodick DW, Limmroth V, Lipton RB, Pascual J, Wang SJ (2008) Guidelines for controlled trials of prophylactic treatment of chronic migraine in adults. Cephalalgia 28(5):484–495

25. Dworkin RH, Turk DC, Wyrwich KW, Beaton D, Cleeland CS, Farrar JT, Hertz S, Heyse JF, Iyengar S, Jadad AR, Jay GW, Jermano JA, Katz NP, Manning DC, Martin S, Max MB, McGrath P, McQuay HJ, Quessy S, Rappaport BA, Revicki DA, Rothman M, Stauffer JW, Svensson O, White RE, Witter J (2008) Interpreting the clinical importance of treatment outcomes in chronic pain clinical trials: IMMPACT recommendations. J Pain 9(2):105–121

26. Morotti M, Remorgida V, Venturini PL, Ferrero S (2014) Progestin-only contraception compared with extended combined oral contraceptive in women with migraine without aura: a retrospective pilot study. Eur J Obstet Gynecol Reprod Biol 183:178–182

27. Nappi RE, Sances G, Allais G, Terreno E, Benedetto C, Vaccaro V, Facchinetti F (2011) Effects of an estrogen-free, desogestrel-containing oral contraceptive in women with migraine with aura: a prospective diary-based pilot study. Contraception 83(3):223–228

28. Calhoun A, Ford S, Pruitt A (2012) The impact of extended-cycle vaginal ring contraception on migraine aura: a retrospective case series. Headache 52(8):1246–1253

29. De Leo V, Scolaro V, Musacchio MC, Di Sabatino A, Morgante G, Cianci A (2011) Combined oral contraceptives in women with menstrual migraine without aura. Fertil Steril 96(4):917–920

30. Sulak P, Willis S, Kuehl T, Coffee A, Clark J (2007) Headaches and oral contraceptives: impact of eliminating the standard 7-day placebo interval. Headache 47(1):27–37

31. MacGregor EA, Guillebaud J (1998) Combined oral contraceptives, migraine and ischaemic stroke. Clinical and Scientific Committee of the Faculty of Family Planning and Reproductive Health Care and the Family Planning Association. Br J Fam Plann 24(2):55–60

32. Lidegaard O, Nielsen LH, Skovlund CW, Lokkegaard E (2012) Venous thrombosis in users of non-oral hormonal contraception: follow-up study, Denmark 2001–10. BMJ 344:e2990

33. Merki-Feld GS, Breitschmid N, Seifert B, Kreft M (2014) A survey on Swiss women's preferred menstrual/withdrawal bleeding pattern over different phases of reproductive life and with use of hormonal contraception. Eur J Contracept Reprod Health Care 19(4):266–275

34. Cutrer FM, Moskowitz MA (1996) Wolff Award 1996. The actions of valproate and neurosteroids in a model of trigeminal pain. Headache 36(10):579–585

35. Multon S, Pardutz A, Mosen J, Hua MT, Defays C, Honda S, Harada N, Bohotin C, Franzen R, Schoenen J (2005) Lack of estrogen increases pain in the trigeminal formalin model: a behavioural and immunocytochemical study of transgenic ArKO mice. Pain 114(1–2):257–265

36. Bolay H, Berman NE, Akcali D (2011) Sex-related differences in animal models of migraine headache. Headache 51(6):891–904

37. Joshi G, Pradhan S, Mittal B (2010) Role of the oestrogen receptor (ESR1 Pvull and ESR1 325 C- > G) and progesterone receptor (PROGINS) polymorphisms in genetic susceptibility to migraine in a North Indian population. Cephalalgia 30(3):311–320

38. Liu A, Margaill I, Zhang S, Labombarda F, Coqueran B, Delespierre B, Marchand-Leroux C, O'Malley BW, Lydon JP, De Nicola AF, Sitruk-Ware R, Mattern C, Plotkine M, Schumacher M, Guennoun R (2012) Progesterone receptors: a key for neuroprotection in experimental stroke. Endocrinology 153(8):3747–3757

39. Schumacher M, Mattern C, Ghoumari A, Oudinet JP, Liere P, Labombarda F, Sitruk-Ware R, De Nicola AF, Guennoun R (2013) Revisiting the roles of progesterone and allopregnanolone in the nervous system: Resurgence of the progesterone receptors. Prog Neurobiol 113:6–39

40. Kokate TG, Svensson BE, Rogawski MA (1994) Anticonvulsant activity of neurosteroids: correlation with gamma-aminobutyric acid-evoked chloride current potentiation. J Pharmacol Exp Ther 270(3):1223–1229

21

Improvement of migraine symptoms with a proprietary supplement containing riboflavin, magnesium and Q10

Charly Gaul[1,2*], Hans-Christoph Diener[2], Ulrich Danesch[3] and on behalf of the Migravent® Study Group

Abstract

Background: Non-medical, non-pharmacological and pharmacological treatments are recommended for the prevention of migraine. The purpose of this randomized double-blind placebo controlled, multicenter trial was to evaluate the efficacy of a proprietary nutritional supplement containing a fixed combination of magnesium, riboflavin and Q10 as prophylactic treatment for migraine.

Methods: 130 adult migraineurs (age 18 – 65 years) with ≥ three migraine attacks per month were randomized into two treatment groups: dietary supplementation or placebo in a double-blind fashion. The treatment period was 3 months following a 4 week baseline period without prophylactic treatment. Patients were assessed before randomization and at the end of the 3-month-treatment-phase for days with migraine, migraine pain, burden of disease (HIT-6) and subjective evaluation of efficacy.

Results: Migraine days per month declined from 6.2 days during the baseline period to 4.4 days at the end of the treatment with the supplement and from 6.2 days to 5.2 days in the placebo group (p = 0.23 compared to placebo). The intensity of migraine pain was significantly reduced in the supplement group compared to placebo (p = 0.03). The sum score of the HIT-6 questionnaire was reduced by 4.8 points from 61.9 to 57.1 compared to 2 points in the placebo-group (p = 0.01). The evaluation of efficacy by the patient was better in the supplementation group compared to placebo (p = 0.01).

Conclusions: Treatment with a proprietary supplement containing magnesium, riboflavin and Q10 (Migravent® in Germany, Dolovent® in USA) had an impact on migraine frequency which showed a trend towards statistical significance. Migraine symptoms and burden of disease, however, were statistically significantly reduced compared to placebo in patients with migraine attacks.

Keywords: Migraine; Prevention; Nutritional Supplement

Background

Migraine is a functional disorder of the brain. The pathophysiology of migraine involves many different mechanisms including modulation of central and peripheral pain structures and release of vasoactive peptides. Patients typically experience episodes of headaches, mostly throbbing, unilateral and severe which vary within and among patients. Headaches are frequently accompanied by other symptoms like nausea, phonophobia and/or photophobia [1].

Acute attacks are treated with different analgesics or triptans. Only a minority of migraineurs take preventive medication to decrease the frequency, duration and severity of migraine attacks. Prophylactic drug treatment of migraine should be considered when the quality of life is severely impaired, when two or more attacks occur per month, when migraine attacks do not respond to acute drug treatment or in case of intolerance to or side effects of acute treatment [2].

* Correspondence: c.gaul@migraene-klinik.de
[1]Migraine and Headache Clinic, Königstein im Taunus, Germany
[2]Department of Neurology, University Hospital Essen, Essen, Germany

The guidelines of the German Headache and Migraine Society and the American Academy of Neurology recommend primarily beta-blockers, antiepileptics (topiramate or valproic acid), and antidepressants (e.g. amitriptyline) for migraine prevention [3,4]. Vitamin B2 (riboflavin), magnesium and coenzyme Q10 are alternatives to drugs and appeal to patients with a desire for more natural treatment. In addition, micronutrients are seen by the patients as a "mild" form of treatment with no or minor side effects [5,6].

Studies revealed decreased levels of the micronutrients riboflavin, magnesium and coenzyme in plasma and in the brain of migraine patients [7-9]. A deficit of these nutrients could play a role in the pathophysiology of migraine. Mitochondrial dysfunction is associated with migraine [10,11]. Riboflavin, magnesium and coenzyme Q10 play an important role in the production of energy in the mitochondria [12]. Magnesium is needed in various physiological processes which influence the pathophysiology of migraine (vasoconstriction, platelet inhibition, secretion of serotonin). Magnesium is also needed as a co-factor for proper functioning of the ATP-synthase which produces ATP. Furthermore, Mg is the physiological antagonist at the NMDA-channel which is involved in the regulation of neuronal excitability. Riboflavin is a precursor for flavin-mononucleotide (FMN) and flavin-adenine-dinucleotide (FAD). Both are essential components of complex I and complex II responsible for electron-transport in the mitochondrial membrane. Coenzyme Q10 is a vitamin-like compound which can be synthesized by the body from phenylalanine and tyrosine. Coenzyme Q10 is needed for all cellular processes requiring energy. Coenzyme Q10 is an electron-carrier, transferring electrons from complex I/complex II to cytochrome C. Based on these observations, it seems plausible that a substitution of these micronutrients in migraine patients might be able to prevent or reduce the intensity of migraine attacks. Migraine treatment with a nutritional supplement might be of benefit for patients with recurrent migraine who cannot tolerate chemical drugs due to side effects or contra-indications due to concomitant diseases.

The commercially available food supplement Migravent® in Germany (Dolovent® in the USA) contains riboflavin, magnesium and coenzyme in high doses along with low-dose multi-vitamins for support of general health. This supplement has already been tested in an open clinical study with 31 migraine patients in Germany [13]. The present trial was conducted to prove the efficacy of Migravent®/Dolovent® compared to placebo in a larger number of patients and under randomized, double-blind and multicenter conditions.

Methods
Participants and recruitment
Otherwise healthy adults aged 18 to 65 years of either sex were recruited by neurologists practicing in Germany. All participants had migraine with and without aura diagnosed according to the IHS-criteria ICHD-II 1.1 und 1.2 [14]. The age at onset of migraine was less than 50 years of age and diagnosis of migraine was at least one year before study entry. The participants were required to have at least 3 migraine attacks per month in the last 3 months before recruitment and not more than 10 headache days. Patients were excluded if they used migraine prevention (drugs, nutritional supplements or psychotherapy) as well as antipsychotic or antidepressant medication during the last 3 months prior to study entry and throughout the study. Patients with medication overuse were excluded. Patients who had failed to respond to more than 2 different prophylactic agents in the past and patients resistant to all acute migraine drugs were not included.

The study was approved by the Institutional Review Board for each center. All participants gave written informed consent. The study was conducted according to the ethics principles of the Declaration of Helsinki. The trial was registered in the German Clinical Trial Register DRKS00004565.

Interventions
The investigational nutritional product (INP) is a dietary food for special medical purposes (according to EU regulations) containing 400 mg riboflavin (vitamin B2), 600 mg magnesium, 150 mg coenzyme Q10 along with a multivitamin/trace elements combination per 4 capsules (Migravent®, Dolovent®). The amount of additional multivitamin/trace elements per 4 capsules is as follows: 750 µg vitamin A, 200 mg vitamin C, 134 mg vitamin E, 5 mg thiamin, 20 mg niacin, 5 mg vitamin B6, 6 µg vitamin B12, 400 µg folic acid, 5 µg vitamin D, 10 mg pantothenic acid, 165 µg biotin, 0.8 mg iron, 5 mg zinc, 2 mg manganese, 0.5 mg copper, 30 µg chromium, 60 µg molybdenum, 50 µg selenium, 5 mg bioflavonoides. Placebo capsules indistinguishable from verum were used as control. Patients were instructed to take two capsules orally in the morning and two capsules in the evening for 3 months. Treatments for other conditions which may have an effect on migraine prevention were not allowed. These were mainly beta-blockers (e.g. propranolol, bisoprolol, metoprolol), calcium-antagonists (e.g. flunarizine), antiepileptics (e.g. topiramate, valproate), antidepressants (e.g. amitryptiline), supplements containing petasites (butterbur) or tanacetum (feverfew), magnesium, riboflavin or coenzyme Q10 in doses above 50 mg. Non-medical/non-nutritional treatment for migraine prevention like acupuncture or psychotherapy were also not permitted. However, participants were allowed to treat migraine attacks with their usual rescue pain medication and anti-emetics.

Study design
The study was conducted as a randomized, placebo-controlled, parallel-arm, double-blind, prospective multi-

center study. After screening, patients underwent a one-month baseline period without treatment to verify that they had more than 3 migraine attacks but not more than 10 days with migraine or non-migraine headaches. The baseline phase also served as a baseline for the evaluation of efficacy parameters. Before entering the baseline phase patients had to meet inclusion and exclusion criteria (see Participants and recruitment). Demographic data, concomitant medication, medical history, migraine diagnosis as well as previous migraine preventive measures were documented by the investigator. Following the baseline phase and provided no inclusion/exclusion criteria were violated, eligible patients were randomized in double-blind fashion to verum or to placebo (1:1). In this follow-up visit patients were also asked to fill in an HIT-6 questionnaire. Randomization was done by computer and randomization lists were prepared. Randomization was done by blocks of four per center. The investigator sequentially allocated the random numbers to patients, starting from the lowest number. A blockwise randomization was used. The sequential order was verified by fax sent to a blinded person at the sponsor and from entries in the screening logs. Both investigator and patient were blinded to the treatments. Treatment with either verum or placebo was for 3 months. Migraine parameters and intake of the investigational products were recorded daily by the patients throughout the baseline and the treatment phase in an electronic diary accessed online via the internet. Compliance (documentation, intake of investigational products) was monitored regularly by the investigator and delegates of the sponsor. Patients were immediately contacted by the investigator if regular documentation was missing for more than a week. At the follow-up visit at the end of the treatment the patients again had to fill in an HIT-6 questionnaire and they were asked to evaluate the tolerability and efficacy of the treatment from their view. Concomitant medication and occurrence of adverse events were checked at each follow-up visit. Compliance was assessed by a pill count of the returned investigational product.

Efficacy parameters

The primary efficacy endpoint was defined as days with migraine as recorded in the online diary by the patient. Secondary endpoints were maximal pain of migraine headaches as recorded in the online diary, migraine burden as assessed through the HIT-6 questionnaire [15] and subjective patient evaluation of efficacy.

Days with migraine and migraine pain intensity were compared between the one-month baseline period and the last month of the 3-month treatment. A migraine day was defined as a day with at least 4 hours of migraine pain or a day with migraine pain and concomitant intake of pain medication. For each migraine day, pain intensity was rated as mild, moderate or severe by the patient. The HIT-6

questionnaire (headache impact test), which measures the impact of headache on a patient´s life, was filled out by the patient at the start of the treatment (randomization) and at the end of the 3-month treatment. This validated questionnaire consists of 6 questions, each question or item has the following response options: never (6 points), rare (8 points), sometimes (10 points), very often (11 points) and always (13 points) [14]. Headache impact on this scale ranges from 36 (no headache) to 78 (very severe headache). All checked points are added for the analysis. Efficacy of the treatment as a subjective evaluation by each patient was recorded at the end of the study as very good, good, moderate or poor.

Statistical methods

The sample size estimation was performed with the Test of the Ratio of Two Poisson Means module of PASS 11 software (NCSS, LLC. Kaysville, Utah, USA). A reduction by at least 50% in the number of migraine days should be achieved in the verum group because this was considered a clinically relevant improvement and a 30% reduction in the placebo group was assumed as the worst case scenario since placebo effects of around 30% have been seen in trials. Based on these assumptions, the estimated sample size without compensation for drop-out is $39.2 \approx 40$ patients per treatment group, i.e. 80 patients in total. The sample size was increased to 104 patients in total to compensate for overdispersion and a 15% drop-out rate.

The statistical analysis was based on the ICH Topic E9 Note for guidance on statistical principles for clinical trials (CPMP/ICH/363/96). A detailed description of the statistical evaluation was provided in a Statistical Analysis Plan (SAP).

The primary endpoint migraine days was compared statistically in a confirmatory test approach on superiority of Migravent® compared to placebo. The respective statistical test was performed using the generalized linear model in the following form: it was assumed that the number of migraine days during the last month of the 3-month treatment period can be described by Poisson distributions. The migraine day rate depends on treatment and disease severity at baseline, which is defined as the number of migraine days during the one-month baseline period. This was modeled through a Poisson regression with covariate "number of migraine days during the one-month baseline period" and with the factors "treatment" and "center". The null hypothesis to be tested was whether the rate ratio for treatment ($\rho = \lambda_{Placebo}/\lambda_{Verum}$) is smaller or equal to 1 (i.e. log rate ratio is smaller or equal to 0). The type-I error rate was set to $\alpha = 0.025$ (one-sided). Confounding factors were not controlled for.

The maximal intensity of migraine pain per migraine day during the last month of the 3-month treatment was compared between treatment groups by an ANCOVA with the maximal intensity of migraine pain during the baseline period as baseline covariate.

The burden of disease measured by HIT-6 sum scores for the end of treatment was compared between treatment groups by an ANCOVA with the burden of disease sum scores for the start of treatment as baseline covariate.

Subjective evaluation of efficacy by the patient at the end of therapy was displayed by default descriptive statistics for continuous data as well as for categorical data. The treatment groups were compared by van-Elteren's test.

Results

Recruitment

173 migraine patients fulfilled the inclusion- and exclusion criteria and were enrolled in the baseline phase. The enrollment took place in 12 neurological centers in Germany from October 2012 to November 2013. The baseline phase consisted of a 30-day period without prophylactic migraine treatment. 34 patients could not be randomized into the treatment groups because they failed inclusion and fulfilled exclusion criteria after baseline; of the 34 patients, 4 had no migraine attack at all, 21 had between 1 and 2 migraine attacks per month and 9 had more than 10 days with migraine. Nine patients

were lost during the baseline phase, mostly due to non-compliance with the use of the online diary. The number of patients with prior migraine prevention was slightly higher in the placebo group (40 vs 36), however, 3 vs 1 patients in the verum group had used more than 3 migraine preventions in the past. The same, to a slightly more extent, is observed regarding medical history and concomitant medications. Of the 130 patients randomized, one patient provided no efficacy data since he did not open the diary during the treatment phase and did not show up for the final visit. Due to major protocol violations, 9 patients in the active-group and 8 patients in the placebo-group were excluded from efficacy analysis (Figure 1).

The baseline characteristics of all patients included in the efficacy analysis are described in Table 1. There was no significant difference in baseline parameters. 37 patients (64.9%) in the placebo group had migraines without aura compared to 28 patients (50.9%) in the active group. The number of patients without any prophylactic migraine treatments in their medical history was similar in both groups. However, the number of patients with up to 3 different prophylactic treatments in the past was higher in the placebo group (35.0%) than in the active group (21.8%). Number of concomitant diseases and medications was higher in the placebo group.

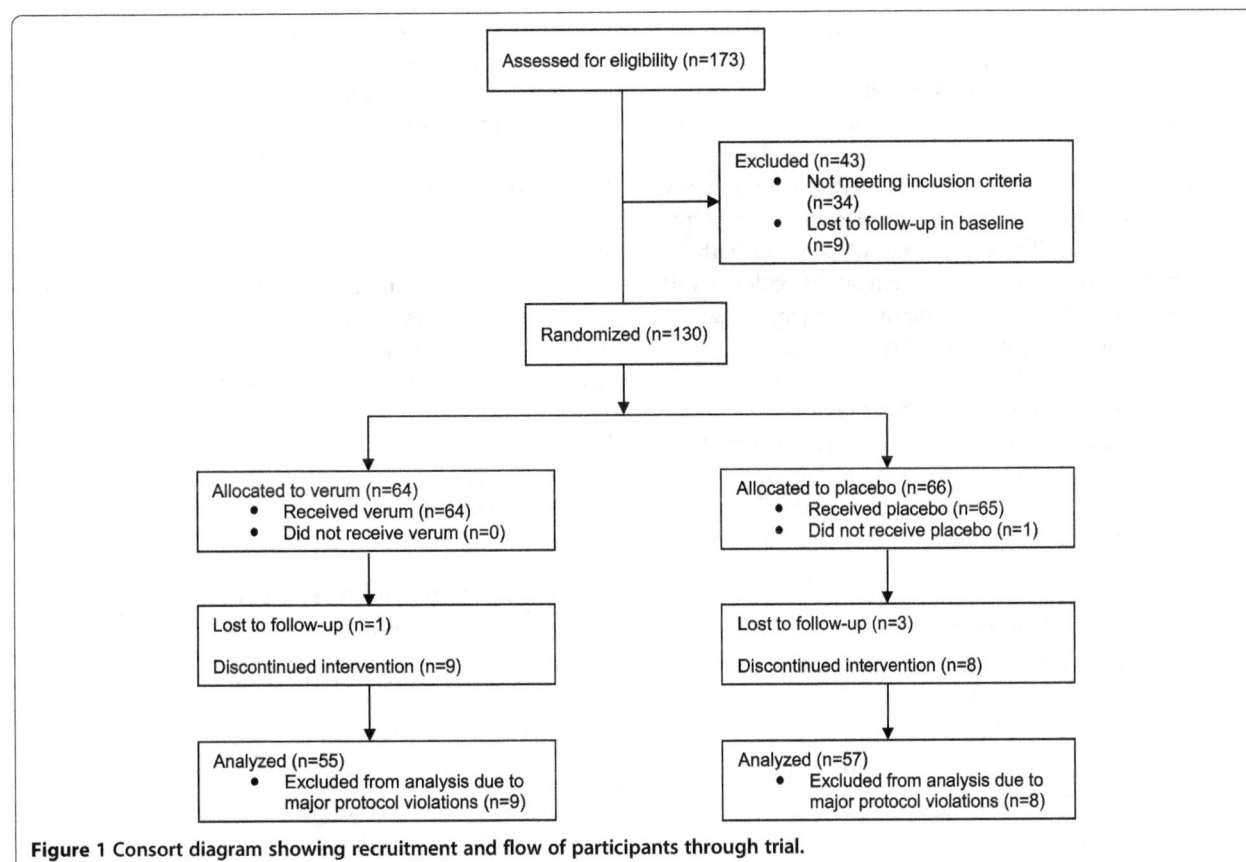

Figure 1 Consort diagram showing recruitment and flow of participants through trial.

Table 1 Baseline characteristics of evaluable participants

Characteristic	Verum	Placebo
	N = 55	N = 57
Female n (%)	48 (87.3)	49 (86.0)
Age y (SD)	40.4 (13.39)	36.4 (11.14)
BMI (SD)	23.16 (3.57)	23.17 (3.55)
Migraine type		
With aura n (%)	22 (40.0)	16 (28.1)
Without aura n (%)	28 (50.9)	37 (64.9)
Previous migraine prevention		
Participants with no previous preventions n (%)	40 (72.7)	36 (63.2)
Participants with 1-3 previous preventions n (%)	12 (21.8)	20 (35.0)
Participants with more than 3 previous preventions n (%)	3 (5.4)	1 (1.8)
Medical history, diseases n (%)	43 (42.1)	59 (57.8)
Concomitant medication n (%)	24 (36.3)	42 (63.6)

n denotes numbers, events or medication, respectively.

Reduction of migraine days

Active treatment was able to reduce the number of days with migraine from 6.2 days in the baseline-phase to 4.4 days after 3 month of treatment by 1.8 days (Table 2). However, this reduction of migraine days compared to placebo was not statistically significant (p = 0.23).

Maximal pain intensity per migraine day

Verum reduced the mean maximal pain intensity of a migraine day based on a 3-point-scale by 0.24 points at the end of the 3-month treatment. This reduction was statistically significant compared to placebo (0.06 points, p = 0.03) (Table 3). The percentage of patients with severe pain was lower and the percentage of patients with mild pain at the end of the 3-month treatment phase was higher in the active group compared to placebo.

HIT-6 Questionnaire (headache impact test)

Verum reduced the sum score of the HIT-6 questionnaire by 4.8 points (from 61.9 points at baseline to 57.1 points at the end of the 3-month treatment). This reduction was statistically significant compared to placebo

Table 3 Reduction of maximal pain per migraine day

Intensity (SD)	Verum	Placebo	P value
	N = 55	N = 57	
Baseline	2.71 (0.458)	2.70 (0.533)	-
Treatment 1st month	2.55 (0.503)	2.63 (0.620)	0.17
Treatment 2nd month	2.44 (0.572)	2.53 (0.630)	0.53
Treatment 3rd month	2.47 (0.639)	2.64 (0.520)	0.03
Patients (%)	**Verum**	**Placebo**	**P value**
	N = 55	N = 57	
Baseline			-
- mild	0 (0)	2 (3.5)	
- moderate	16 (29.1)	13 (22.8)	
- severe	39 (70.9)	42 (73.7)	
Treatment 3rd month			0.03
- mild	4 (7.3)	1 (1.8)	
- moderate	20 (36.4)	18 (31.6)	
- severe	29 (52.7)	37 (64.9)	

(p = 0.01). The reduction of HIT-6 sum scores in the placebo group was 2 points (from 61.9 points to 59.9).

Evaluation of efficacy by the patient

At the end of the 3-month treatment, the efficacy as evaluated by the patient was statistically significantly superior compared to placebo (p = 0.01) (Table 4). No patient in the placebo group rated the efficacy as very good, whereas 18% of the patients treated with verum rated the efficacy as very good. Nearly half of the patients in the placebo group rated the efficacy as poor (43.9%) compared to only 29.1% in the active treatment group.

Safety

Adverse events were classified by System Organ Class (SOC) and Preferred Term (PT) of the MedDRA-coding system. The safety population consisted of n = 63 patients in the verum group as well as in the placebo group. No serious adverse events (SAE) were observed in this trial. The incidence of adverse events (AE) was higher under active treatment (34 AE in 21 (33.3%) of 63 patients) compared to placebo (9 AE in 7 (11.1%) of 63 patients). All adverse events whose causal relationship to the study

Table 2 Reduction of migraine days

Days with migraine (SD)	Verum	Placebo	P value
	N = 55	N = 57	
Baseline	6.2 (1.95)	6.5 (1.78)	-
Treatment 1st month	5.0 (3.39)	5.7 (3.03)	0.37
Treatment 2nd month	4.8 (3.29)	5.5 (3.01)	0.39
Treatment 3rd month	4.4 (2.99)	5.2 (3.22)	0.23

Table 4 Evaluation of efficacy by patient

	Verum	Placebo	P value
	N = 55	N = 57	
Mean (SD)	2.6 (1.09)	3,2 (0.81)	0.01
very good n (%)	10 (18.2)	0 (0)	
good n (%)	16 (29.1)	14 (24.6)	
moderate n (%)	13 (23.6)	18 (31.6)	
poor n (%)	16 (29.1)	25 (43.9)	

treatment was assessed by the investigator as at least possibly related were classified as adverse reactions (AR). The incidence of adverse reactions was higher under active treatment (24 AR in 15 (23.8%) of 63 patients) compared to (3 AR in 3 (4.8%) of 63 patients). The two most frequent adverse reactions were gastrointestinal disorders (verum: 10 AR in 8 (12.7%) of 63 patients; placebo: 2 AR in 2 (3.2%) of 63 patients) mainly diarrhea and chromaturia (verum: 8 AR in 8 (12.7%) of 63 patients; placebo: 0 AR in 0 (0%) patients).

The majority of adverse reactions observed under active treatment were completely recovered before the end of the study (21 (87.5%) of 24 AR). While most adverse reactions (13 AR (54.2%)) did not lead to any action regarding the study treatment, 3 (12.5%) adverse reactions led to dose change, 6 (25%) adverse reactions to permanent discontinuation of the active treatment and 2 (8.3%) adverse reactions to another treatment.

Discussion

Drugs like metoprolol, propranolol, flunarizine, valproic acid or topiramate have been shown in clinical trials to be effective in reducing migraine symptoms when administered as prophylactic agents in episodic migraine [16-22]. All of these drugs have potential side effects, sometimes of severe nature. For this reason many patients look for a natural preventive treatment of migraine. In fact, some clinical trials have been performed with magnesium [23-29], riboflavin (vitamin B2) [30-35] or ubiquinone (ubichinon, coenzyme Q10) [36-38] mostly as single agents. One RCT used a combination of magnesium, riboflavin and the botanical feverfew [31] which revealed no advantage over the control group (intake of 25 mg riboflavin), most likely due to the fact that 25% - 38% of the patients in the verum and control group took concomitant migraine prophylaxis during the study. To the best of our knowledge, there is no report of a randomized, double-blind and controlled trial with a triple combination of magnesium, riboflavin and coenzyme Q10. It is interesting to note, that a pharmacogenomic study demonstrated the importance of the mitochondrial genetic background on response to riboflavin [39]. This underlines the role of the mitochondrion in migraine and the potential role of magnesium, coenzyme Q10 and riboflavin in alleviating migraine symptoms. It can also explain why certain patients are non-responders.

Baseline values were comparable between the treatment groups. The number of patients who used migraine prevention before study entry was slightly higher in the placebo group. The numbers are too small to be significant and to have had an impact on the primary endpoint. The same, to a slightly more extent is observed regarding medical history and concomitant medications. Since patients were allocated in a strict randomized fashion to both treatment arms this observation might be pure chance. It is not justified to suggest that patients in one group who seem to be slightly more ill than patients in the other group would show a difference in the prevention of migraine.

In this clinical trial, a combination of three natural nutritional substances, magnesium, riboflavin and Q10, was tested against placebo in the treatment of migraine in adult patients. Treatment for 3 months with this proprietary nutritional supplement was able to reduce the number of days with migraine by almost 2 days (1.8), which is considered to be a clinically relevant reduction. The reduction by placebo was 1.3 days. However, the reduction in migraine days was not statistically significant.

A very similar reduction was achieved in a randomized, placebo-controlled study (MIGR-003) with topiramate [19]. Migraine days were reduced by 1.8 days by topiramate 100 mg/day and by 1.1 days by placebo. This result was statistically significant (p = 0.026). However, the number of patients in the 100 mg topiramate arm was 139 compared to 55 in the arm of this trial with the nutritional supplement containing a fixed combination of magnesium, riboflavin and Q10. This suggests that the trial might have been underpowered with regard to the primary endpoint migraine days. The fact that the 200 mg topiramate arm in the MIGR-003 study did not reach statistical significance even with 143 patients (probably due to many early drop-outs) suggests that 55 patients are simply not enough to show statistical significance of any treatment in reducing migraine days.

Otherwise, the secondary endpoints that were analyzed in addition to the reduction of migraine days in this trial demonstrated a statistically significant benefit of the triple combination compared to placebo. Patients treated with verum had a statistically significantly greater reduction in the maximally experienced pain per migraine day compared to placebo (p = 0.03). In the verum group, 70.9% of the patients reported severe migraine pain prior to treatment. At the end of the treatment, only 52.7% had severe pain, 7.3% had mild pain. In the placebo group, 73.7% patients had severe pain in the baseline period, 64.9% patients had severe pain at the end of treatment and only 1.8% patients had mild pain.

The beneficial efficacy of verum was also shown by a statistically significant reduction in the score of the headache impact test questionnaire HIT-6 (p = 0.01). The sum score of the questionnaire was reduced in the active group after 3 months of treatment by a mean of 4.8 points. A primary care population of migraine patients was analyzed in the publication by Smelt. A within-person minimal important change (MIC) was established between -2.5 and -5.5 points depending on the statistical approach [40]. The within-person MIC is defined as the smallest change in the score which patients perceive as important. The reduction of -4.8 points in this trial is therefore a clinically relevant improvement which shows statistical significance compared to placebo. The HIT-6 questionnaire is a scale with 5 response options. The response options never (6 points), rarely (8 points) and always (13 points) are not represented in the study population because those patients were excluded from participation based on the inclusion and exclusion criteria. Therefore, sometimes (10 points) and very often (11 points) are left as the only possible answers for the study population, with only a 1-point difference between them. This 1-point difference in the questionnaire corresponds to a relevant difference in medical terms or in terms of disease burden/headache impact. A 4.8 point reduction translates into nearly 5 items (questions in the questionnaire) being improved from very often to sometimes. Smelt also established a between-group minimally important difference (MID) of -1.5 points [40]. Similar to the within-person MIC, the between-group MID is the smallest difference between scores of groups of patients that is considered important. The difference between the placebo group and the verum group was -2.8 points in this trial.

In agreement with the above result, the evaluation of efficacy of the preventive treatment was better for verum than for placebo. The difference was statistically significant (p = 0.01). 18.2% of the patients in the active group rated the efficacy as very good, none in the placebo group. Nearly 50% (47.3%) of the patients rated the efficacy "very good" or "good" which was twice as many as in the placebo group. Also, the number of patients rating efficacy as poor was higher in the placebo group.

These results indicate that the study preparation might have had an impact on the frequency of migraine days and improved clinically relevant prespecified secondary endpoints such as pain intensity, headache impact on life (HIT-6) and subjective evaluation of effectiveness.

The triple combination had a favorable adverse event profile. Adverse events usually observed with drugs like weight gain, depression, tiredness or dizziness were not observed.

A shortcoming is the possibility of unblinding patients in the verum group due to chromaturia. However, every patient was told at the beginning of the trial that a discoloration of the urin might appear in order to rule out that chromaturia would be associated with verum only. The only way to avoid this would have been to add riboflavin to placebo.

The strength of this study is the prospective, double-blind and placebo-controlled design. The study was powered to show a possible difference for the primary endpoint. The study used validated endpoints.

Conclusions

A fixed combination in a daily dose of 600 mg magnesium, 400 mg riboflavin and 150 mg Q10 in a proprietary nutritional supplement including also various low-dose multivitamins did not show statistically significant efficacy in the reduction of migraine days probably due to being underpowered. It did, however, prove to be superior for several secondary outcomes in the treatment of migraine. After 3 months of treatment with the supplement, a reduction of migraine pain and burden of disease was seen. Patients rated the efficacy of the treatment significantly superior to placebo. Adverse events associated with the supplement were mainly abdominal discomfort and diarrhea due to high amounts of magnesium. There were no serious adverse events reported in this trial.

Competing interests

CG has received honoraria for advisory boards, lectures or clinical studies (payment to the center) from Allergan, Berlin Chemie, MSD, elctroCore, St. Jude, Grünenthal, Bayer, Boehringer Ingelheim, ATI, and Hormosan. CG has no ownership interest and does not own stocks of any pharmaceutical company.

HCD received honoraria for participation in clinical trials, contribution to advisory boards or oral presentations from: Addex Pharma, Alder, Allergan, Almirall, Amgen, Autonomic Technology, AstraZeneca, Bayer Vital, Berlin Chemie, Böhringer Ingelheim, Bristol-Myers Squibb, Chordate, Coherex, CoLucid, Electrocore, GlaxoSmithKline, Grünenthal, Janssen-Cilag, Labrys Bioloogicals, Lilly, La Roche, 3 M Medica , Medtronic, Menerini, Minster, MSD, Neuroscore, Novartis, Johnson & Johnson, Pierre Fabre, Pfizer, Schaper and Brümmer, Sanofi, St. Jude and Weber & Weber. Financial support for research projects was provided by Allergan, Almirall, AstraZeneca, Bayer, Electrocore, GSK, Janssen-Cilag, MSD and Pfizer. Headache research at the Department of Neurology in Essen is supported by the German Research Council (DFG), the German Ministry of Education and Research (BMBF) and the European Union. H.C. Diener has no ownership interest and does not own stocks of any pharmaceutical company. Members of the Migravent Study Group: AP received honoraria for contribution to advisory boards or oral presentations from Novartis and Allergan. He has no ownership interest and does not own stocks of any pharmaceutical company. AS received honoraria for contribution to advisory boards, lectures or study participation from Allergan, Böhringer Ingelheim, Cerbromed, electroCore, Novatis, Hormosan. AS has no ownership interests and does hold stocks of Bayer/Germany). RS, HK, SU, MT-M, MW, SR, KOS, and WA declared non-competing interests.

UD is employed by the sponsor of the trial.

The sponsor of the trial is Weber & Weber Gmbh & Co.KG, Herrschinger Strasse 33, 82266 Inning.

Authors' contributions

The study was designed by UD together with CG and HCD, UD coordinated center recruitment, monitoring and statistical analysis. CG, HCD were principal investigators participating in the study and are authors of the manuscript together with UD. All authors read and approved the manuscript.

Acknowledgements

The authors gratefully acknowledge Dr. Merten Menke for data management and Holger Stammer and Christoph Glasmacher for statistical analysis. Marion Seybold assisted in project management.

Members of the study group (in order of the number of included patients)

Members of the Migravent Study Group (all sides are located in Germany) (patients recruited/randomized): Andreas Peikert, Bremen (21/14); Holger Kaube, München (20/16); Susanne Urban, Frankfurt a. M. (19/13); Walter Albrecht, Ellwangen (17/16); Rüdiger Schellenberg, Hüttenberg (13/12); Manuela Thinesse-Mallwitz, München (12/12); Andreas Straube, München (10/7); Stefan Ries, Erbach (10/5); Karl-Otto Sigel, Unterhaching (10/5); Martin L.J. Wimmer, München (6/5).

Author details

[1]Migraine and Headache Clinic, Königstein im Taunus, Germany.
[2]Department of Neurology, University Hospital Essen, Essen, Germany.
[3]Weber & Weber GmbH & Co.KG, Clinical Research, Inning, Germany.

References

1. Goadsby PJ, Lipton RB, Ferrari MD (2002) Migraine - current understanding and treatment. N Engl J Med 346:257–270

2. Silberstein SD, Holland S, Freitag F, Dodick DW, Argoff C, Ashman E (2012) Evidence-based guideline update: Pharmacologic treatment for episodic migraine prevention in adults: Report of the Quality Standards Subcommittee of the American Academy of Neurology and the American Headache Society. Neurology 78:1337–1345

3. Diener HC, Evers S, Förderreuther S, Freilinger T, Fritsche G, Gaul C, Göbel H, Haag G, Heinze A, Holle D, Jürgens T, Katsarava Z, Kropp P, Limmroth V, Malzacher R, Marziniak M, May A, Meier U, Obermann M, Ruschewya R, Straube A, Sandor P, Gantenbein A, Lampl C, Brössner G (2012) Therapie der Migräne. In: Diener HC, Weimar C, Berlit P, Deuschl G, Elger C, Gold R, Hacke W, Hufschmidt A, Mattle H, Meier U, Oertel WH, Reichmann H, Schmutzhard E, Wallesch C-W, Weller M (eds) Leitlinien für Diagnostik und Therapie in der Neurologie, 5th edn. Thieme, Stuttgart, pp 688–717

4. Tfelt-Hansen PC (2013) Evidence-based guideline update: pharmacologic treatment for episodic migraine prevention in adults: report of the Quality Standards subcommittee of the American Academy of Neurology and the American Headache Society. Neurology 26:869–870

5. Diener HC, Danesch U (2009) Wirksamkeit chemischer, pflanzlicher und diätetischer Migräneprophylaktika. MMW Fortschr Med 151:42–45

6. Gaul C, Eismann R, Schmidt T, May A, Leinisch E, Wieser T, Evers S, Henkel K, Franz G, Zierz S (2009) Use of complementary and alternative medicine in patients suffering from primary headache disorders. Cephalalgia 29:1069–1078

7. Hershey AD, Powers SW, Benntti AL, deGrauw TJ (1999) Chronic daily headaches (CDH) in children: characteristics and treatment response. Headache 39:358

8. Hershey AD, Powers SW, Vockell AL, Lecates SL, Ellinor PL, Segers A, Burdine D, Manning P, Kabbouche MA (2007) Coenzyme Q10 deficiency and response to supplementation in pediatric and adolescent migraine. Headache 47:73–80

9. Mauskop A, Altura BM (1998) Role of magnesium in the pathogenesis and treatment of migraines. Clin Neurosci 5:24–27

10. Sparaco M, Feleppa M, Lipton RB, Rapoport AM, Bigal ME (2006) Mitochondrial dysfunction and migraine: evidence and hypotheses. Cephalalgia 26:361–372

11. Lodi R, Iotti S, Cortelli P, Pierangeli G, Cevoli S, Clementi V, Soriani S, Montagna P, Barbiroli B (2001) Deficient energy metabolism is associated with low free magnesium in the brains of patients with migraine and cluster headache. Brain Res Bull 54:437–441

12. Bianchi A, Salomone S, Caraci F, Pizza V, Bernardini R, D'Amato CC (2004) Role of magnesium, coenzyme Q10, riboflavin, and vitamin B12 in migraine prophylaxis. Vitam Horm 69:297–312

13. Schellenberg R (2011) Mit bilanzierter Diät erfolgreich gegen die Migräne? Schmerztherapie 3:17

14. Headache Classification Subcommittee (2004) The international classification of headache disorders. 2nd edition. Cephalalgia 24(Suppl 1):1–160

15. Kosinski M, Bayliss MS, Bjorner JB, Ware JE Jr, Garber WH, Batenhorst A, Cady R, Dahlöf CG, Dowson A, Tepper S (2003) A six-item short-form survey for measuring headache impact: the HIT-6. Qual Life Res 12:963–974

16. Diener HC, Hartung E, Chrubasik J, Evers S, Schoenen J, Eikermann A, Latta G, Hauke W, Group S (2001) A comparative study of oral acetylsalicyclic acid and metoprolol for the prophylactic treatment of migraine. A randomized, controlled, double-blind, parallel group phase III study. Cephalalgia 21:120–128

17. Linde K, Rossnagel K (2004) Propranolol for migraine prophylaxis. Cochrane Database Syst Rev, Issue 2. Art. No.: CD003225. doi:10.1002/14651858. CD003225.pub2

18. Diener HC, Matias-Guiu J, Hartung E, Pfaffenrath V, Ludin HP, Nappi G, De Beukelaar F (2002) Efficacy and tolerability in migraine prophylaxis of flunarizine in reduced doses: a comparison with propranolol 160 mg daily. Cephalalgia 22:209–221

19. Diener HC, Tfelt-Hansen P, Dahlöf C, Láinez MJ, Sandrini G, Wang SJ, Neto W, Vijapurkar U, Doyle A, Jacobs D, MIGR-003 Study Group (2004) Topiramate in migraine prophylaxis–results from a placebo-controlled trial with propranolol as an active control. J Neurol 251:943–950

20. Linde M, Mulleners WM, Chronicle EP, McCrory DC (2013) Valproate (valproic acid or sodium valproate or a combination of the two) for the prophylaxis of episodic migraine in adults. Cochrane Database Syst Rev Issue 6. Art. No.: CD010611. doi:10.1002/14651858.CD010611

21. Silberstein SD, Neto W, Schmitt J, Jacobs D, MIGR-001 Study Group (2004) Topiramate in migraine prevention: results of a large controlled trial. Arch Neurol 61:490–495

22. Linde M, Mulleners WM, Chronicle EP, McCrory DC (2013) Topiramate for the prophylaxis of episodic migraine in adults. Cochrane Database Syst Rev Issue 6. Art. No.: CD010610. doi:10.1002/14651858.CD010610

23. Peikert A, Wilimzig C, Kohne-Volland R (1996) Prophylaxis of migraine with oral magnesium: results from a prospective, multi-center, placebo-controlled and double-blind randomized study. Cephalalgia 16:257–263

24. Taubert K (1994) Magnesium in migraine. Results of a multicentre pilot study. Fortschr Med 112:328–330

25. Köseoglu E, Talaslioglu A, Gönül AS, Kula M (2008) The effects of magnesium prophylaxis in migraine without aura. Magnes Res 21:101–108

26. Castelli S, Meossi C, Domenici R, Fontana F, Stefani G (1993) Magnesium in the prophylaxis of primary headache and other periodic disorders in children. Pediatr Med Chir 15:481–488

27. Facchinetti F, Sances G, Borella P, Genazzani AR, Nappi G (1991) Magnesium prophylaxis of menstrual migraine: effects on intracellular magnesium. Headache 31:298–301

28. Pfaffenrath V, Wessely P, Meyer C, Isler HR, Evers S, Grotemeyer KH, Taneri Z, Soyka D, Gobel H, Fischer M (1996) Magnesium in the prophylaxis of migraine–a double-blind placebo-controlled study. Cephalalgia 16:436–440

29. Wang F, Van Den Eeden SK, Ackerson LM, Salk SE, Reince RH, Elin RJ (2003) Oral magnesium oxide prophylaxis of frequent migrainous headache in children: a randomized, double-blind, placebo-controlled trial. Headache 43:601–610

30. Schoenen J, Jacquy J, Lenaerts M (1998) Effectiveness of high-dose riboflavin in migraine prophylaxis. A randomized controlled trial Neurology 50:466–470

31. Maizels M, Blumenfeld A, Burchette R (2004) A combination of riboflavin, magnesium, and feverfew for migraine prophylaxis: a randomized trial. Headache 44:885–890

32. Boehnke C, Reuter U, Flach U, Schuh-Hofer S, Einhäupl KM, Arnold G (2004) High-dose riboflavin treatment is efficacious in migraine prophylaxis: an open study in a tertiary care centre. Eur J Neurol 11:475–477

33. Schoenen J, Lenaerts M, Bastings E (1994) High-dose riboflavin as a prophylactic treatment of migraine: results of an open pilot study. Cephalalgia 14:328–329

34. Bruijn J, Duivenvoorden H, Passchier J, Locher H, Dijkstra N, Arts WF (2010) Medium-dose riboflavin as a prophylactic agent in children with migraine: a preliminary placebo-controlled, randomised, double-blind, cross-over trial. Cephalalgia 3012:1426–1434

35. MacLennan SC, Wade FM, Forrest KM, Ratanayake PD, Fagan E, Antony J (2008) High-dose riboflavin for migraine prophylaxis in children: a double-blind, randomized, placebo-controlled trial. J Child Neurol 23:1300–1304

36. Rozen TD, Oshinsky ML, Gebeline CA, Bradley KC, Young WB, Shechter AL, Silberstein SD (2002) Open label trial of coenzyme Q10 as a migraine preventive. Cephalalgia 22:137–141

37. Sándor PS, Di Clemente L, Coppola G, Saenger U, Fumal A, Magis D, Seidel L, Agosti RM, Schoenen J (2005) Efficacy of coenzyme Q10 in migraine prophylaxis: a randomized controlled trial. Neurology 64:713–715

38. Slater SK, Nelson TD, Kabbouche MA, LeCates SL, Horn P, Segers A, Manning P, Powers SW, Hershey AD (2011) A randomized, double-blinded, placebo-controlled, crossover, add-on study of CoEnzyme Q10 in the prevention of pediatric and adolescent migraine. Cephalalgia 31:897–905

39. Di Lorenzo C, Pierelli F, Coppola G, Grieco GS, Rengo C, Ciccolella M, Magis D, Bolla M, Casali C, Santorelli FM, Schoenen J (2009) Mitochondrial DNA haplogroups influence the therapeutic response to riboflavin in migraineurs. Neurology 72:1588–1594

40. Smelt AF, Assendelft WJ, Terwee CB, Ferrari MD, Blom JW (2014) What is a clinically relevant change on the HIT-6 questionnaire? An estimation in a primary-care population of migraine patients. Cephalalgia 34:29–36

22

OnabotulinumtoxinA for Hemicrania Continua: open label experience in 9 patients

Sarah Miller[1], Fernando Correia[1,2], Susie Lagrata[1] and Manjit S Matharu[1*]

Abstract

Background: Hemicrania continua is a strictly unilateral, continuous headache, typically mild to moderate in severity, with severe exacerbations commonly accompanied by cranial autonomic features and migrainous symptoms. It is exquisitely responsive to Indomethacin. However, some patients cannot tolerate treatment, often due to gastrointestinal side effects. Therapeutic alternatives are limited and controlled evidence lacking.

Methods: We present our experience of nine patients treated with OnabotulinumtoxinA for hemicrania continua. All patients were injected using the PREEMPT (Phase 3 REsearch Evaluating Migraine Prophylaxis Therapy) protocol for migraine.

Results: Five of nine patients demonstrated a 50% or more reduction in moderate to severe headache days with OnabotulinumtoxinA with a median reduction in moderate to severe headache days of 80%. Patient estimate of response was 80% or more in five subjects. The median and mean duration of response in the five responders was 11 and 12 weeks (range 6–20 weeks). Improvements were also seen in headache-associated disability

Conclusions: OnabotulinumtoxinA adds a potential option to the limited therapeutic alternatives available in hemicrania continua.

Keywords: Botulinum toxin-A; Hemicrania continua; Treatment; Indomethacin

Background

Hemicrania continua (HC) is a strictly unilateral, continuous headache that is exquisitely responsive to Indomethacin [1]. It is more prevalent in women and usually begins in adulthood [2,3]. The pain is typically of mild to moderate intensity and often involves the forehead, temporal, orbital and occipital regions [3]. Exacerbations of pain are seen in the majority and are commonly accompanied by cranial autonomic features and migrainous symptoms [2,3].

Hemicrania continua is, by definition, exquisitely responsive to Indomethacin [1]. Despite the efficacy of Indomethacin in HC, more than 30% of patients experience adverse effects and 20% have to discontinue the drug [4]. Finding possible therapeutic alternatives to Indomethacin is, thus, of great clinical relevance.

Several other drugs have been reported to be at least partially effective in open-label reports including:

* Correspondence: m.matharu@uclmail.net
[1]Headache Group, Institute of Neurology and The National Hospital for Neurology and Neurosurgery Queen Square, London WC1N 3BG, UK
Full list of author information is available at the end of the article

cyclooxygenase-2 inhibitors, aspirin, ibuprofen, naproxen, topiramate, melatonin, valproic acid, gabapentin, verapamil and methylprednisolone. Other options are greater occipital nerve blocks (GONB) and neuromodulation. However, none appear to be as effective as Indomethacin.

Even though the exact mechanism of action of OnabotulinumtoxinA (BoNT-A) remains unclear, it is thought to involve multiple mechanisms. Theories include inhibition of neurotransmitter release from motor and sensory nociceptive neurons resulting in interruption of the inflammatory loop promoting peripheral and central sensitization or direct inhibition of central sensitization in the CNS, via axonal transport [5].

The efficacy of BoNT-A in chronic migraine prophylaxis is now well established [6]. Experience in trigeminal autonomic cephalalgias (TACs) is scarce; experience in 14 cluster headache and one Short-lasting Unilateral Neuralgiform Headache with Conjunctival Injection and Tearing (SUNCT) patients have been published [7-11]. In HC, there are two single subject case reports on the use of BoNT-A [12,13]. In the first case, painless autonomic attacks continued, whereas in the second case, autonomic features fully resolved. In this open label study we examine the outcome of nine patients undergoing BoNT-A treatment for HC.

Methods

Patients receiving BoNT-A with the Headache Group at the National Hospital for Neurology and Neurosurgery were analyzed. Patients were diagnosed with HC in accordance to International Classification of Headache Disorder criteria (ICHD-3beta) [1]. All had unilateral headaches that had responded fully to an indomethacin trial (oral or intramuscular trials, detailed in Table 1). All patients were injected with BoNT-A as per the Phase 3 REsearch Evaluating Migraine Prophylaxis Therapy (PREEMPT) regime for chronic migraine, with patients having a modified regime (exclusion of occipital and cervical paraspinal sites) if they had an occipital nerve stimulator (ONS) in situ [6].

All data was collected prospectively with the use of headache diaries. Average monthly scores were calculated from a month pre-treatment and a three-month post-final treatment diary. Headache days were recorded as any day on which the subject recorded HC pain. Subjects were asked to score pain intensity on two scales: 1) pain free, mild, moderate and severe; and 2) verbal rating scale (VRS). Headache load (HAL) was calculated from diaries using the formula: Σ (severity (VRS) × pain duration (hours). Disability scores consisting of Headache Impact Test (HIT-6), Migraine Disability Assessment (MIDAS) and Hospital Anxiety and Depression scale (HAD) were collected before and after treatment.

Responders to treatment were classified as those achieving a 50% or greater improvement in headache days rated as moderate to severe. Other outcomes included those achieving a 30% and 50% or greater improvement in HAL and 30% or more improvement in headache days rated as moderate to severe.

Median values pre- and post-treatment were compared using Wilcoxon Signed Ranks tests and a statistically significant result set at the 95% level ($p = 0.05$). Data was processed using IBM SPSS Version 22 for Windows.

The study was approved by Northwick Park Hospital Research Ethics Committee, Hampstead, London, and written consent obtained from all patients.

Results

A total of nine patients with HC received treatment with BoNT-A, of whom six were females and three males (see Table 1). Median age at time of treatment was 48 years (19–61 years) and median duration of HC was 8 years (1–34 years). During exacerbations, migrainous features were present in six and autonomic features in all subjects. Three patients reported visual auras during exacerbations.

Four patients had concomitant episodic migraine (EM) and one co-existent idiopathic stabbing headache. All patients were able to differentiate their co-existent headaches from HC and none of the co-existent headaches had responded to indomethacin trials.

Subjects had failed to respond to a median of seven previous treatments for HC. Two subjects had failed to respond to ONS and one was awaiting ONS implantation.

Reasons for treatment with BoNT-A are summarized in Table 1. Eight patients could not tolerate therapeutic doses of indomethacin due to gastro-intestinal (GI) side effects. Two patients complained of worsening of their EM with indomethacin doses required to suppress HC. Patients had a median of two treatments (range 2–6) with a median BoNT-A dose of 167 units (range 110–185 units) injected at each treatment.

The results of BoNT-A treatment are summarized in Table 2. Five subjects demonstrated a response of 50% or more in reduction of moderate or severe headache days to mild headache days or pain free and were classified as responders to treatment. Six subjects reported a 30% or greater response in reduction of moderate or severe headache days to mild headache days or pain free. The median reduction in total headache days was 90% (range 0–100) ($p = 0.026$) and in moderate to severe headache days 80% (range 0–100) ($p = 0.012$). Headache load showed a median improvement of 62% (range 0–100) with six patients demonstrating a 30% and 50% or more improvement. Significant improvements were also seen in average headache hours and average VRS (Table 2). The median subjective duration of response in the five responders post treatment was 11 weeks (range 6–20 weeks, mean 12 weeks). Five subjects reported a subjective benefit of 80% or more in their HC.

Four subjects were taking indomethacin prior to BoNT-A and all were able to stop regular use after treatment with two using indomethacin as required at a frequency of less than three times a month.

Headache disability scores showed a trend to improvement after BoNT-A (Table 3). HIT-6 showed a median change of 12 points ($p = 0.069$). This is above the three-point change suggestive of minimal clinical difference. MIDAS improved by a median of 51 points ($p = 0.063$).

Adverse events were reported in three subjects: one eyebrow ptosis, one frontalis over-activity and one transient worsening in headache before improvement was noted. All adverse events were rated as mild by patients and transient in nature.

Discussion

This series is the largest so far of BoNT-A treatment for HC. Five out of nine patients showed a greater than 50% reduction in moderate or severe headache days to mild headache days or pain free with a median reduction in

Table 1 Demographic details of patients and treatment

	Sex	Age at treatment (years)	Duration of HC at treatment (years)	Phenotype of HC			Indomethacin dose required to suppress HC	Co-existent headache	Previous number of treatments trialled	Reasons for administering BoNT-A	No of sessions of BoNT-A treatments	Average units injected
				Location	Autonomic symptoms*	Migrainous symptoms†						
1	M	19	1	Right	Yes	Nil	225 mg daily	EMWOA (Bilateral)	4	Worsening EM on Indometacin	4	168
2	F	61	1	Left	Yes	Yes Visual Aura	150 mg daily	Nil	4	GI-upset	3	165
3	M	59	12	Right	Yes	Nil	IM Indometacin test**	Nil	13	Unable tolerate Indometacin; Refractory to other treatments; ONS in-situ	2	175
4	M	48	2	Right	Yes	Yes Visual Aura (occasional)	150 mg daily	EMWA (bilateral, once month)	9	GI-upset; peptic ulcer disease; refractory to other treatments - awaiting ONS	2	165
5	F	47	9	Right	Yes	Yes	225 mg daily	Past EMWOA (stopped 2004)	3	GI-upset	5	167
6	F	49	34	Right	Yes	Yes	150 mg daily	EMWA (bilateral, once month)	6	GI-upset; refractory to other treatments; ONS in-situ	2	110
7	F	48	18	Left	Yes	Yes	IM Indometacin test**	ISH	13	GI-upset	2	155
8	F	41	8	Right	Yes	No Visual Aura	150 mg daily	EMWOA (side variable/bilateral)	7	GI-upset; wheeze; dizziness; worsening EM	6	168
9	F	54	4	Right	Yes	Yes	225 mg daily	Nil	9	GI-upset	2	185
Mean		**47**	**10**						**8**		**3**	**162**
Median (Range)		48 (19–61)	8 (1–34)						7 (3–13)		2 (2–6)	167 (110–185)

M, Male; F, Female; HC, Hemicrania continua; EMWA, Episodic migraine with aura; EMWOA, Episodic migraine without aura ISH, Idiopathic stabbing headache; BoNT-A, Onabotulinumtoxin A; GI, Gastrointenstinal; ONS, Occipital nerve stimulator; IQR, Inter-quartile range; *Autonomic symptoms including ptosis, lacrimation, conjunctival injection, meiosis, nasal blockage, rhinorrhea, facial redness, facial sweating, eyelid oedema, restlessness; †Migrainous symptoms including nausea, vomiting, photophobia, phonophobia, osmophobia, motion sensitivity; **IM Indometacin test blinded placebo test of 100 mg IM Indometacin v normal saline.

Table 2 Headache scores pre- and post- treatment with OnabotulinumtoxinA

ID	Average headache days/month			Average moderate -severe days/month*			Average daily headache hours			Average daily VRS			Change in headache load (%)	Subjective estimate of response	Estimated duration of response (weeks)
	Pre	Post	Change %	Pre	Post	Change %	Pre	Post	Change %	Pre	Post	Change %			
1	30	0	100	20	0	100	24	0	100	5	0	100	100	>90%	16
2	30	0	100	15	0	100	24	0	100	5	0	100	100	>90%	20
3	30	30	0	30	19	37	24	24	0	8	6	25	20	30-50%	5
4	30	30	0	30	30	0	24	24	0	7	6	14	0	0	0
5	30	3	90	30	3	90	24	6	75	7	10	0	98	80-90%	12
6	30	30	0	30	23	23	15	16	0	7	6	14	0	15-25%	4
7	30	22	27	21	13	27	24	7	71	7	4	43	55	40%	6
8	30	2	93	30	0	100	24	8	67	9	2	78	99	80-90%	6
9	30	0	100	30	0	100	24	0	100	8	0	100	100	>90%	9
Mean	**30**	**13**	**57**	**25**	**10**	**64**	**23**	**9**	**57**	**7**	**4**	**51**	**62**		**8**
Median (Range)	**30 (30)**	**3 (0–30)**	**90 (0–100)**	**30 (15–30)**	**3 (0–30)**	**80 (0–100)**	**24 (15–24)**	**7 (0–24)**	**71 (0–100)**	**7 (5–9)**	**4 (0–10)**	**43 (0–100)**	**98 (0–100)**		**6 (0–20)**

*Response defined as 50% or more improvement in average moderate-severe headache days/month; VRS, Verbal Rating Scale; Pre, Pre-treatment; Post, Post-final treatment.

Table 3 Headache-associated disability scores pre- and post- treatment with OnabotulinumtoxinA

ID	HIT-6			MIDAS			HAD-A			HAD-D		
	Pre	Post	Change in score	Pre	Post	Change in score	Pre	Post	Change in score	Pre	Post	Change in score
1	65	58	7	73	0	73	10	8	2	9	3	6
2	57	36	21	24	0	24	1	0	1	0	0	0
3	56	68	-12	52	52	0	3	9	-6	2	12	-10
4	68	67	1	105	130	-25	12	6	6	10	8	2
5	67	44	23	120	0	120	9	2	7	9	1	8
6	63	60	3	121	13	108	16	18	-2	15	15	0
7	63	54	9	24	13	9	2	3	-1	5	7	-2
8	64	62	2	240	4	236	0	0	0	3	0	3
9	76	24	52	51	0	51	12	0	12	4	0	4
Mean	**64**	**53**	**12**	**90**	**24**	**66**	**7**	**5**	**2**	**6**	**5**	**1**
Median (Range)	**64 (56–76)**	**58 (24–68)**	**7 (–12 to 52)**	**73 (24–240)**	**4 (0–130)**	**51 (–25 to 236)**	**9 (0–16)**	**3 (0–18)**	**1 (–6 to 12)**	**5 (0–15)**	**3 (0–15)**	**2 (–10 to 8)**

HIT-6, Headache Impact Test; MIDAS, Migraine Disability Assessment; HAD-A, Hospital Anxiety and Depression scale (Anxiety); HAD-D, Hospital Anxiety and Depression Scale (Depression); Pre, Pre-treatment; Post, Post-final treatment.

moderate and severe days of 80%. All four subjects taking daily indomethacin prior to treatment were able to stop regular use. Five patients reporting an 80% or more improvement in their HC and clinically significant improvements were seen in both HIT-6 and MIDAS.

The patient group had tried a median of seven previous preventatives and had suffered from HC for a median of 8 years at the time of BoNT-A treatment. The refractory nature of the group means that it is doubtful that our observations are due to spontaneous remission. Despite four patients reporting co-existing episodic migraine, all were clearly able to differentiate this from their HC. The phenotype of HC was secure in all subjects and all meet ICHD-3beta criteria including a complete response of their side-locked headache to an adequate indometacin trial. Although a number of subjects report migrainous symptoms associated with HC, this is an accepted feature commented on in epidemiological studies and the ICHD-3beta criteria [1,3]. Given that all patients were carefully phenotyped and could clearly differentiate their episodic migraine attacks from hemicrania continua taken together with the sparse evidence for the efficacy of botulinum toxin in episodic migraine, our data are consistent with a change in HC and not the co-existent episodic migraine.

This series is still small, and this must be considered when interpreting the results. Previous studies of BoNT-A have reported a significant placebo response and we cannot eliminate this as a potential confounding factor in our outcomes. However, the relatively high response rates taken together with the consistent efficacy of repeated BoNT-A injections and a mean duration of effect similar to that seen in other reports in TAC as well as chronic migraine suggest that the response to BoNT-A in this series cannot be attributed entirely to the placebo response [10,12,13].

The exact mechanisms by which BoNT-A produces therapeutic benefit remains unclear, but the neurotoxin is likely to function by multiple mechanisms, suppressing events associated with peripheral and central sensitization. Both migraine and TACs are believed to share a common pathophysiology comprising of the activation of the trigeminovascular system and involvement of neuroactive peptides such as calcitonin gene-related peptide (CGRP), vasoactive peptide (VIP) and glutamate [14]. Animal studies have provided evidence of BoNT-A suppressing nociception in peripheral trigeminovascular neurons and also suppressing CGRP and VIP release from these neurons [5] There is also data to support the hypothesis that the toxin may act via central mechanisms with studies showing retrograde axonal transport of active BoNT-A [15,16]. The potential target of BoNT-A in chronic migraine is the direct blockage of trigeminal neurons providing nociception to the head and face. Suppression of neuro-inflammatory mediator release leads to decreased activation of second-order neurons within the trigemino-cervical complex and brainstem. BoNT-A may therefore be assumed to exert its benefit by repressing the neuro-inflammatory mediators responsible for the maintenance of peripheral and central sensitization [17,18]. It is therefore possible that BoNT-A has a wider therapeutic potential than chronic migraine. It is interesting to speculate that the clinical and functional imaging similarities between migraine and HC may mean that BoNT-A has more of an impact in HC than the other TACs which are much more clinically distinct to migraine [19].

Conclusion

OnabotulinumtoxinA may be a promising alternative to Indomethacin in patients with HC who do not tolerate the drug. Treatment appears to be associated with a significant improvement in moderate to severe headache days and related disability. It may add another potential therapeutic agent for HC to the limited number available. However, further controlled studies are necessary to clarify the efficacy of BoNT-A in HC.

Competing interests

SM has received educational grants from St Jude Medical and Medtronic and has received payment for educational presentations from Allergan. FC has no competing interests. SL has received payment for educational sessions from Allergan. MSM serves on the advisory board for Allergan and St Jude Medical, and has received payment for the development of educational presentations from Allergan, Merck Sharpe and Dohme Ltd and Medtronic.

Authors' contributions

SM carried out data collection and analysis and drafted the manuscript. FC helped to collect data and draft the manuscript. SL carried out data collection and helped to draft the manuscript. MSM conceived the study, phenotyped the patients and participated in data collection and interpretation and revising the manuscript. All authors read and approved the final manuscript.

Author details

[1]Headache Group, Institute of Neurology and The National Hospital for Neurology and Neurosurgery Queen Square, London WC1N 3BG, UK.
[2]Department of Neurology, Centro Hospitalar do Porto, Oporto, Portugal.

References

1. Headache Classification Committee of the International Headache S (2013) The International Classification of Headache Disorders, 3rd edition (beta version). Cephalalgia 33(9):629–808, PubMed
2. Peres MF, Silberstein SD, Nahmias S, Shechter AL, Youssef I, Rozen TD et al (2001) Hemicrania continua is not that rare. Neurology 25(6):948–951, PubMed
3. Cittadini E, Goadsby PJ (2010) Hemicrania continua: a clinical study of 39 patients with diagnostic implications. Brain 133(Pt 7):1973–1986, PubMed Epub 2010/06/19. eng
4. Dodick DW (2004) Indomethacin-responsive headache syndromes. Curr Pain Headache Rep 8(1):19–26, PubMed
5. Durham PL, Cady R (2011) Insights into the mechanism of onabotulinumtoxinA in chronic migraine. Headache 51(10):1573–1577, PubMed Pubmed Central PMCID: 3306767. Epub 2011/11/16. eng
6. Dodick DW, Turkel CC, DeGryse RE, Aurora SK, Silberstein SD, Lipton RB et al (2010) OnabotulinumtoxinA for treatment of chronic migraine: pooled results from the double-blind, randomized, placebo-controlled phases of the PREEMPT clinical program. Headache 50(6):921–936, PubMed Epub 2010/05/22. eng

7.   Robbins L (2001) Botulinum Toxin A (Botox) for cluster headache: 6 cases. Cephalalgia 21:492–503
8.   Smuts JA, Barnard PWA (2000) Botulinum toxin type A in the treatment of headache syndromes: a clinical report on 79 patients. Cephalalgia 20:332–337
9.   Sostak P, Krause P, Forderreuther S, Reinisch V, Straube A (2007) Botulinum toxin type-A therapy in cluster headache: an open study. J Headache Pain 8 (4):236–241, PubMed Epub 2007/09/29. eng
10. Freund BJ, Schwartz M (2000) The use of Botulinum toxin-A in the treatment of refractory cluster headache: case reports. Cephalalgia 20:235–331
11. Zabalza RJ (2012) Sustained response to botulinum toxin in SUNCT syndrome. Cephalalgia 32(11):869–872, PubMed Epub 2012/06/27. eng
12. Garza I, Cutrer FM (2010) Pain relief and persistence of dysautonomic features in a patient with hemicrania continua responsive to botulinum toxin type A. Cephalalgia 30(4):500–503, PubMed Epub 2009/06/12. eng
13. Khalil M, Ahmed F (2013) Hemicrania continua responsive to botulinum toxin type a: a case report. Headache 53(5):831–833, PubMed Epub 2013/03/29. eng
14. May A, Goadsby PJ (1999) The trigeminovascular system in humans: pathophysiologic implications for primary headache syndromes of the neural influences on the cerebral circulation. J Cereb Blood Flow Metab 19(2):115–127, PubMed Epub 1999/02/23. eng
15. Matak I, Bach-Rojecky L, Filipovic B, Lackovic Z (2011) Behavioral and immunohistochemical evidence for central antinociceptive activity of botulinum toxin A. Neuroscience 186:201–207
16. Meng J, Ovsepian SV, Wang J, Pickering M, Sasse A, Aoki KR et al (2009) Activation of TRPV1 mediates calcitonin gene-related peptide release, which excites trigeminal sensory neurons and is attenuated by a retargeted botulinum toxin with anti-nociceptive potential. J Neurosci 29(15):4981–4992
17. Aoki KR (2003) Evidence for antinociceptive activity of botulinum toxin type A in pain management. Headache 43(Suppl 1):S9–S15
18. Seybold VS (2009) The role of peptides in central sensitization. Handb Exp Pharmacol 194:451–491
19. Matharu MS, Cohen AS, McGonigle DJ, Ward N, Frackowiak RS, Goadsby PJ (2004) Posterior hypothalamic and brainstem activation in hemicrania continua. Headache 44(8):747–761, PubMed Epub 2004/08/28. eng

Permissions

The contributors of this book come from diverse backgrounds, making this book a truly international effort. This book will bring forth new frontiers with its revolutionizing research information and detailed analysis of the nascent developments around the world.

We would like to thank all the contributing authors for lending their expertise to make the book truly unique. They have played a crucial role in the development of this book. Without their invaluable contributions this book wouldn't have been possible. They have made vital efforts to compile up to date information on the varied aspects of this subject to make this book a valuable addition to the collection of many professionals and students.

This book was conceptualized with the vision of imparting up-to-date information and advanced data in this field. To ensure the same, a matchless editorial board was set up. Every individual on the board went through rigorous rounds of assessment to prove their worth. After which they invested a large part of their time researching and compiling the most relevant data for our readers.

The editorial board has been involved in producing this book since its inception. They have spent rigorous hours researching and exploring the diverse topics which have resulted in the successful publishing of this book. They have passed on their knowledge of decades through this book. To expedite this challenging task, the publisher supported the team at every step. A small team of assistant editors was also appointed to further simplify the editing procedure and attain best results for the readers.

Apart from the editorial board, the designing team has also invested a significant amount of their time in understanding the subject and creating the most relevant covers. They scrutinized every image to scout for the most suitable representation of the subject and create an appropriate cover for the book.

The publishing team has been an ardent support to the editorial, designing and production team. Their endless efforts to recruit the best for this project, has resulted in the accomplishment of this book. They are a veteran in the field of academics and their pool of knowledge is as vast as their experience in printing. Their expertise and guidance has proved useful at every step. Their uncompromising quality standards have made this book an exceptional effort. Their encouragement from time to time has been an inspiration for everyone.

The publisher and the editorial board hope that this book will prove to be a valuable piece of knowledge for researchers, students, practitioners and scholars across the globe.

List of Contributors

Sabina Cevoli
IRCCS Institute of Neurological Sciences of Bologna, UOC Clinica Neurologica, Bellaria Hospital, Via Altura 3, 40139 Bologna, Italy

Giulia Giannini, Valentina Favoni, Rossana Terlizzi, Giulia Pierangeli and Pietro Cortelli
IRCCS Institute of Neurological Sciences of Bologna, UOC Clinica Neurologica, Bellaria Hospital, Via Altura 3, 40139 Bologna, Italy
Department of Biomedical and NeuroMotor Sciences (DiBiNeM), Alma Mater Studiorum - University of Bologna Italy, Bologna, Italy

Elisa Sancisi
Neurology, AUSL (Local Health Service) of Ferrara, Ferrara, Italy

Marianna Nicodemo
Division of Neurology, Maggiore Hospital, IRCCS Institute of Neurological Sciences of Bologna, Bologna, Italy

Stefano Zanigni
Functional MR Unit, Policlinico S.Orsola-Malpighi, Bologna, Italy
Department of Biomedical and NeuroMotor Sciences (DiBiNeM), Alma Mater Studiorum - University of Bologna Italy, Bologna, Italy

Maria Letizia Bacchi Reggiani
Department of Experimental, Diagnostic and Specialty Medicine (DIMES), Alma Mater Studiorum, University of Bologna, Bologna, Italy

Jacob Edvinsson and Lars Edvinsson
Department of Medicine, Lund University, Lund, Sweden

Karin Warfvinge
Department of Clinical Experimental Research, Glostrup Research Institute, Glostrup Hospital, Glostrup, Denmark
Department of Medicine, Lund University, Lund, Sweden

Lars Neeb, Ulrich Dirnagl and Uwe Reuter
Department of Neurology and Experimental Neurology, Charité Universitätsmedizin Berlin, Charitéplatz 1, 10117 Berlin, Germany

Peter Hellen
Department of Neuroradiology, Universitätsmedizin Göttingen, Robert-Koch-Straße 40, 37075 Göttingen, Germany

Jan Hoffmann
Department of Systems Neuroscience, University Medical Center Hamburg-Eppendorf, Martinistrasse 52, D-20246 Hamburg, Germany
Department of Neurology and Experimental Neurology, Charité Universitätsmedizin Berlin, Charitéplatz 1, 10117 Berlin, Germany

Yuanchao Li, Qin Zhang, Dandan Qi, Li Zhang, Lian Yi, Qianqian Li and Zhongling Zhang
Department of Neurology, The First Affiliated Hospital of Harbin Medical University, No. 23 Youzheng Road, Harbin 150001, People's Republic of China

Saras Menon, Bushra Nasir, Nesli Avgan, Rodney Lea and Lyn Griffiths
Genomics Research Centre, Institute of Health and Biomedical Innovation, Queensland University of Technology, Kelvin Grove, QLD, Australia

Maree Smith and Sussan Ghassabian
Centre for Integrated Preclinical Drug Development Faculty of Medicine and Biomedical Sciences, University of Queensland, Brisbane, QLD, Australia

Christopher Oliver
Blackmores Institute, 20 Jubilee Avenue, Warriewood NSW 2102, Australia

Pietro Cortelli and Giulia Pierangeli
Department of Biomedical and Neuromotor Sciences DIBINEM, University of Bologna, Bologna, Italy
Padiglione G, Bellaria Hospital, IRCCS Institute of Neurological Sciences of Bologna, Via Altura 3, 40139 Bologna, Italy

Luana Lazzerini
Service for the Diagnosis and Treatment of Eating Disorders, Service for the Diagnosis and Treatment of Anxiety and Psychosomatic Disorders, Centro Gruber, Bologna, Italy

Marialuisa Rausa
Service for the Diagnosis and Treatment of Eating Disorders, Service for the Diagnosis and Treatment of Anxiety and Psychosomatic Disorders, Centro Gruber, Bologna, Italy
Department of Biomedical and Neuromotor Sciences DIBINEM, University of Bologna, Bologna, Italy

Daniela Palomba
Department of General Psychology, University of Padova, Padova, Italy
Service for the Diagnosis and Treatment of Eating Disorders, Service for the Diagnosis and Treatment of Anxiety and Psychosomatic Disorders, Centro Gruber, Bologna, Italy

Sabina Cevoli
Padiglione G, Bellaria Hospital, IRCCS Institute of Neurological Sciences of Bologna, Via Altura 3, 40139 Bologna, Italy

Elisa Sancisi
Neurology, AUSL (Local Health Service) of Ferrara, Ferrara, Italy

Clinton Lauritsen and Santiago Mazuera
Department of Neurology, Thomas Jefferson University, Jefferson Headache Center, Philadelphia, PA, USA

Richard B. Lipton
Department of Neurology, Montefiore Headache Center, Albert Einstein College of Medicine, Bronx, NY, USA

Sait Ashina
Department of Neurology, New York University School of Medicine, NYU Langone Medical Center, NYU Lutheran Headache Center, New York, NY, USA

Haiyang Xu, Wei Han, Jinghua Wang and Mingxian Li
The First hospital of Jilin University, No. 71 Xinmin Street, Changchun 130021, Jilin, China

Mengqi Liu, Shuangfeng Liu and Lin Ma
Department of Radiology, Chinese PLA General Hospital, 28 Fuxing Road, Beijing 100853, China

Zhiye Chen
Department of Radiology, Chinese PLA General Hospital, 28 Fuxing Road, Beijing 100853, China
Department of Neurology, Chinese PLA General Hospital, 28 Fuxing Road, Beijing 100853, China

Xiaoyan Chen and Shengyuan Yu
Department of Neurology, Chinese PLA General Hospital, 28 Fuxing Road, Beijing 100853, China

Roger K. Cady, Ryan J. Cady and Heather R. Manley
Clinvest/A Division of Banyan Inc., 3805 S Kansas Expy, Springfield, MO 65807, USA

Elimor Brand-Schieber and Sagar Munjal
Dr. Reddy's Laboratories Ltd., 107 College Road East, Princeton, NJ 08540, USA

Aijie He
Department of Neurosurgery, the Affiliated Yantai Yuhuangding Hospital of Qingdao University, 264000 Yantai, Shandong, China

Dehua Song
Department of Radiotherapy, the Affiliated Yantai Yuhuangding Hospital of Qingdao University, 264000 Yantai, Shandong, China

Lei Zhang
Department of Pharmacy, Yantai Hospital of Traditional Chinese Medicine, 264000 Yantai, Shandong, China

Chen Li
Department of Anesthesia, Yantai Hospital of Traditional Chinese Medicine, No. 39 Xingfu Road, Zhifu Disctrict, 264000 Yantai, Shandong, China

Elif Ilgaz Aydinlar, Pinar Yalinay Dikmen, Seda Kosak and Ayse Sagduyu Kocaman
Department of Neurology, Acibadem University School of Medicine, Içerenkoy, Kayisdagi Cd, 34752 Atasehir/Istanbul, Turkey

Licia Grazzi and Domenico D'Amico
Neurological Institute "C. Besta" IRCCS Foundation, Headache and Neuroalgology Unit, Via Celoria 11, 20133 Milan, Italy

Laura De Torres, Matilde Leonardi, Emanuela Sansone and Alberto Raggi
Neurological Institute "C. Besta" IRCCS Foundation, Neurology, Public Health and Disability Unit, Milan, Italy

Andrea De Giorgio
eCampus University, Faculty of Psychology, Novedrate, Italy

Francisco Salgado-García and Frank Andrasik
Department of Psychology, Univeristy of Memphis, Memphis, TN, USA

Danièle Ranoux and François Caire
Department of Neurosurgery, Centre Hospitalier Universitaire de Limoges, Limoges, France

Gaelle Martiné and Gaëlle Espagne-Dubreuilh
Pain Center, Centre Hospitalier Universitaire de Limoges, Limoges, France

Marlène Amilhaud-Bordier
Pain Center, Centre Hospitalier de Guéret, Guéret, France

Laurent Magy
Department of Neurology, Centre Hospitalier Universitaire de Limoges, Limoges, France

Julia M. Hebestreit and Arne May
Department of Systems Neuroscience, Center for Experimental Medicine, University Medical Center Eppendorf, Martinistr. 52, 20246 Hamburg, Germany

Juana Marin
Wellcome Foundation Building, King's College Hospital, London SE5 9PJ, UK

Nicola Giffin
Royal United Hospital, Coombe Park, Bath BA1 3NG, UK

Elizabeth Consiglio
Interface Clinical Services, Gate Way Drive, Yeadon, Leeds LS19 7XY, UK

Candace McClure
North American Science Associates, Inc., 400 US-169, Minneapolis, MN 55441, USA

Eric Liebler
electroCore, Inc., 150 Allen Road, Suite 201, Basking Ridge, NJ 07920, USA

Brendan Davies
University Hospitals of North Midlands, Newcastle Road, Stoke-on-Trent ST4 6QG, UK

Jasem Y. Al-Hashel
Department of Neurology, Ibn Sina Hospital, Safat, 13115 Kuwait City, Kuwait
Department of Medicine, Faculty of Medicine, Health Sciences Centre, Kuwait University, Kuwait City, Kuwait

Samar Farouk Ahmed
Department of Neurology and Psychiatry, Al-Minia University, Minia, Egypt
Department of Neurology, Ibn Sina Hospital, Safat, 13115 Kuwait City, Kuwait

Fatemah J Alshawaf
Mubarak Al- Kabeer Hospital, Jabriya, Hawalli, Kuwait

Raed Alroughani
Division of Neurology, Amiri Hospital, Qurtoba, 73767 Kuwait City, Kuwait

Stefanie Förderreuther
Department of Neurology, Ludwig Maximilian University, Munich, Bavaria, Germany

Qi Zhang
Sanofi, Bridgewater, NJ, USA

Virginia L. Stauffer and Sheena K. Aurora
Eli Lilly and Company, Lilly Corporate Center, Indianapolis, IN 46285, USA

Miguel J. A. Láinez
Hospital Clínico Universitario, Universidad Católica de Valencia, Valencia, Spain

Andreas Straube, O. Eren, B. Blum and R. Ruscheweyh
Klinik und Poliklinik für Neurologie, Oberbayerisches Kopfschmerzzentrum, Klinikum Großhadern, Ludwig-Maximilians-Universität München, Marchioninistr. 15, 81377 Munich, Germany

J. Ellrich
Department of Health Science and Technology, Aalborg University, Fredrik Bajers Vej 7D2, DK-9220 Aalborg, Denmark Cerbomed GmbH, Medical Valley Center, Henkestr. 91, 91052 Erlangen, Germany

Gabriele S Merki-Feld and Bruno Imthurn
Department of Reproductive Endocrinology, University Hospital Zürich, Rämistrasse 100, CH - 8091 Zürich, Switzerland

Ronald Langner
Headache Clinic Hirslanden Zürich, Zurich, Switzerland

Burkhardt Seifert
Epidemiology, Biostatistics and Prevention Institute, Department of Biostatistics, University of Zürich, Zurich, Switzerland

Andreas R Gantenbein
Neurorehabilitation, RehaClinic, Bad Zurzach, Switzerland

Charly Gaul
Migraine and Headache Clinic, Königstein im Taunus, Germany
Department of Neurology, University Hospital Essen, Essen, Germany

Hans-Christoph Diener
Department of Neurology, University Hospital Essen, Essen, Germany

Ulrich Danesch
Weber & Weber GmbH & Co.KG, Clinical Research, Inning, Germany

Sarah Miller, Susie Lagrata and Manjit S Matharu
Headache Group, Institute of Neurology and The National Hospital for Neurology and Neurosurgery Queen Square, London WC1N 3BG, UK

Fernando Correia
Department of Neurology, Centro Hospitalar do Porto, Oporto, Portugal
Headache Group, Institute of Neurology and The National Hospital for Neurology and Neurosurgery Queen Square, London WC1N 3BG, UK

Index

www.ingramcontent.com/pod-product-compliance
Lightning Source LLC
Chambersburg PA
CBHW082021190326
41458CB00010B/3231